Pathology of the Medical Kidney

Editor

ANTHONY CHANG

SURGICAL PATHOLOGY CLINICS

www.surgpath.theclinics.com

Consulting Editor
JOHN R. GOLDBLUM

September 2014 • Volume 7 • Number 3

ELSEVIER

1600 John F. Kennedy Boulevard • Suite 1800 • Philadelphia, Pennsylvania, 19103-2899

http://www.theclinics.com

SURGICAL PATHOLOGY CLINICS Volume 7, Number 3
September 2014 ISSN 1875-9181, ISBN-13: 978-0-323-32347-5

Editor: Joanne Husovski
Developmental Editor: Donald Mumford

Surgical Pathology Clinics (ISSN 1875-9181) is published quarterly by Elsevier Inc., 360 Park Avenue South, New York, NY 10010. Months of issue are March, June, September, and December. Business and Editorial Office: Elsevier Inc., 1600 John F. Kennedy Blvd., Ste. 1800, Philadelphia, PA 19103-2899. Accounting and Circulation Offices: Elsevier Inc., 3251 Riverport Lane, Maryland Heights, MO 63043. Periodicals postage paid at New York, NY and at additional mailing offices. Subscription prices are $200.00 per year (US individuals), $233.00 per year (US institutions), $100.00 per year (US students/residents), $250.00 per year (Canadian individuals), $266.00 per year (Canadian Institutions), $250.00 per year (foreign individuals), $266.00 per year (foreign institutions), and $120.00 per year (international & Canadian students/residents). Foreign air speed delivery is included in all *Clinics'* subscription prices. All prices are subject to change without notice. **POSTMASTER:** Send address changes to *Surgical Pathology Clinics*, Elsevier, 3251 Riverport Lane, Maryland Heights, MO 63043. Customer Service: 1-800-654-2452 (US). From outside the United States, call 1-314-447-8871. Fax: 1-314-447-8029. E-mail: JournalsCustomerServiceusa@elsevier.com (for print support) and JournalsOnlineSupport-usa@elsevier.com (for online support).

Reprints. For copies of 100 or more, of articles in this publication, please contact the Commercial Reprints Department, Elsevier Inc., 360 Park Avenue South, New York, NY 10010-1710. Tel. 212-633-3874; Fax: 212-633-3820; E-mail: reprints@elsevier.com.

Contributors

CONSULTING EDITOR

JOHN R. GOLDBLUM, MD
Chairman, Professor of Pathology, Department
of Anatomic Pathology, Cleveland Clinics
Lerner College of Medicine, Cleveland Clinic,
Cleveland, Ohio

EDITOR

ANTHONY CHANG, MD
Associate Professor of Pathology, University of
Chicago Medical Center, Chicago, Illinois

AUTHORS

IBRAHIM BATAL, MD
Instructor, Department of Pathology, Brigham
and Women's Hospital, Harvard Medical
School, Boston, Massachusetts

VANESA BIJOL, MD
Assistant Professor, Department of Pathology,
Brigham and Women's Hospital, Harvard
Medical School, Boston, Massachusetts

LYNN D. CORNELL, MD
Associate Professor of Laboratory Medicine
and Pathology, Division of Anatomic
Pathology, Department of Laboratory Medicine
and Pathology, Mayo Clinic, Rochester,
Minnesota

AGNES B. FOGO
John L. Shapiro Professor of Pathology,
Microbiology and Immunology; Professor of
Medicine and Pediatrics; Director of Renal/EM
Division of Pathology; Director, Renal
Pathology Fellowship Program; Department of
Pathology, Microbiology, and Immunology,
Vanderbilt University Medical Center,
Nashville, Tennessee

JOSEPH P. GAUT, MD, PhD
Nephropathology Associates, Little Rock,
Arkansas

MARK HAAS, MD, PhD
Department of Pathology and Laboratory
Medicine, Cedars-Sinai Medical Center,
Los Angeles, California

LEAL C. HERLITZ, MD
Associate Professor, Division of Renal
Pathology, Department of Pathology and Cell
Biology, Columbia University Medical Center,
New York Presbyterian Hospital, New York,
New York

JEAN HOU, MD
Department of Pathology and Cell Biology,
Columbia University Medical Center, New York
Presbyterian Hospital, New York, New York

DONALD C. HOUGHTON, MD
Department of Pathology, Oregon Health and
Science University, Portland, Oregon

MICHAEL MENGEL, MD
Department of Laboratory Medicine and
Pathology, University of Alberta Hospital,
Edmonton, Canada

NASREEN MOHAMED, MD, FRCPA
Consultant Nephropathologist, Department of
Pathology and Laboratory Medicine, King
Fahad Specialist Hospital-Dammam,
Dammam, Kingdom of Saudi Arabia

SAMIH H. NASR, MD
Department of Laboratory Medicine and
Pathology, Mayo Clinic, Rochester,
Minnesota

PAISIT PAUEKSAKON, MD
Associate Professor of Pathology,
Microbiology, and Immunology; Associate
Director of Renal/EM Division of Pathology;
Associate Director, Renal Pathology
Fellowship Program; Department of
Pathology, Microbiology, and Immunology,
Vanderbilt University Medical Center,
Nashville, Tennessee

M. BARRY STOKES, MD
Associate Professor of Clinical Pathology
and Cell Biology, Department of Pathology,
Columbia University College of Physicians
and Surgeons, New York, New York

MEGAN L. TROXELL, MD, PhD
Department of Pathology, Oregon Health and
Science University, Portland, Oregon

Contents

Risk factors for kidney cancers and medical kidney diseases are similar; therefore, it is not surprising that up to 25% of renal cell carcinoma patients have chronic kidney disease prior to nephrectomy and a significant number of patients with normal pre-nephrectomy renal function markers progress to chronic kidney disease over time. Evaluation of non-neoplastic parenchyma in tumor nephrectomy specimens can identify patients at risk for progression to chronic kidney disease, which is a critical step for early intervention and potential improvement of morbidity and mortality rates in this patient population.

This review discusses the pathology of non-neoplastic kidney disease that pathologists may encounter as nephrectomy specimens. The spectrum of pediatric disease is emphasized. Histopathologic assessment of non-neoplastic nephrectomy specimens must be interpreted in the clinical context for accurate diagnosis. Although molecular pathology is not the primary focus of this review, the genetics underlying several of these diseases are also touched on.

We provide an overview of assessment of the kidneys at autopsy, with special considerations for pediatric versus adult kidneys. We describe the approach to gross examination, tissue allocation when needed for additional studies of potential medical renal disease, the spectrum of congenital abnormalities of the kidneys and urinary tract, and approach to cystic diseases of the kidney. We also discuss common lesions seen at autopsy, including acute tubular injury, ischemic versus toxic contributions to this injury, interstitial nephritis, and common vascular diseases. Infections commonly involve the kidney at autopsy, and the key features and differential diagnoses are also discussed.

In patients with end-stage renal disease, kidney transplantation is the best means to extend survival and offer a better quality of life. The current shortage of organs available for transplantation has led to an effort to expand the kidney donor pool, including the use of nonideal donor kidneys. Assessment of the quality of the donated kidney is essential, and would facilitate the decision to transplant a potential organ or discard it. Multiple clinical and histologic parameters have been examined to evaluate the donor kidney and relate the findings to the graft outcome, but clear-cut criteria are yet to be defined.

The Basics of Renal Allograft Pathology   367

Megan L. Troxell and Donald C. Houghton

Renal allograft biopsy provides critical information in the management of renal transplant patients, and must be analyzed in close collaboration with the clinical team. The histologic correlates of acute T-cell mediated rejection are interstitial inflammation, tubulitis, and endothelialitis; polyomavirus nephropathy is a potential mimic. Evidence of antibody-mediated rejection includes C4d deposition; morphologic acute tissue injury; and donor specific antibodies. Acute tubular injury/necrosis is a reversible cause of impaired graft function, especially in the immediate post-transplant period. Drug toxicity, recurrent disease, chronic injury, and other entities affecting both native and transplant kidneys must also be evaluated.

Renal Infections   389

Jean Hou and Leal C. Herlitz

This review discusses the various gross and histologic findings seen in renal infections due to bacteria, viruses, fungi, and mycobacteria. It is crucially important to separate infectious processes in the kidney from other inflammatory or neoplastic processes, as this will have a major impact on therapy. We describe the diagnostic features of renal infections with a specific focus on the differential diagnosis and other processes that may mimic infection. The topics discussed include acute bacterial pyelonephritis, chronic bacterial pyelonephritis, xanthogranulomatous pyelonephritis, malacoplakia, viral infections in the kidney, fungal pyelonephritis and mycobacterial infection of the kidney.

Renal Amyloidosis   409

Nasreen Mohamed and Samih H. Nasr

Amyloidosis is an uncommon group of diseases in which soluble proteins aggregate and deposit extracellularly in tissue as insoluble fibrils, leading to tissue destruction and progressive organ dysfunction. More than 25 proteins have been identified as amyloid precursor proteins. Amyloid fibrils have a characteristic appearance on ultrastructural examination and generate anomalous colors under polarized light. Amyloidosis can be systemic or localized. The kidney is a prime site for amyloid deposition. Immunofluorescence, immunoperoxidase, and more recently laser microdissection and mass spectrometry are important tools used in the typing of renal amyloidosis.

Classification Systems in Renal Pathology: Promises and Problems   427

M. Barry Stokes

Kidney diseases are morphologically heterogeneous. Pathologic classifications of renal disease permit standardization of diagnosis and may identify clinical-pathologic subgroups with different outcomes and/or responses to treatment. To date, classifications have been proposed for lupus nephritis, allograft rejection, IgA nephropathy, focal segmental glomerulosclerosis, antineutrophil cytoplasmic antibody-related glomerulonephritis, and diabetic glomerulosclerosis. These classifications share several limitations related to lack of specificity, reproducibility, validation, and relevance to clinical practice. They offer a standardized approach to diagnosis, however, which should facilitate communication and clinical research.

In this article, various omics technologies and their applications in renal pathology (native and transplant biopsies) are reviewed and discussed. Despite significant progress and novel insights derived from these applications, extensive adoption of molecular diagnostics in renal pathology has not been accomplished. Further validation of specific applications leading to increased diagnostic precision in a clinically relevant way is ongoing.

The consensus classification of antibody-mediated rejection (AMR) of renal allografts developed at the Sixth Banff Conference on Allograft Pathology, in 2001, identified three findings necessary for the diagnosis of active AMR: histologic evidence, antibodies against the graft, and capillary C4d deposition. Morphologic and molecular studies have noted evidence of microvascular injury, which, in the presence of donor-specific antibodies (DSAs) but the absence of C4d deposition, is associated with development of transplant glomerulopathy and graft loss. Recent studies suggest that intimal arteritis may in some cases be a manifestation of DSA-induced graft injury. These newly recognized lesions of AMR have now been incorporated into a revised Banff diagnostic schema.

SURGICAL PATHOLOGY CLINICS

FORTHCOMING ISSUES

Thyroid Pathology
Peter Sadow, *Editor*

Neuropathology
Tarik Tihan, *Editor*

Pathology Informatics
Anil Parwani, *Editor*

Genitourinary Pathology
Michelle Hirsch, *Editor*

RECENT ISSUES

Cutaneous Lymphomas
Antonio Subtil, *Editor*

Cytopathology
Tarik ElSheikh, *Editor*

Hematopoietic Neoplasms: Controversies in Diagnosis and Classification
Tracy George and Daniel Arber, *Editors*

Gastrointestinal Pathology: Classification, Diagnosis, Emerging Entities
Jason L. Hornick, *Editor*

RELATED INTEREST

Endocrinology and Metabolism Clinics of North America
June 2012; Volume 41, Issue 2
Insulin-Like Growth Factors in Normal and Diseased Kidney
Daniela Kiepe and Burkhard Tönshoff, *Authors*
Claire M. Perks and Jeff M.P. Holly, *Editors*

Preface
"Urine" the "Medulla" of the Kidney: Concentrate!

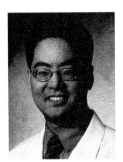

Anthony Chang, MD
Editor

The introduction of the modern technique for percutaneous kidney biopsy 60 years ago in Chicago was a landmark event for nephropathology. Shortly thereafter, the incorporation of immunofluorescence and electron microscopy in the evaluation of these small tissue samples accelerated the characterization and our understanding of a wide variety of kidney diseases, which was critical for establishing the framework of knowledge that exists today. More recent investigative tools to study genomic and proteomic data will continue to reveal additional insights.

The inception of dialysis over a half century ago represents a remarkable achievement in modern medicine, which has extended the lives of countless individuals. However, as a consequence of this amazing invention, the importance of preservation of renal function has gradually faded from the minds of the general public and even physicians. There is a false presumption that dialysis provides a safety net and represents a perfect replacement for failed kidneys, but this could not be further from the truth, as end-stage renal disease due to any cause is more deadly than the vast majority of cancers. In the United States, more than 90,000 Americans die from kidney diseases annually, which exceed the number of combined deaths from breast and prostate cancer. Similar to cancer, early detection of renal diseases provides better opportunities for medical interventions that can alter disease progression and improve clinical outcomes. In particular, this scenario is becoming more commonplace for patients with kidney cancer for whom the status of the non-neoplastic kidney is emerging as the most important predictor of clinical outcome.

The current practice of renal pathology is challenging and routinely requires the complex integration of clinical and laboratory data with light, immunofluorescence, and electron microscopic findings. Fellowship-trained nephropathologists are already in short supply and this problem is likely to worsen, so general surgical pathologists increasingly will be called on to evaluate kidney specimens. These scenarios already occur routinely for autopsies, tumor nephrectomies, and donor kidney evaluation.

The practice of general surgical pathology has become increasingly difficult, as the amount of knowledge that must be absorbed to maintain competency within any given subspecialty increases at an exponential rate. Most pathology residency training programs have either ignored or placed minimal emphasis on teaching nephropathology, so this issue of "Pathology of the Medical Kidney" has been created to provide guidance for the common diagnostic dilemmas that the general surgical pathologist may occasionally encounter in the nonneoplastic kidney specimen.

I wish to thank my contributors for providing excellent reviews for this special issue of *Surgical Pathology Clinics* and to acknowledge their hard work and superb effort. I would also like to express my gratitude to Joanne Husovski for her guidance, and I am indebted to John Goldblum for the opportunity to be a guest editor. I would not have been

Surgical Pathology 7 (2014) ix–x
http://dx.doi.org/10.1016/j.path.2014.06.001
1875-9181/14/$ – see front matter © 2014 Elsevier Inc. All rights reserved.

surgpath.theclinics.com

introduced to the wonderful world of renal pathology without my mentor, Charles Alpers, or a brief, yet unforgettable, session at the microscope with Fred Silva during my second year of residency at the University of Washington. I also want to express my appreciation for my pathology colleagues at the University of Chicago as they have been an essential component of the nurturing and supportive environment that has been critical for my professional development. Finally, none of this would be possible without the enduring love and support from my parents, Mee-Tsung and Shu-Er, my wife, Brittany, and children, Brandon and Brianna.

Anthony Chang, MD
Associate Professor of Pathology
University of Chicago Medical Center
5841 S. Maryland Avenue
Chicago, IL 60637, USA

E-mail address:
anthony.chang@uchospitals.edu

Non-neoplastic Pathology in Tumor Nephrectomy Specimens

Vanesa Bijol, MD*, Ibrahim Batal, MD

KEYWORDS

- Nephrectomy • Normal kidney • Solitary kidney • Renal tumor • Vascular sclerosis
- Diabetic glomerulosclerosis

ABSTRACT

Risk factors for kidney cancers and medical kidney diseases are similar; therefore, it is not surprising that up to 25% of renal cell carcinoma patients have chronic kidney disease prior to nephrectomy and a significant number of patients with normal prenephrectomy renal function markers progress to chronic kidney disease over time. Evaluation of non-neoplastic parenchyma in tumor nephrectomy specimens can identify patients at risk for progression to chronic kidney disease, which is a critical step for early intervention and potential improvement of morbidity and mortality rates in this patient population.

most important risk factors having an impact on the mortality and morbidity among these patients. Several recent studies highlighted the great value of thorough evaluation of non-neoplastic pathology in tumor nephrectomy specimens. Understanding the importance of such evaluation is the first step in establishing routine protocols and systematic approaches to this problem. This article (1) addresses the most important aspects of medical kidney disease after nephrectomy procedure, (2) reviews the relevant literature on non-neoplastic pathology evaluation for better management of patients after nephrectomy procedures, and (3) describes the most common non-neoplastic histopathologic lesions and best practices for evaluation of kidney parenchyma in tumor nephrectomy specimens.

OVERVIEW

Nephrectomy, radical or partial, is still a standard treatment of renal neoplasms, many times providing the only hope for cure from cancer; however, these procedures may be associated with an increased risk of chronic kidney disease (CKD), sometimes with progression to end stage kidney disease (ESKD). Development of better imaging and surgical techniques has led to early cancer diagnosis and improved oncologic outcomes in patients with renal malignancies. This recent trend and stage migration placed even more emphasis on recognizing those at risk for developing CKD and ESKD, since they have become one of the

CHRONIC KIDNEY DISEASE AFTER NEPHRECTOMY PROCEDURE

The most common consequence of nephrectomy procedure on the remaining nephronal mass is a decrease in glomerular filtration rate, hypertension, and proteinuria.[1,2] The mechanisms behind the development of CKD after the nephrectomy procedure fall into the category of structural and functional adaptations of the surviving nephrons after nephronal loss, with development of adaptive hypertrophy and glomerular exhaustion leading to focal sclerosis. A nephrectomy is an obvious example of nephronal loss, but other causes

Disclosures: None.
Department of Pathology, Brigham and Women's Hospital, Harvard Medical School, 75 Francis Street, Boston, MA 02115, USA
* Corresponding author.
E-mail address: VBijol@partners.org

surgpath.theclinics.com

include a variety of glomerular, tubulointerstitial, and vascular diseases. Among glomerular diseases, glomerulosclerosis is frequently associated with inflammatory glomerulopathies, such as IgA nephropathy, lupus nephritis and other immune complex–mediated glomerulopathies, and crescentic glomerulonephritides, to name a few. Primary tubulointerstitial diseases are frequently drug induced and may sometimes lead to pronounced chronic damage, particularly in prolonged, ongoing, and repetitive injury; other tubulointerstitial nephropathies commonly resulting in scarring and chronic damage include various infections, sarcoidosis, toxic injury (such as Chinese herb nephropathy or heavy metal toxicity), and metabolic diseases, among others. Urologic conditions (nephrolithiasis, chronic pyelonephritis, and reflux nephropathy), cystic diseases (eg, polycystic kidney disease and medullary cystic kidney disease), and developmental abnormalities (unilateral renal agenesis, hypoplasia, and dysplasia) can also result in significant nephronal loss. Vascular diseases are an important and frequent cause of nephronal loss and may sometimes result in extensive damage and catastrophic events. Focal infarcts, cortical necrosis, thrombotic microangiopathies, atheroembolic kidney disease, and vasculitides are some examples commonly seen in practice. In some of these conditions, nephronal loss may develop over a prolonged period of time and follow a smoldering course; in other situations, the nephronal loss may be sudden, as seen in nephrectomy procedures. Regardless of the cause and the rate of progression, the surviving nephrons undergo adaptive changes.

Over a short period of time after the nephrectomy, the surviving nephrons undergo compensatory hypertrophy and develop hyperfiltration, driven in part by intracapillary hypertension, to compensate for the initial loss of function.[3,4] The effect of nephronal loss on surviving nephrons has been studied in animal models and similar changes have been observed in humans as well. These adaptive changes and hyperfiltration injury were observed in the classic 5/6 nephrectomy animal model.[5] Although this particular model demonstrates dramatic changes after a substantial loss of nephronal mass, such a severe circumstance is not commonly expected in humans after nephrectomy procedures. It is reasonable to assume, however, that patients undergoing the nephrectomy procedure for tumor, who have preexisting and independent reduction of functional nephrons due to vascular sclerosing disease or diabetic nephropathy, for example, may follow a similar pattern over time and exhibit the same mechanisms of injury and adaptive changes.

Hypertension, smoking, obesity, diabetes mellitus, and increasing age are risk factors for renal malignancy and, independently, they all have strong impact on renal function as well.[6–10] It seems that the same population of patients at increased risk of undergoing nephrectomy is also at increased risk of chronic renal failure. Therefore, renal insufficiency can be expected in a significant proportion of patients with renal cancer undergoing total nephrectomy and such patients may benefit from early recognition and prompt institution of treatment measures.

The rationale behind nephron-sparing surgery (NSS) was criticized at first, because of the notion that a solitary kidney can maintain an adequate glomerular filtration rate, based on data derived from healthy kidney transplant donors.[11–13] The difference between the healthy transplant donor population and typical renal cell carcinoma (RCC) patients, however, who carry several risk factors and comorbidities, from cigarette smoking to hypertension and diabetes, became obvious when several studies showed a significant risk of postnephrectomy renal failure in RCC patients. Also, up to 25% of RCC patients have CKD prior to nephrectomy and additional loss of nephronal mass in nephrectomy procedures may be critical for these patients; moreover, those with normal renal function are more likely to develop CKD after a radical nephrectomy (RN) procedure compared with partial nephrectomy (PN).[14–16] Lau and colleagues[17] compared the renal function in matched cohorts of patients undergoing RN and PN with a normal contralateral kidney and at 10-year follow-up found similar overall and cancer-specific survival and the rate of cancer recurrence and metastasis between the 2 groups; however, the incidence of CKD was 22.4% and 11.6%, respectively, for the RN and PN groups (risk ratio, 3.7; 95% CI, 1.2–11.2; $P = .01$). Similar results were obtained in a large study by Weight and colleagues,[18] where it was confirmed that PN offered cancer-specific survival equivalent to that of RN, whereas the renal function was better preserved in patients after PN compared with RN; this study also demonstrated an increased risk of cardiovascular death and overall death in patients who progressed to CKD after nephrectomy. The rate of progression to CKD after nephrectomy can be variable and may either be accelerated, requiring earlier renal replacement therapy, or hopefully delayed, if the use of renal protective regimen is initiated immediately after surgery; this pattern is dependent on preexisting conditions, the presence of CKD prior to surgery, and the extent of renal mass reduction.[19]

With better surgical techniques, the body of literature on safety and efficacy of NSS expanded concurrently with improvement in imaging and marked increase in the incidence of small renal masses. Minimally invasive techniques, cryoablation, and radiofrequency ablation have developed with promising results.[20] Such trends resulted in a dramatic change in the presentation and treatment of RCC in recent years, with a greater proportion of newly diagnosed patients presenting with stage I disease compared with earlier years. RCC is increasingly diagnosed as incidental small renal masses in asymptomatic patients, resulting in improved oncologic outcomes.[21] Factors that determine the selection of a particular surgical technique include the tumor size and location within the kidney and patient age, comorbidities, and general condition.

As cancer becomes a less likely factor in dictating overall survival and morbidity rates in early stage RCC, non-neoplastic parenchymal diseases and their evaluation in nephrectomy samples have become more important than ever before, because patient morbidity, quality of life, and overall cost of long-term health care depend on medical kidney disease diagnosis and treatment, including cases with limited nephronal loss in NSS. To achieve excellence in patient care by improving medical renal outcomes and patient quality of life, while minimizing the need for renal replacement therapy (dialysis and kidney transplantation), the most important focus should be the recognition of patients at risk and those in need for early intervention. Most patients with medical kidney diseases who undergo tumor nephrectomy have not had a kidney biopsy diagnosis in the past, and few would have it performed in the postnephrectomy period, because biopsy of a solitary kidney is not a common practice due to risk of complications, including the loss of the kidney. Therefore, examination of the non-neoplastic part of the kidney in the tumor nephrectomy sample is a unique opportunity to identify the exact pathology and ultimately modify management of these patients. Early detection and institution of renoprotective measures is paramount in the preservation of renal function and may significantly improve the quality of life and delay the need for renal replacement therapy in individual patients. The role of surgical pathologists has become essential in this regard, because the evaluation of non-neoplastic parenchyma in tumor nephrectomy samples is key and a great predictor of decline in kidney function.[22,23]

EVALUATION OF NON-NEOPLASTIC PATHOLOGY IN TUMOR NEPHRECTOMY SPECIMENS

In the past decade, several studies have pointed out that the accurate evaluation of non-neoplastic pathology in tumor nephrectomy specimens is essential for early recognition and prompt management of patients at risk for developing CKD and ESKD or medical kidney disease in general (**Table 1**).[22–26] In a combined retrospective and prospective study by Bijol and colleagues,[22] pathologic abnormalities were present In greater than 60% of tumor nephrectomy cases; most commonly, these included vascular sclerosing disease with parenchymal scarring and various stages of diabetic renal disease. Subsequent studies confirmed the high incidence of non-neoplastic pathology in tumor nephrectomy specimens and underlined the need for thorough evaluation of these samples.[23–25]

Henriksen and colleagues[24] retrospectively reviewed 246 tumor nephrectomy cases and found non-neoplastic pathologic diagnoses in 24 cases, comprising mostly diabetic renal disease and vascular pathology, including thrombotic microangiopathy and atheroembolic disease. The investigators also pointed out that 88% of these diagnoses were initially missed. Salvatore and colleagues[23] performed a 10-year retrospective review of 456 consecutive tumor nephrectomy cases; of those, approximately 30% had minimal pathologic alterations as defined by less than 5% global glomerulosclerosis, less than 10% tubulointerstitial scarring, and mild or no significant vascular sclerosis. The remaining 70% of cases displayed significant pathologic changes in one of the main compartments of renal parenchyma, with 15% of cases with definitive medical renal diagnoses that were not recognized or diagnosed at the time of initial nephrectomy specimen evaluation in greater than 60% of cases. In spite of high incidence and clinical significance, non-neoplastic renal lesions are frequently missed. This is likely due to a combination of underappreciation of their importance, lack of expertise in kidney pathology among general pathologists due to limited exposure and current training practices in pathology residency programs, and the increasing complexity of neoplastic pathology diagnostic evaluation, which inevitably shifts the focus away from non-neoplastic kidney pathology evaluation. These observations have collectively led to important practice recommendations and the establishment of further steps to ensure the highest quality care in this patient population at

Table 1
Selected studies of histopathologic evaluation of non-neoplastic parenchyma in tumor nephrectomy specimens

Study	No. Patients	Main Findings	Other Important Findings/Comments
Bijol et al,[22] 2006	110	Only 10% cases had unremarkable parenchyma and no vascular sclerosis; >60% of cases with some parenchymal chronic damage or disease.	39 patients had 6 mo follow-up; those with >20% GS and advanced diabetic renal disease had statistically significant worsening in serum creatinine pre- and postnephrectomy.
Henriksen et al,[24] 2007	246	24 of 246 cases had non-neoplastic pathologic diagnoses—diabetic renal disease, TMA, sickle cell nephropathy, and FSGS; 88% of these diagnoses were initially missed.	Survey of pathology residency programs shows 36% have mandatory renal pathology training and 29% residency programs offer no formal training in renal pathology.
Gautam et al,[28] 2010	49	Severity of GS can predict the rate of renal function decrease after RN; for each 10% increase in GS, the estimated glomerular filtration rate decreased by 9% from baseline.	The study included follow up of 3–60.8 mo.
Garcia-Roig et al,[25] 2013	45	Study on PN samples to evaluate non-neoplastic sampling adequacy; pathologic evaluation was adequate in 91.8% samples.	Non-neoplastic pathologic changes observed in 42.2% of samples, mostly arterial sclerosis, mesangial expansion, and interstitial fibrosis.
Salvatore et al,[23] 2013	456	Retrospective 10-year review. Medical renal disease was identified in 15% of cases; these diagnoses were initially missed in >60% cases. The degrees of vascular sclerosis, GS, and IFTA are predictive of elevated creatinine levels in postnephrectomy patients	70% of cases displayed significant pathologic changes in one of the main compartments of renal parenchyma. This study has the largest and longest follow-up data (156 patients, minimum 12 mo)

Abbreviations: FSGS, focal and segmental glomerulsoclerosis; GS, glomerulosclerosis; IFTA, interstitial fibrosis and tubular atrophy; TMA, thrombotic microangiopathy.

high risk for CKD, ESKD, and other serious complications.[27]

The most convincing evidence for the great value of non-neoplastic tissue evaluation in tumor nephrectomy specimens comes from the data correlating the pathologic findings with postnephrectomy clinical outcomes. Although this experience is limited to a few studies, they all suggest a significant decline in renal function in patients with preexisting medical kidney disease.[22,23,28] In patients with greater than 20% parenchymal scarring and advanced diabetic renal disease, a statistically significant change in serum creatinine can be seen even 6 months after nephrectomy.[22] In their study of 49 patients with approximately 20 months of follow-up data, Gautam and colleagues[28] showed that the severity of glomerulosclerosis can predict the rate of renal function

decrease after RN. In the largest study of 156 patients with a minimum follow-up of 12 months (mean 49.2 ± 34.8 months), Salvatore and colleagues[23] showed that the degrees of vascular sclerosis, glomerulosclerosis, and tubulointerstitial scarring are predictive of elevated creatinine levels in postnephrectomy patients. Overall, identifying patients with significant medical kidney disease has an important prognostic value and helps in determining the best management practices in this vulnerable patient population.

PRACTICAL RECOMMENDATIONS

Current protocol from the College of American Pathologists requires the assessment of non-neoplastic kidney in nephrectomy or nephroureterectomy specimens; it is suggested that evaluation for medical renal disease should be performed in each case, with application of periodic acid–Schiff (PAS) and/or Jones methenamine silver (JMS) stain, if necessary, as well as consultation with a nephropathologist as needed.[29] Systematic evaluation is further emphasized, to include a thorough examination of all compartments of renal parenchyma, from glomeruli to tubules, interstitium, and vessels. The Association of Directors of Anatomic and Surgical Pathology made similar recommendation for additional PAS or JMS stain to enhance the histologic review and serve as a prompt to address the condition of the non-neoplastic kidney.[30]

In general, for evaluation of non-neoplastic tissue in tumor nephrectomy specimens, it is recommended that all samples should be reviewed at least by light microscopy. A representative section of non-neoplastic tissue should be sampled as far away from the tumor as possible, to avoid the tumor compression artifact. This practice may be difficult in PN samples, although a recent report suggests adequate sampling in nearly 92% of PN specimens.[25] As recommended by several investigators, at least PAS and/or JMS (possibly in addition to trichrome) stain should be used in this evaluation; PAS and JMS stains help better visualize fine details of basement membranes as well as general parenchymal architecture.[23,27,29,30] The parenchyma should be evaluated systematically. When looking at the glomeruli, those that appear well perfused should be used for further evaluation of size, architecture, and cellularity. The presence of endoluminal thrombi or hypercellularity should be noted and further characterized. If the membranes are thickened, PAS and JMS stains may help further establish whether there are basement membrane spikes or double contours contributing to the thickness, in which case there should be suspicion of membranous nephropathy or a membranoproliferative pattern of injury, respectively. The amount of mesangial matrix and the presence of nodular mesangial expansion should also be noted. Extracapillary proliferative lesions should be further characterized as crescents or collapsing lesions. Many of the glomerular lesions (discussed previously) may be focal; therefore, a larger section and thorough examination help greatly in the diagnostic process. The tubulointerstitium should be evaluated for the presence of atrophy and fibrosis as well as inflammation; these are the most common changes in the nephrectomy samples and can also be very focal. In the preserved areas, signs of inflammation, edema, crystal deposition, tubular epithelial

injury, and necrosis should be looked for. The vascular compartment frequently exhibits some level of arterial and arteriolar sclerosis or hyalinosis. There are no generally accepted criteria for grading arterial and arteriolar sclerosis. Most practices include classification into mild, moderate, or severe sclerosis. Bijol and colleagues[22] proposed these definitions: mild vessel sclerosis is a subintimal sclerosis without significant occlusion of the vessel lumen (<10%), involving occasional vessels (**Fig. 1**); subintimal arterial sclerosis with involvement of most vessels, with occlusion of 50% or less of the lumen is graded as moderate (**Fig. 2**); and, if the occlusion is greater than 50%, then it is defined as severe sclerosis, typically involving a majority of vessels (**Fig. 3**). Gautam and colleagues[28] use a semiquantitative grading system that they defined by the extent of luminal occlusion and graded as 1 (0%–5% occlusion), 2 (6%–25% occlusion), 3 (26%–50% occlusion), and 4 (>50% occlusion). Signs of vasculitis or fibrinoid necrosis are rare but important because they may suggest the most severe forms of kidney injury in general.

If a thorough light microscopic examination suggests significant pathologic changes, further characterization is needed and other stains (eg, Congo red or immunohistochemistry stain) and/or studies (electron and immunofluorescence microscopy) can be helpful and important in unveiling the pathologic process. Immunofluorescence and electron microscopy studies should ideally be performed on tissue saved at the time of gross examination, in appropriate media or fixatives (Michel or Zeus medium for immunofluorescence microscopy sample and glutaraldehyde fixative for electron microscopy sample). In a majority of cases, samples saved for potential studies are not used and, therefore, are discarded after the final report is issued, making this practice time consuming and costly.[27] Both electron and immunofluorescence microscopy studies can be optimized for use on paraffin-embedded tissue, although this is less ideal due to processing artifacts.[31–33]

COMMON NON-NEOPLASTIC RENAL PARENCHYMAL LESIONS SEEN IN TUMOR NEPHRECTOMY SPECIMENS

Changes related to neoplastic growth (compression artifact and obstructive uropathy) need to be considered when evaluating non-neoplastic pathology. These changes may be focal or unilateral and may, therefore, have less clinical impact and

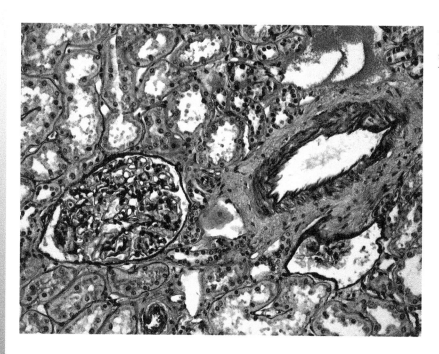

Fig. 1. Mild arterial subintimal sclerosis without significant occlusion of the vessel lumen (PAS, ×200).

significance compared with non-localized medical kidney diseases, such as vascular sclerosing disease, with or without parenchymal scarring, and diabetic renal disease. Although prevalent, these changes are frequently overlooked, dismissed as irrelevant, or attributed to normal aging, particularly when it comes to vascular sclerosis; therefore, most of this discussion is devoted to these categories of medical kidney disease. A variety of other conditions may be also noted in nephrectomy specimens and they are addressed briefly later.

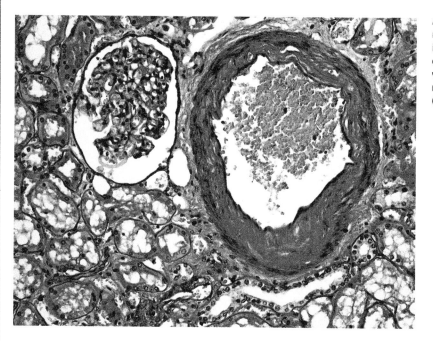

Fig. 2. Moderate subintimal arterial sclerosis with involvement of entire circumference of the vessel wall but with mild narrowing of the lumen (PAS, ×200).

Fig. 3. Severe arterial sclerosis with greater than 50% of luminal narrowing (PAS, ×200).

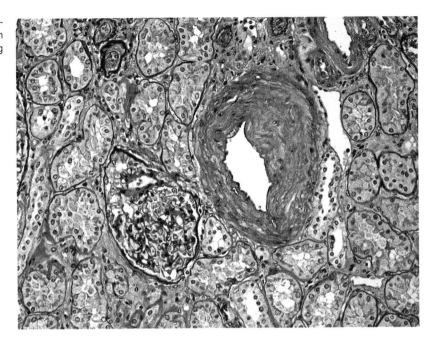

CHANGES RELATED TO NEOPLASTIC GROWTH

Many renal tumors are surrounded by a zone of compressed renal parenchyma, usually referred to as renal peritumoral pseudocapsule (**Figs. 4** and **5**). The changes are focal and related to the tumor growth and, therefore, usually are of no clinical importance. Some tumors, such as oncocytomas, angiomyolipomas, and chromophobe RCCs, tend not to have pseudocapsule even when large. Conventional clear cell RCC may have a pesudocapsule even when small, suggesting that direct tumor-related factors may contribute to the observed changes.[34]

Large renal cell neoplasms, in particular those arising in medulla or urothelial cell carcinomas, may result in obstructive uropathy. The location

Fig. 4. Tumor pseudocapsule forms as the tumor growth compresses the surrounding non-neoplastic parenchyma; this compression artifact is seen in the band of tissue between the white and black arrows in this image. More pronounced dense fibrosis, without recognizable kidney parenchyma, is seen at the bottom, below the white arrow (PAS, ×100).

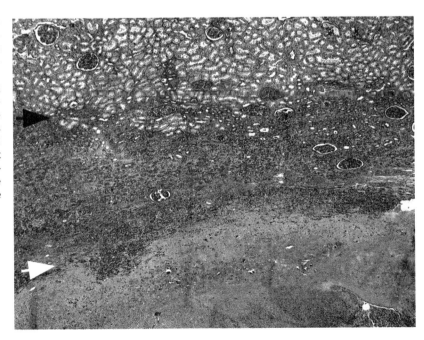

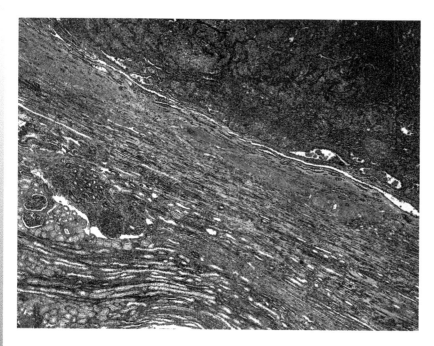

Fig. 5. Tumor pseudo-capsule; papillary renal carcinoma is seen in the top aspect of the image, and compressed renal parenchyma with formation of renal pseudocapsule is seen below the tumor (PAS, ×100).

and size of such tumors usually warrant a total nephrectomy or nephroureterectomy procedure. Because such lesions are commonly unilateral, they do not have impact on the renal function of the contralateral kidney. When significant, obstruction can cause hydronephrosis and dilatation of proximal structures, with compression of the parenchyma (**Fig. 6**); such changes can be easily visualized by ultrasound and other radiologic techniques. Intraparenchymal focal obstruction of tubules by tumor growth, at the level of individual nephrons, without clinical or radiologic evidence of obstruction, may, however, result in histopathologic changes suggestive of obstruction, including tubular distension, sometimes with microcystic formation, a low epithelial lining, and tubular inspissation by Tamm-Horsfall protein with or without focal extravasation into interstitium and

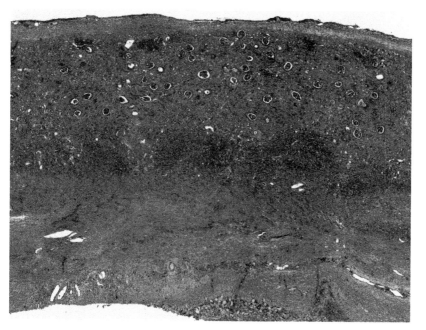

Fig. 6. Urinary obstruction and hydronephrosis due to tumor growth causes dilatation of pelvicaliceal system with compression of renal parenchyma. The image reveals diffuse tubular atrophy and interstitial fibrosis with patchy inflammation (PAS, ×40).

inflammatory reaction (**Fig. 7**). Such changes should be recorded, but their interpretation depends on the extent and distribution of the changes as well as clinical and laboratory parameters in individual patients.

CHANGES RELATED TO MEDICAL KIDNEY DISEASE, INDEPENDENT OF TUMOR GROWTH

Vascular Sclerosing Disease

Only approximately 10% of tumor nephrectomy specimens show no parenchymal scarring or vascular sclerosis and, in an additional 20% to 30% of patients, there are various degrees of vascular sclerosis found in the absence of parenchymal scarring. This leaves 60% to 70% of cases with parenchymal pathologic changes, of which up to half demonstrate various degrees of vascular sclerosis and parenchymal scarring.[22,23] Therefore, vascular sclerosing disease, with or without parenchymal scarring, is the most common lesion seen in the renal parenchyma of tumor nephrectomy specimens.

Hypertensive nephropathy and hypertensive and benign nephrosclerosis are all synonyms for parenchymal scarring in the context of vascular sclerosing disease. Arterionephrosclerosis is a term used to describe arterial sclerosis in the kidney, although the changes are not specific or different compared with vascular sclerosis seen in other tissues or organs. The authors prefer more nonspecific terminology, such as parenchymal scarring in vascular sclerosing disease, because it effectively describes the pathologic lesion, in the authors' opinion, without creating a sense of definitive or specific diagnosis, which may be the case with the use of other terminology. A variety of primary vascular diseases and endothelial cell injury may result in similar histopathologic changes that may lead to hypertension. Endothelial cell injury and vascular sclerosing disease in the kidney are poorly studied and characterized, and they are frequently ascribed to hypertension, although most of the time factors other than hypertension have not been ruled out with any level of certainty. Hypertension is common in patients with RCC undergoing nephrectomy procedures and found in 25% to 60% of patients.[3,15,35–38]

Apart from hypertension, normal aging is another factor that may be attributed to vascular sclerosing disease. Increased frequency of vascular changes is commonly seen in older patients; however, it is difficult to assign these changes only to a normal aging process because it is hard to separate them from effects of accumulated injury through comorbid states that occur with increased frequency in elderly people. Many structural changes in the kidney have been observed as a result of aging (decreased organ weight, increased glomerulosclerosis, and tubulointerstitial fibrosis).[39] There is a general agreement that in people younger than 50 years, the "acceptable" percentage of global glomerulosclerosis is below 10%, but in people older than 50 years, the distinction of "normal" and "abnormal" becomes less well defined, and there

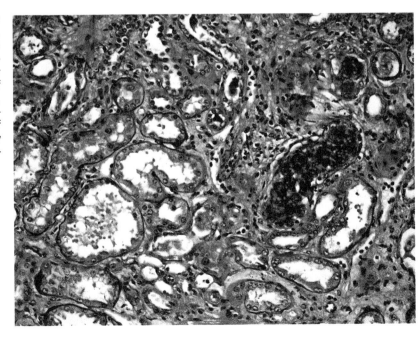

Fig. 7. Focal tubular distension, to the left, and tubular inspissation by Tamm-Horsfall protein, to the right, may suggest obstruction; if the changes are focal, they may represent obstruction at the level of a single tubule and may not be clinically significant (PAS, ×400).

is more disagreement regarding an acceptable magic number for a particular age group.

Glomerular endothelial cell injury, with glomerular capillary wall remodeling and vascular sclerosis, is a common finding on a kidney biopsy. In the authors' opinion, these findings fall into the spectrum of change below the clinical threshold of recognition for thrombotic microangiopathies, with mild or subtle phenotypes that do not reach enough acute injury to precipitate the easily recognizable clinical picture of acute thrombotic microangiopathy with hemolytic anemia and thrombocytopenia. Such injury, however, may be important enough to cause subtle and frequently repetitive endothelial cell damage that results in remodeling of the glomerular capillaries, ischemic injury with consequent chronic changes and focal global and segmental glomerulosclerosis, tubulointerstitial scarring, and vascular sclerosis. Similar to these nonspecific histopathologic findings, these patients also have nonspecific clinical presentation with hypertension, proteinuria, and CKD. Acute thrombotic microangiopathy represents only a tip of the iceberg and is a rare occurrence in everyday renal pathology practice. It is important to keep these concepts in mind and suggest a potential primary vascular injury in patients with pronounced vascular sclerosis and parenchymal scarring, regardless of their age and the history of hypertension. Such vascular injury shares the differential diagnosis of thrombotic angiopathies and includes hemolytic-uremic syndrome, thrombotic thrombocytopenic purpura, malignant hypertension, scleroderma, and antiphospholipid antibody syndrome, to name a few. Severe arterial and arteriolar sclerosis, with onionskin lesions (multilayering and hypertrophy of the muscle layer with obliteration of the lumen) and remodeling of glomerular capillaries are characteristic of severe chronic thrombotic microangiopathies (**Fig. 8**).

Atheroembolic disease (AED) is another important vascular lesion to look for in nephrectomy samples; cholesterol clefts in the vascular walls and/or glomeruli may be a focal but important finding to unveil the cause of renal failure in some patients (**Fig. 9**). AED most commonly follows catheterization procedures or, in general, manipulations of the atheromatous plaque. In such circumstances, dislocation of the plaque material is much more efficient than in spontaneous embolization; however, the latter is probably not infrequent in reality, likely more subclinical.

Diabetic Renal Disease

Diabetes mellitus is a risk factor for RCC and approximately 10% to 20% of RCC patients have diabetes mellitus.[15,35] Diabetes is a microvascular disease, affecting many organ systems and cell types, with profound effects on the kidney. Diabetic nephropathy is a specific clinical term defined by the presence of albuminuria, hypertension, and glomerular filtration rate; however, the term has been used loosely in practice and frequently by pathologists to suggest the presence of diffuse and nodular diabetic glomerulosclerosis.

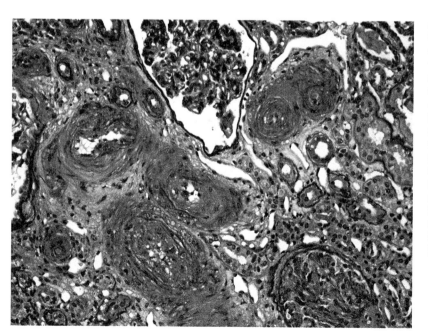

Fig. 8. In chronic thrombotic microangiopathy, changes in the vasculature are severe, with multilayering of the muscle layer and thickening of the vessel walls (onionskin lesions), and obliteration of the lumens. A portion of a glomerulus is seen at the top of the image, showing thickening and remodeling of the capillary walls. A globally sclerosed glomerulus is seen in the lower right corner (PAS, ×200).

Fig. 9. Atheroembolic kidney disease is characterized by the presence of cholesterol clefts in the vascular lumens, usually associated with reactive changes and proliferation of the endothelial cells (PAS, ×100).

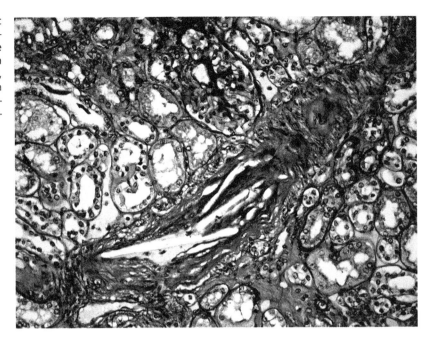

Glomerular hypertrophy occurs as an early diabetic lesion due to insulin effects. The glomerular filtration rate is increased in early diabetic renal disease and, over time, leads to hyperfiltration injury, at least in part responsible for thickening of the basement membranes. Due to hyperglycemia, the mesangial cells overproduce matrix, resulting in mesangial expansion, forming Kimmelstiel-Wilson nodules (**Fig. 10**). These are typically seen in patients with diabetes, but they are not entirely specific, because the nodular glomerulopathy may be seen in heavy smoking, paraprotein deposition diseases, healed mesangyiolytic lesions, and old immune complex–mediated glomerulopathies. Amyloidosis can also present with nodular expansion of the mesangium by acellular and amorphous material. This material is of different texture and argyrophilic properties

Fig. 10. Moderate diabetic nodular glomerulosclerosis, with expansion of the mesangial matrix and only mild increase in mesangial cellularity (PAS, ×400).

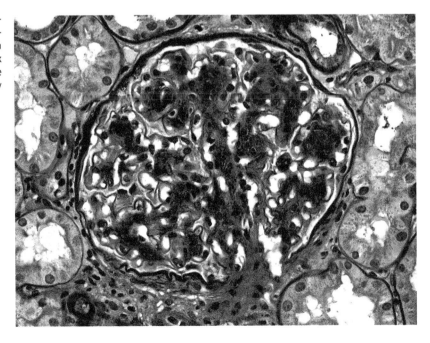

than nodular diabetic glomerulosclerosis; however, when in doubt, a Congo red stain should always be performed to confirm or rule out renal amyloidosis. Diabetic patients frequently develop significant endothelial cell injury and vascular sclerosis and hyalinosis. Various degrees of diabetic renal disease can be seen in tumor nephrectomy specimens and the presence of advanced changes and diabetic nodular glomerulosclerosis predicts progression of CKD. Early recognition of such changes is important because strict control of diabetes and blood glucose levels may result in reversal of initial changes and may significantly slow down the progression of the disease.

Tubulointerstitial Disease

The most common changes of the tubulointerstitial compartment include tubular atrophy and interstitial fibrosis. These chronic changes are invariably associated with some, usually mild-to-moderate level, chronic and probably nonspecific inflammation. Inflammatory infiltrate in the areas of preservation, associated with interstitial edema and tubulitis, is a finding characteristic of an acute interstitial nephritis, commonly drug induced (**Fig. 11**). The infiltrate may or may not reveal the presence of eosinophils. Other causes of acute interstitial nephritis include direct infections, immune complex–mediated diseases, and other deposition diseases, in the context of autoimmune diseases, cryoglobulinemia, or paraprotein deposition diseases. Such findings are unusual in tumor nephrectomy samples; however, a thorough work-up is suggested in an overt inflammatory condition. Infiltration with atypical lymphoplasmacytic cells should be adequately worked up for lymphomas and other lymphoproliferative disorders.

Granulomatous interstitial nephritides (GIN) can also be seen in tumor nephrectomy samples; bacillus Calmette-Guérin (BCG)–related GIN should be suspected in patients with urothelial malignancies treated with BCG, where numerous granulomas may be seen in the non-neoplastic parenchyma.[40] The true nature of this process is still unknown; some investigators suspect a hypersensitivity reaction and others suggest direct infection by attenuated microorganisms. Regardless of the true mechanism, the presence of acid-fast bacteria has not been confirmed in these lesions and necrotizing changes are not common in this form of GIN. Xanthogranulomatous pyelonephritis has been described with both urothelial carcinomas and RCC. Prominent foamy macrophages admixed with lymphocytes and plasma cells are characteristically seen in this lesion.[41]

Nonspecific acute tubular injury and epithelial necrosis are occasionally noted in tumor nephrectomy samples, but these can be difficult to distinguish from autolysis and preservation artifacts. The presence of reactive nuclear changes, mitotic figures, and interstitial edema and inflammation are helpful associated findings. Crystal deposition is frequently seen in the kidney, including urate crystals in gout, calcium oxalate crystals in hyperoxaluric states, and calcium phosphate crystals in phosphate nephropathy.

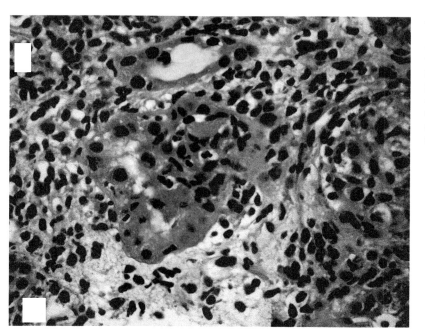

Fig. 11. Acute interstitial nephritis, with acute tubulitis and invasion of tubular epithelium by lymphocytes and neutrophils; interstitial edema and mixed infiltrate with eosinophils, lymphocytes, and neutrophils is also seen (hematoxylin-eosin ×400).

Other Medical Renal Diseases

Other medical renal diseases can also be present in tumor nephrectomy samples; IgA nephropathy, amyloidosis, membranous nephropathy, thin glomerular basement membranes, crescentic glomerulonephritis, and even fibrillary glomerulopathy have all been reported.[22,24,42–46] Describing each of these entities is not the focus of this review; rather, the possibility of these lesions is pointed out and pathologists urged to carefully look for glomerular and other changes in the parenchyma—thickening of the basement membranes, inflammatory changes, mesangial expansion, crystal deposits, and so forth. Further characterization by performing special stains and techniques, including PAS, Congo red, immunofluorescence, and electron microscopy, is suggested in any suspicious case.

Recommendation Summary
FOR NON-NEOPLASTIC KIDNEY PATHOLOGY EVALUATION

1. Sample non-neoplastic tissue as far away from the tumor as possible. Up-front ordering of PAS and/or JMS stain on this section may serve as a reminder to include the non-neoplastic pathology evaluation in the final report.

2. If there is clinical history of proteinuria or significant renal dysfunction at the time of gross examination of the nephrectomy specimen, it is prudent to harvest the non-neoplastic renal cortex for potential immunofluorescence and electron microscopy studies.

3. Evaluation of the renal parenchyma should be systematic and include all compartments: glomeruli, tubulointerstitium, and vessels.

4. Glomeruli should be counted and globally sclerosed glomeruli should be expressed as a percent. A percentage of hypoperfused glomeruli can also be a useful measure of nonfunctional nephrons. Better perfused glomeruli should be evaluated for mesangial expansion and/or hypercellularity, capillary wall changes, endocapillary or extracapillary proliferation, segmental necrosis, thrombosis, or collapse.

5. Preserved tubules should be evaluated for the presence of inflammation, crystal deposition, epithelial necrosis, protein reabsorption granules, or degenerative changes. In healthy cortical parenchyma, tubules are back to back and the interstitium is delicate.

6. In tubular atrophy, tubules are small and separated from each other by interstitial inflammation and fibrosis.

7. Arteries and arterioles should be evaluated for subintimal and/or medial sclerosis. AED is rare but occasionally may be seen in nephrectomy samples. Vasculitides are exceedingly rare.

Diagnostic Pitfalls
IN NON-NEOPLASTIC KIDNEY PATHOLOGY EVALUATION
IN TUMOR NEPHRECTOMY SPECIMENS

! Glomerular cellularity is frequently overestimated. If there is no clear mesangial expansion and hypercellularity, endocapillary proliferation and occlusion of capillaries by inflammatory cells, or cellular crescents, then pathologists should be cautious of making a diagnosis of acute glomerulonephritis. The cellularity should be estimated on a low or intermediate magnification and compared with the tubular or overall cellularity.

! Interstitial inflammation is interpreted as active interstitial nephritis. Interstitial inflammation is common and usually associated with tubular atrophy and interstitial fibrosis. Sometimes, even few neutrophils and eosinophils may be seen in these infiltrates. If such inflammation is present in the preserved parenchyma, pushing apart nonatrophic tubules and invading their epithelium, usually in association with interstitial edema, then this should be noted as acute interstitial nephritis. Such findings are rare in nephrectomy samples.

! Vascular sclerosis is ignored or attributed to old age. Even if present in elderly patients, these findings although common are not normal and should be recorded.

REFERENCES

1. Hakim RM, Goldszer RC, Brenner BM. Hypertension and proteinuria: long-term sequelae of uninephrectomy in humans. Kidney Int 1984;25(6):930–6.

2. Ohishi A, Suzuki H, Nakamoto H, et al. Status of patients who underwent uninephrectomy in adulthood more than 20 years ago. Am J Kidney Dis 1995; 26(6):889–97.

3. Shirasaki Y, Tsushima T, Saika T, et al. Kidney function after nephrectomy for renal cell carcinoma. Urology 2004;64(1):43–7.

4. Sugaya K, Ogawa Y, Hatano T, et al. Compensatory renal hypertrophy and changes of renal function following nephrectomy. Hinyokika Kiyo 2000;46(4): 235–40.

5. Hostetter TH, Olson JL, Rennke HG, et al. Hyperfiltration in remnant nephrons: a potentially adverse response to renal ablation. Am J Physiol 1981; 241(1):F85–93.

6. Lindblad P, Chow WH, Chan J, et al. The role of diabetes mellitus in the aetiology of renal cell cancer. Diabetologia 1999;42(1):107–12.

7. Shapiro JA, Williams MA, Weiss NS. Body mass index and risk of renal cell carcinoma. Epidemiology 1999;10(2):188–91.

8. Shapiro JA, Williams MA, Weiss NS, et al. Hypertension, antihypertensive medication use, and risk of renal cell carcinoma. Am J Epidemiol 1999;149(6): 521–30.

9. Yuan JM, Castelao JE, Gago-Dominguez M, et al. Tobacco use in relation to renal cell carcinoma. Cancer Epidemiol Biomarkers Prev 1998;7(5):429–33.

10. Chow WH, Gridley G, Fraumeni JF Jr, et al. Obesity, hypertension, and the risk of kidney cancer in men. N Engl J Med 2000;343(18):1305–11.

11. Najarian JS, Chavers BM, McHugh LE, et al. 20 years or more of follow-up of living kidney donors. Lancet 1992;340(8823):807–10.

12. Ibrahim HN, Foley R, Tan L, et al. Long-term consequences of kidney donation. N Engl J Med 2009; 360(5):459–69.

13. Fehrman-Ekholm I, Elinder CG, Stenbeck M, et al. Kidney donors live longer. Transplantation 1997; 64(7):976–8.

14. McKiernan J, Simmons R, Katz J, et al. Natural history of chronic renal insufficiency after partial and radical nephrectomy. Urology 2002;59(6):816–20.

15. Huang WC, Levey AS, Serio AM, et al. Chronic kidney disease after nephrectomy in patients with renal cortical tumours: a retrospective cohort study. Lancet Oncol 2006;7(9):735–40.

16. Jeon HG, Jeong IG, Lee JW, et al. Prognostic factors for chronic kidney disease after curative surgery in patients with small renal tumors. Urology 2009; 74(5):1064–8.

17. Lau WK, Blute ML, Weaver AL, et al. Matched comparison of radical nephrectomy vs nephron-sparing surgery in patients with unilateral renal cell carcinoma and a normal contralateral kidney. Mayo Clin Proc 2000;75(12):1236–42.

18. Weight CJ, Larson BT, Fergany AF, et al. Nephrectomy induced chronic renal insufficiency is associated with increased risk of cardiovascular death and death from any cause in patients with localized cT1b renal masses. J Urol 2010;183(4):1317–23.

19. Chapman D, Moore R, Klarenbach S, et al. Residual renal function after partial or radical nephrectomy for renal cell carcinoma. Can Urol Assoc J 2010;4(5): 337–43.

20. Jorns JJ, Thiel DD, Castle EP. Update on contemporary management of clinically localized renal cell carcinoma. Minerva Urol Nefrol 2012;64(4):261–72.

21. Kane CJ, Mallin K, Ritchey J, et al. Renal cell cancer stage migration: analysis of the National Cancer Data Base. Cancer 2008;113(1):78–83.

22. Bijol V, Mendez GP, Hurwitz S, et al. Evaluation of the nonneoplastic pathology in tumor nephrectomy specimens: predicting the risk of progressive renal failure. Am J Surg Pathol 2006;30(5):575–84.

23. Salvatore SP, Cha EK, Rosoff JS, et al. Nonneoplastic renal cortical scarring at tumor nephrectomy predicts decline in kidney function. Arch Pathol Lab Med 2013;137(4):531–40.

24. Henriksen KJ, Meehan SM, Chang A. Nonneoplastic renal diseases are often unrecognized in adult tumor nephrectomy specimens: a review of 246 cases. Am J Surg Pathol 2007;31(11):1703–8.

25. Garcia-Roig M, Gorin MA, Parra-Herran C, et al. Pathologic evaluation of non-neoplastic renal parenchyma in partial nephrectomy specimens. World J Urol 2013;31(4):835–9.

26. Truong LD, Shen SS, Park MH, et al. Diagnosing nonneoplastic lesions in nephrectomy specimens. Arch Pathol Lab Med 2009;133(2):189–200.

27. Henriksen KJ, Meehan SM, Chang A. Nonneoplastic kidney diseases in adult tumor nephrectomy and nephroureterectomy specimens: common, harmful, yet underappreciated. Arch Pathol Lab Med 2009; 133(7):1012–25.

28. Gautam G, Lifshitz D, Shikanov S, et al. Histopathological predictors of renal function decrease after laparoscopic radical nephrectomy. J Urol 2010; 184(5):1872–6.

29. Srigley JR, Amin MB, Delahunt B, et al. Protocol for the examination of specimens from patients with invasive carcinoma of renal tubular origin. Arch Pathol Lab Med 2010;134(4):e25–30.

30. Association of Directors of Anatomic and Surgical Pathology. Recommendations for the reporting of surgically resected specimens of renal cell carcinoma. Am J Clin Pathol 2009;131(5):623–30.

31. Nasr SH, Galgano SJ, Markowitz GS, et al. Immuno-fluorescence on pronase-digested paraffin sections: a valuable salvage technique for renal biopsies. Kidney Int 2006;70(12):2148–51.

32. Molne J, Breimer ME, Svalander CT. Immunoperoxi-dase versus immunofluorescence in the assessment of human renal biopsies. Am J Kidney Dis 2005; 45(4):674–83.

33. Nasr SH, Markowitz GS, Valeri AM, et al. Thin basement membrane nephropathy cannot be diagnosed reliably in deparaffinized, formalin-fixed tissue. Nephrol Dial Transplant 2007;22(4):1228–32.

34. Bonsib SM, Pei Y. The non-neoplastic kidney in tumor nephrectomy specimens: what can it show and what is important? Adv Anat Pathol 2010;17(4):235–50.

35. Hepps D, Chernoff A. Risk of renal insufficiency in African-Americans after radical nephrectomy for kidney cancer. Urol Oncol 2006;24(5):391–5.

36. Shirasaki Y, Tsushima T, Nasu Y, et al. Long-term consequence of renal function following nephrectomy for renal cell cancer. Int J Urol 2004;11(9):704–8.

37. Melman A, Grim CE, Weinberger MH. Increased incidence of renal cell carcinoma with hypertension. Journal Urol 1977;118(4):531–2.

38. Kirchner FK Jr. Incidence of renal cell carcinoma with hypertension. J Urol 1978;119(4):579.

39. Epstein M. Aging and the kidney. J Am Soc Nephrol 1996;7(8):1106–22.

40. Modesto A, Marty L, Suc JM, et al. Renal complications of intravesical bacillus Calmette-Guerin therapy. Am J Nephrol 1991;11(6):501–4.

41. Li L, Parwani AV. Xanthogranulomatous pyelonephritis. Arch Pathol Lab Med 2011;135(5):671–4.

42. Fujita Y, Kashiwagi T, Takei H, et al. Membranous nephropathy complicated by renal cell carcinoma. Clin Exp Nephrol 2004;8(1):59–62.

43. Kapoulas S, Liakos S, Karkavelas G, et al. Membranous glomerulonephritis associated with renal cell carcinoma. Clin Nephrol 2004;62(6):476–7.

44. Magyarlaki T, Kiss B, Buzogany I, et al. Renal cell carcinoma and paraneoplastic IgA nephropathy. Nephron 1999;82(2):127–30.

45. Sessa A, Volpi A, Tetta C, et al. IgA mesangial nephropathy associated with renal cell carcinoma. Appl Pathol 1989;7(3):188–91.

46. Jain S, Kakkar N, Joshi K, et al. Crescentic glomerulonephritis associated with renal cell carcinoma. Ren Fail 2001;23(2):287–90.

Nephrectomy for Non-neoplastic Kidney Diseases

Joseph P. Gaut, MD, PhD

KEYWORDS

- Chronic pyelonephritis • Dysplasia • ADPKD • ARPKD • Xanthogranulomatous pyelonephritis
- Reflux nephropathy • Obstructive nephropathy

ABSTRACT

This review discusses the pathology of non-neoplastic kidney disease that pathologists may encounter as nephrectomy specimens. The spectrum of pediatric disease is emphasized. Histopathologic assessment of non-neoplastic nephrectomy specimens must be interpreted in the clinical context for accurate diagnosis. Although molecular pathology is not the primary focus of this review, the genetics underlying several of these diseases are also touched on.

OVERVIEW

Nephrectomy is the mainstay of treatment of non-neoplastic renal diseases of various causes. A search of the pathology archives of the Barnes Hospital Lauren V. Ackerman Laboratory of Surgical Pathology revealed a majority, 175 of 295 (59%), of partial or total nephrectomies in the pediatric (<18 years) population were performed for non-neoplastic causes. The most common pathologic diagnoses in such cases were obstructive nephropathy, renal dysplasia, and chronic pyelonephritis (**Table 1**). Reflux nephropathy was frequently diagnosed in combination with renal dysplasia and/or obstruction. Trauma, autosomal recessive polycystic kidney disease (ARPKD), congenital nephrotic syndrome with intractable proteinuria, venous thrombosis, severe oxalosis, lithiasis, renal hypoplasia, and agenesis were also identified as diagnoses rendered in pediatric nephrectomies but were considerably less common. Of the patients with chronic pyelonephritis, vesicoureteric reflux (VUR) and obstruction were the most common associated causes. A summary of the major causes and the key diagnostic features is outlined in **Table 2**. Previous studies showed a similarly high incidence of non-neoplastic entities among pediatric nephrectomy specimens.[1,2] Several of these entities may coexist. For example, patients with reflux nephropathy may also have chronic pyelonephritis.

CHRONIC PYELONEPHRITIS

Chronic pyelonephritis as a descriptive term refers to the presence of chronic tubulointerstitial inflammation and scarring secondary to bacterial infection; it can be associated with urine reflux from the lower urinary tract or urine flow obstruction. A precise diagnosis requires clinical and radiographic correlation and involvement of the renal pelvis by inflammation. It may be broken into obstructive and nonobstructive pyelonephritis. Urine reflux is most commonly due to an incompetent ureterovesical valve located at the entry of the ureter into the bladder, known as the *ureterovesical junction*, and is referred to as VUR. VUR is the underlying cause of disease in many children with chronic nonobstructive pyelonephritis. The term, *reflux nephropathy*, was introduced and is distinguished from pyelonephritis by the presence of discrete scars in a lobar distribution. Because reflux nephropathy does not require history of bacterial infection, it may be used in cases of sterile reflux. Similarly, the term, *obstructive nephropathy*, is used when a definitive cause of obstruction, either functional or structural, can be identified. The terms, *reflux nephropathy* and *obstructive nephropathy*, have caused considerable confusion

Nephropathology Associates, 10810 Executive Center Drive, Suite 100, Little Rock, AR 72211, USA
E-mail address: joe.gaut@nephropath.com

Surgical Pathology 7 (2014) 307–319
http://dx.doi.org/10.1016/j.path.2014.04.010
1875-9181/14/$ – see front matter

surgpath.theclinics.com

Table 1
Review of pathology case records from the Barnes Hospital Lauren V. Ackerman Laboratory of Surgical Pathology

Cause	Number of Cases
Non-neoplastic	175 (59%)
Obstruction ± reflux ± chronic pyelonephritis	63 (36%)
Dysplasia ± reflux ± obstruction	58 (33%)
Chronic pyelonephritis	19 (11%)
Trauma	12 (7%)
Reflux nephropathy	7 (4%)
Congenital nephrotic syndrome	3 (2%)
Venous thrombosis	2 (1%)
ARPKD	1 (<1%)
Oxalosis	1 (<1%)
Hypoplasia	1 (<1%)
Agenesis	1 (<1%)
Lithiasis	1 (<1%)
ESRD, unknown	6 (3%)
Neoplastic	120 (41%)
Wilms tumor	76 (63%)
Other	44 (37%)

Case records were reviewed between 1989 and 2013. Patients under the age of 18 who underwent partial or total nephrectomy were included. A total of 295 nontransplant cases were identified.

but a good rule for applying the term, *chronic pyelonephritis*, is history of recurrent urinary tract infections (UTIs) irrespective of the presence or absence of VUR and/or obstruction.

GROSS FEATURES OF CHRONIC PYELONEPHRITIS

Grossly, kidneys with chronic pyelonephritis are small with irregular parenchymal scarring. The number and location of scars vary, but the renal poles tend to be preferentially involved. The cortical surface may be smooth, particularly in cases of congenital VUR, or granular when associated with arterionephrosclerosis. Hydronephrosis (dilatation of the pelvis and or calyces) is present to varying degrees. In general, cases associated with obstruction show more severe hydronephrosis (**Fig. 1A**). Cystic changes are frequent and the cortex is thinned (atrophic). There are no specific gross findings to distinguish infectious from non-infectious renal cortical scarring.

MICROSCOPIC FEATURES

Histologic examination of nephrectomy specimens from patients with chronic pyelonephritis demonstrates scarring that is most prominent at the renal poles. The tubules are atrophic and have a thyroidization appearance, named for the superficial resemblance to normal thyroid parenchyma (see **Fig. 1B**). Thyroidization is not a pathognomonic finding of past infections but is commonly associated with chronic parenchymal damage of all causes. A patchy chronic inflammatory infiltrate is present within the interstitium of the cortex, the medulla, or both the cortex and medulla. The inflammatory cells are a mixture of lymphocytes, monocytes, and plasma cells. The inflammatory infiltrate may be dense and show germinal center formation (see **Fig. 1C**). If there is a neutrophilic predominant infiltrate with neutrophilic tubular casts, a superimposed acute infection should be

Table 2
Key pathologic features

Diagnosis	Histologic and Associated Findings
ARPKD	Columnar-shaped cysts
ADPKD	Spherical cysts with flat, cuboidal, or papillary lining
Dysplasia	Immature tubules with fibromuscular collars
Congenital VUR	Renal scarring with segmental renal dysplasia; clinical history of reflux
Acquired VUR	Renal scarring without dysplasia; clinical history of reflux
Chronic pyelonephritis	Renal scarring with tubule thyroidization and pelvic inflammation associated with infection
Obstructive nephropathy	Interstitial fibrosis/tubular atrophy associated with functional or mechanical obstruction
XGP	Renal scarring associated with infection. Numerous foamy histiocytes. May mimic tumor
NPHP-MCKD	Corticomedullary cysts, tubular disruption, tubular atrophy

Fig. 1. (*A*) Gross photo of a nephrectomy specimen from a 12-year-old female patient with obstructive nephropathy and marked hydroureteronephrosis. The pelvis and renal calyces are markedly dilated. The maximum cortical width measured 0.5 cm. No mass lesions were identified. The patient had radiographic evidence of obstruction in utero. The patient had repeated episodes of UTIs that were intractable to medical management. (*B*) Histologic examination of the specimen from (*A*) shows extensive tubular thyroidization, a common but nonspecific finding in cases of chronic pyelonephritis (hematoxylin-eosin ×400). (*C*) Interstitial chronic inflammation is commonly observed in cases of chronic pyelonephritis. This inflammatory infiltrate shows prominent germinal center formation (hematoxylin-eosin ×100).

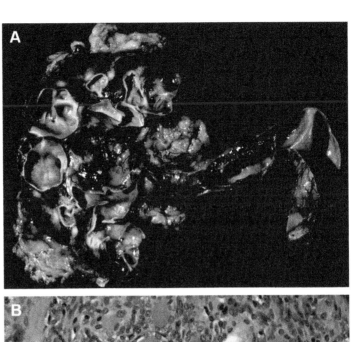

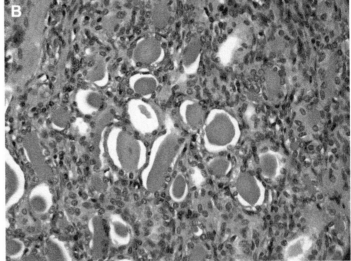

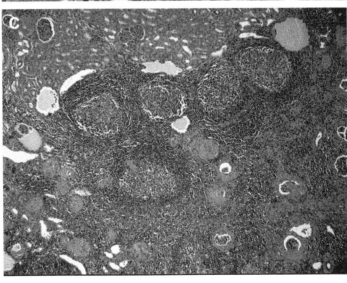

investigated. The cortex interstitium is fibrotic. As the disease advances, arteries become progressively thickened, accounting for the development of hypertension. Usually, there is increased global glomerulosclerosis. The nonsclerotic glomeruli may appear unremarkable or enlarged or show secondary focal segmental glomerulosclerosis.[3]

REFLUX NEPHROPATHY

VUR is the most common congenital urinary tract abnormality of childhood.[4] VUR is defined as the retrograde flow of urine from the lower urinary tract to the upper urinary tract.[5] Several studies indicate that approximately one-third of children who present with UTIs have underlying VUR.[5] The severity of reflux is graded according to the International Reflux Study system on a scale of 1 to 5, with grade 5 representing the most severe form.[6] Although VUR may resolve spontaneously with age, this is not always the case, particularly in patients who present with high-grade disease.

The underlying causes of VUR are divided into congenital and acquired categories. Congenital, or primary, VUR is the result of developmental abnormalities, is more common in male children, presents at an earlier age, and is more likely to be high grade.[4] One or both kidneys may be affected. The scarring associated with reflux may result directly from sterile urine or may be associated with infection. Acquired VUR results from repeated UTIs and is more common in females. Reflux nephropathy reportedly accounts for 12% to 21% of childhood chronic renal failure.[4,7,8] The most common adverse consequences associated with reflux nephropathy are hypertension and proteinuria. Proteinuria is more common in adult patients.[4] Only severe cases of congenital VUR are seen in pathology, usually at fetal autopsy. Typically, the ureters are dilated, sometimes to their entire length, and connect to normal-appearing or grossly malformed kidneys.

GROSS FEATURES

Grossly, kidneys associated with reflux nephropathy appear smaller than normal. The outer surface of the kidney appears irregular due to the presence of renal scarring. The renal cortex is thinned and cystic changes may be present. The ureters are dilated, the degree of which determines the grade of VUR. Duplicate ureters are frequently encountered.[9]

MICROSCOPIC FEATURES

The microscopic appearance of reflux nephropathy is nonspecific renal parenchymal scarring that may be segmental or diffuse. The renal scarring is manifested by interstitial fibrosis, tubular atrophy, loss of cortex, and global glomerulosclerosis. Tubular thyroidization may also be present. The presence of an acute inflammatory interstitial infiltrate should raise suspicion for a coexisting acute infection.

There are few microscopic findings that lend support to a specific cause. A clue to a congenital cause of reflux nephropathy, however, is the presence of segmental renal dysplasia characterized by aborted, primitive-appearing collecting ducts with surrounding fibromuscular collars. The Ask-Upmark kidney is a rare form of reflux nephropathy originally described by Eric Ask-Upmark in 1929. The histologic findings, also known as *segmental hypoplasia*, are identical to reflux nephropathy with the notable exception of the absence of glomeruli. Initially thought congenital, the Ask-Upmark kidney is now believed secondary to VUR.[10] Dysplastic changes are not observed in cases of Ask-Upmark kidney.

OBSTRUCTIVE NEPHROPATHY

Obstructive nephropathy refers to kidney damage secondary to blockade of urine flow at various points along the ureter. Obstructive nephropathy is distinguished from pyelonephritis by the unique presence of infectious agents in the latter. Physical obstruction may result from tumors, stones, prostatic disease, endometriosis, and pregnancy. Obstruction that occurs in the absence of a physical cause is referred to as functional obstruction. Defects of the ureteral peristaltic components, including neuronal and smooth muscle abnormalities, may lead to functional obstruction. The term, ureteropelvic junction obstruction (UPJO), refers to obstruction that occurs at the junction between the ureter and the renal pelvis. Similarly, ureterovesical junction obstruction (UVJO) refers to obstruction located at the junction between the ureter and the bladder. UPJO is the most common cause, affecting 1 in 1000 to 1 in 2000 births.[11] Male infants are more commonly affected than female infants at a 3:1 ratio.[12] Bilateral obstruction occurs in approximately one-fourth of cases.[11] UVJO is more common in males and tends to arise on the left. Similar to UPJO, bilateral UVJO is present in approximately one-fourth of cases.

GROSS FEATURES

The renal pelvis is dilated and the calyces appear flattened. As the disease advances, the kidney becomes progressively atrophic. The renal cortex is diffusely thinned with loss of the corticomedullary junction. Cysts may be present but should raise suspicion for dysplasia and a congenital cause.[9] Gross examination may reveal the underlying cause of obstruction, such as a mass or a stone. In congenital obstructive nephropathy, late obstruction results in hydronephrosis whereas early obstruction leads to renal dysplasia or agenesis.[13]

MICROSCOPIC FEATURES

Microscopic examination of kidneys with obstruction shows nonspecific cortical scarring and inflammation. As in all cases of renal scarring, the histologic appearance is that of interstitial fibrosis and tubular atrophy. The inflammatory infiltrate is typically composed of chronic inflammatory cells. As discussed previously, the presence of an acute inflammatory component should raise the possibility of a coexisting infection. The ureteropelvic junction typically shows smooth muscle fiber disarray and increased muscular thickness.[9]

XANTHOGRANULOMATOUS PYELONEPHRITIS

Xanthogranulomatous pyelonephritis (XGP) is a pyelonephritis variant that is characterized by the presence of predominant foamy, lipid-laden macrophage inflammation. XGP accounts for 0.6% of cases of chronic pyelonephritis.[14,15] XGP has been documented in ages ranging from 2 to 84 years, but individuals in the fifth and sixth decades of life affected are more commonly affected.[15] Women are more commonly affected than men. Patients present with fever, weight loss, flank pain, and hematuria. A palpable mass may be identified. The disease is most commonly unilateral.[15–17] Clinically and radiographically, XGP may be mistaken for a malignancy in both pediatric and adult populations.[16,18] Although no single clinical or radiologic finding is diagnostic, the presence of renal calculi should raise suspicion for XGP.[16]

The etiology underlying the development of XGP is unclear, but bacterial infection, obstruction, and lithiasis have been associated with disease development; 50% to 75% of cases have documented *Escherichia coli* and *Proteus* spp as common infectious culprits.[15–17]

GROSS FEATURES

XGP is typically diffuse, but may present with focal involvement mimicking a renal mass lesion (**Fig. 2A**). The involved kidney is often enlarged

with a thickened capsule. In cases of infection spread beyond the kidney, perirenal fibrosis and adhesions to the perirenal fat are present. The renal pelvis and calyces are frequently dilated and contain staghorn calculi, necrotic debris, and pus. The dilated calyces and renal cortex have a characteristic yellow friable appearance. Focal disease mimics a mass lesion with a yellow-red color, irregular borders, hemorrhage, and necrosis. This focal appearance raises the differential of carcinoma or renal tuberculosis.

MICROSCOPIC FEATURES

The histologic centerpiece of XGP is the presence of nodular inflammation composed of numerous foamy macrophages that appear to engulf the renal parenchyma (see **Fig. 2B**). The microscopic differential diagnosis includes a clear cell renal cell carcinoma. In cases of XGP, however, the cells have a more granular appearance rather than the cleared appearance of clear cell renal cell carcinoma. In challenging cases of little material, immunohistochemical stains for CD68, positive in histiocytes, and for CD10, positive in renal cell carcinoma, should clarify the cell type.[15] Other inflammatory cells, including neutrophils, lymphocytes, eosinophils, and plasma cells, are admixed with the foamy histiocytes. Abscess formation and necrosis may be evident. The glomeruli may appear normal or globally sclerosed. The interstitium may be fibrotic with scattered chronic inflammatory cells. In focal disease, the uninvolved portion of the kidney appears normal. The localized area of XGP shows finding similar to the diffuse form.

RENAL DYSPLASIA

Renal dysplasia is a developmental abnormality within the congenital anomalies of the kidney and urinary tract spectrum that results from aberrant interactions between the ureteric bud and mesenchyme. The result is characteristic abnormal branching of the collecting ducts, nephron loss, and formation of cysts, cartilage, and increased mesenchymal stroma.[19] Genetic factors, exposure to various teratogens, and lower urinary tract obstruction are known causes of renal dysplasia.[19] Given this variable etiology, the diagnosis of renal dysplasia overlaps with obstructive nephropathy and reflux nephropathy.

Renal dysplasia is commonly detected by antenatal ultrasound, affecting approximately 1 in 4300 live births.[20] The disease is increasingly recognized due to advances in ultrasound technology.[21–23] The kidneys typically appear enlarged and bright on ultrasound scan at 20 weeks. Renal

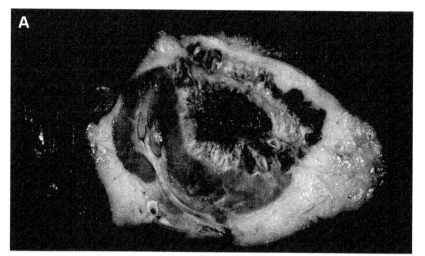

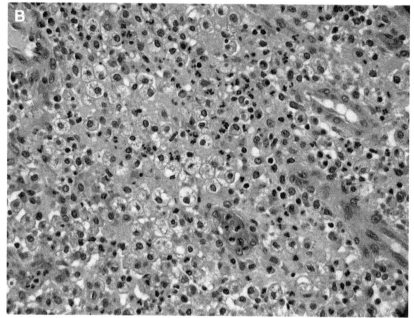

Fig. 2. XGP. (*A*) Cross-section of a nephrectomy from a patient who presented with a left renal mass. The lesion has an irregular yellow border with central hemorrhage and necrosis. The uninvolved renal parenchyma appears grossly normal. (*B*) Histologic examination from the case in (*A*) shows numerous foamy histiocytes admixed with neutrophils, plasma cells, and lymphocytes (hematoxylin-eosin ×400).

dysplasia may affect only one or both kidneys but is more commonly unilateral. Males and females are equally affected. Bilateral renal dysplasia may lead to Potter sequence and death. Children who are born with bilateral renal dysplasia represent the most frequent cause of chronic renal failure in childhood.[24] Patients with unilateral renal dysplasia may be asymptomatic at birth and develop secondary focal segmental glomerulosclerosis in adulthood. A long-term follow-up study by the multicystic dysplastic kidney (MCDK) study group indicated that patients with unilateral MCDK could be conservatively managed given minimal complications associated with the disease. The

investigators suggested that patients routinely require micturating cystourethrogram evaluations if they present at less than 1 year of age with a UTI.[25] Patients with dysplasia frequently have other coexisting abnormalities of the urinary tract and should undergo appropriate screening pre- and postnatally.[26] Of patients with unilateral renal dysplasia, 15% to 28% have VUR in the contralateral kidney.[27]

Progress in understanding of renal dysplasia has been improved by the identification of genetic defects associated with this disease. Approximately 10% of children with dysplasia have a positive family history.[19,28,29] Numerous genes have been identified suggesting key roles for *TCF2*, *PAX2*, and uroplakins in the formation of dysplastic kidneys.[19,30]

GROSS FEATURES

Dysplastic kidneys may be small, normal sized, or slightly enlarged. They contain diffuse or partial cysts that are randomly distributed at the periphery of the kidney. The peripheral cysts outline a central solid core (**Fig. 3A**). The cortex is thinned due to the decreased nephron mass. Ureteral defects, such as duplicate ureters, are frequent. In such cases, the dysplastic portion of the kidney is typically segmental and located just above the duplication.[31]

MICROSCOPIC FEATURES

Microscopically, dysplastic kidneys contain primitive-appearing undifferentiated tubules that have concentric fibromuscular collars (see **Fig. 3B, C**). Dilated tubules with a cystic appearance are common. The organization of the renal cortex is disrupted. Metaplastic cartilage is identified in approximately one-third of cases (see **Fig. 3D**). The glomeruli may show focal or diffuse cystic changes (see **Fig. 3E**), raising the microscopic differential diagnosis of GCKD. In cases of GCKD, however, the glomerular cysts are a dominant finding and secondary to a familial cause.[32,33] Rarely, nephrogenic rests may be seen. The presence of nephrogenic rests has raised suspicion regarding the malignant potential of dysplastic kidneys, but the risk of developing a Wilms tumor in cases of MCDK is essentially nil.[34]

AUTOSOMAL RECESSIVE POLYCYSTIC KIDNEY DISEASE

ARPKD has a reported incidence ranging from 1:10,000 to 40,000 live births.[35–37] Previously known as a perinatal disease, ARPKD is also diagnosed later in childhood or even adulthood. Patients with ARPKD usually have liver involvement that is manifest by a ductal plate malformation culminating in congenital hepatic fibrosis.[37,38] Diagnosis is made late in pregnancy by ultrasound. Neonatal ARPKD is characterized by corticomedullary involvement and has a more rapid decline in renal function.[39] In severe cases, the classic presentation of Potter sequence, markedly enlarged kidneys, and hepatic fibrosis is observed. Many of these patients die as a consequence of pulmonary hypoplasia.[37] Of the 70% to 75% of patients that survive infancy, the reported 5-year survival rate is 75%.[37,40] Physical examination of infants with ARPKD reveals large, palpable flank masses.[37] If not detected in infancy, older children may present with symptoms associated with primary liver disease, such as portal hypertension, esophageal varices, acute cholangitis, and hypersplenism.[38] The differential diagnosis includes autosomal dominant polycystic kidney disease (ADPKD) and MCKD/nephronophthisis (NPHP). ADPKD is discussed later. NPHP-MCKD is rare, affecting 1:50,000 to 1,000,000 live births and is only briefly discussed.[41] The diagnostic dilemma arises when renal cysts are discovered by ultrasound in the neonatal period. NPHP-MCKD cysts are characteristically located at the corticomedullary junction. Patients with NPHP-MCKD, however, may present in the absence of cysts. Mutations in numerous genes related to ciliary function have been identified in NPHP-MCKD (**Table 3**).[42] A host of syndromes have been described in association with mutations in NPHP genes and currently the gold standard for diagnosis is genetic analysis.[41]

ARPKD is due to mutations in the *polycystic kidney and hepatic disease 1 gene (PKHD1)*. *PKHD1* is located on chromosome 6p21 and encodes the transmembrane receptor fibrocystin/polyductin. Similar to polycystin-1 and polycystin-2, fibrocystin/polyductin is expressed in cilia. Cilia are organelles on various cells, including renal tubular and biliary epithelium. The role of cilia is thought to be sensing fluid flow. Because ARPKD is a disease of ciliary dysfunction, it has been placed, along with ADPKD, into a group of disorders, termed *ciliopathies*. Many mutations within the *PKHD1* gene have been identified, without evidence of specific hot spots.[43] The type of mutation affects the severity of disease. Missense mutations are associated with a milder phenotype whereas truncating mutations result in the most severe disease.[43]

GROSS FEATURES

Classically, the kidneys of ARPKD are massively enlarged. The external surface of the kidney retains the reniform shape but harbors numerous translucent cysts that are apparent just underneath the surface. Cross-sectioning of the kidney reveals diffuse cylindrically shaped cysts arranged perpendicular to the cortex (**Fig. 4A**). The size of ARPKD kidneys stabilizes after birth and may even decrease.[44]

MICROSCOPIC FEATURES

The cysts of ARPKD appear as elongated cylinders of medullary and cortical collecting ducts (see **Fig. 4B**). A branching pattern has been

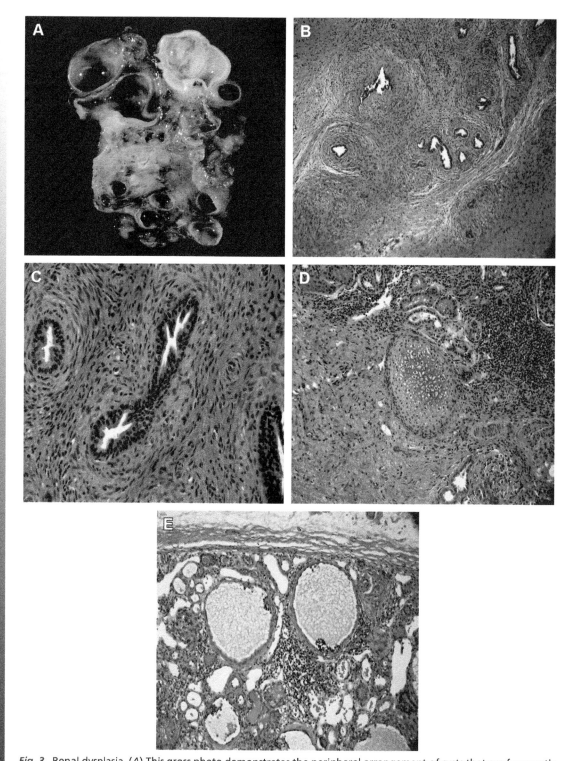

Fig. 3. Renal dysplasia. (*A*) This gross photo demonstrates the peripheral arrangement of cysts that are frequently present in cases of renal dysplasia. The central solid core is white-appearing without any resemblance to normal renal parenchyma. (*B*) Low-power photomicrograph of the case in (*A*) Several dilated, primitive-appearing tubules are identified that have a haphazard arrangement. The characteristic fibromuscular collars are visible at low power (hematoxylin-eosin ×100). (*C*) Higher-power view demonstrating the fibromuscular collars surrounding the irregularly shaped tubule (hematoxylin-eosin ×400). (*D*) Metaplastic cartilage is present in approximately one-third of cases and is considered definitive evidence of renal dysplasia (hematoxylin-eosin ×200). (*E*) Glomerular cysts are often seen in association with dysplastic kidneys. These are not, however, the dominant feature (hematoxylin-eosin ×200).

Table 3
Genes and gene products involved in the major heritable cystic kidney diseases

Diagnosis	Gene(s)	Gene Product
ARPKD	*PKHD1*	Fibrocystin/polyductin
ADPKD	*PKD1, PKD2*	Polycystin-1, polycystin-2
GCKD	*PKD1, HNF1β*	Polycystin-1, LFB3
NPHP-MCKD	*NPHP, MCKD*	Nephrocystins (NPHP1, NPHP3-11), inversin (NPHP2), uromodulin (MCKD2)

described in occasional cases of fetal and neonatal ARPKD.[31] The nephrons situated between the cysts appear microscopically normal. Interstitial fibrosis is variably present. The cysts are lined by a low cuboidal epithelium resembling their collecting duct origin. Renal dysplasia is not present. In contrast, the cysts of NPHP-MCKD appear spherical and, when present, are localized to the corticomedullary junction. A characteristic finding is tubulointerstitial injury with tubular basement membrane duplication, thickening, and chronic interstitial inflammation.[31]

AUTOSOMAL DOMINANT POLYCYSTIC KIDNEY DISEASE

ADPKD is common, with an incidence of 1:400 to 1000 individuals. A majority of cases are inherited, but approximately 5% of patients have spontaneous mutations.[45] Although the disease begins in infancy, patients do not typically present until adulthood. Rare infantile presentations, however, have been reported. Patients may present with various symptoms, including gross or microscopic hematuria, renal failure, UTI, and hypertension.

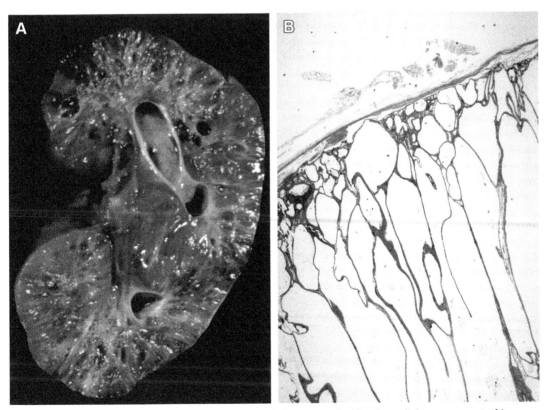

Fig. 4. ARPKD. (*A*) The gross appearance of an ARPKD kidney is typified by the radial arrangement of innumerable cortical and medullary cysts. (*B*) The microscopic appearance of cysts associated with ARPKD recapitulate the gross phenotype. The cysts are radially arranged with intervening nephron segments that appear pushed together by the cysts.

Approximately twice as many patients with ADPKD develop renal stones compared with the general population.[45,46] In addition to renal cysts, patients with ADPKD also have cysts in the pancreas, liver, seminal vesicles, and arachnoid.[47] Women tend to have more severe liver involvement. Approximately 8% of patients have brain aneurysms.[48] There is not a clearly increased risk of renal cell carcinoma in patients with ADPKD, although this has been reported.[49]

The *PKD1* gene, encoding for the protein polycystin-1, is mutated in approximately 85% of cases. Mutations in the *PKD2* gene, encoding the protein polycystin-2, account for the remainder of cases. Patients with *PKD1* mutations are younger by approximately 20 years and present with more severe disease compared with patients who have mutations in *PKD2*. Studies suggest that the polycystin proteins form a complex that is associated with cilia in tubular epithelial cells and other cells in the body, such as those in the liver and pancreas. The polycystin complex is integral for calcium regulation in these cells. Because of the defects in ciliary function, the syndromic forms of polycystic kidney disease have been termed, *ciliopathies*.[47,50]

GROSS FEATURES

The kidneys are markedly enlarged, weighing an average of 2.5 kg, approximately 16 times the weight of a normal kidney. The external surface is completely covered with thin-walled cysts, ranging in size from a few millimeters to several centimeters (**Fig. 5**). The cysts contain clear, hemorrhagic, or gelatinous fluid. Cysts may contain

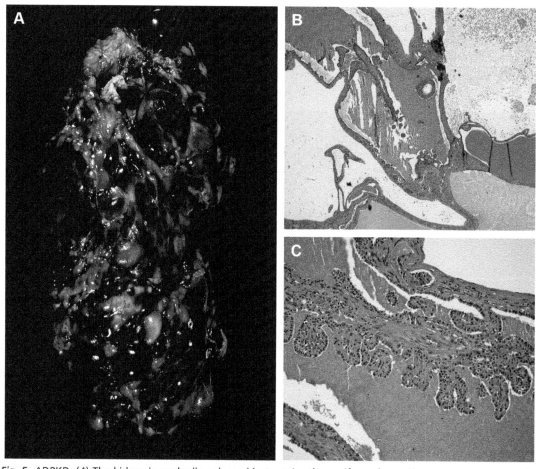

Fig. 5. ADPKD. (*A*) The kidney is markedly enlarged but retains the reniform shape. Numerous cysts occupy the entire kidney. Some cysts appear hemorrhagic and others contain a clear fluid. (*B*) The cut surface of an ADPKD kidney demonstrates the variability in size and shape of the cysts. In contrast to the ARPKD cysts, ADPKD cysts appear spherical and ovoid. The inner lining of the cysts is smooth and translucent. (*C*) Many of the cysts have an attenuated or cuboidal epithelial lining. Granular proteinaceous or colloid-like material fills the cysts. Elongate papillary growths extend into the cyst lumen. An attenuated cyst lining is seen in the upper right portion of the photomicrograph (hematoxylin-eosin ×100).

turbid-appearing fluid in cases that are secondarily infected. In contrast to the radial arrangement of ARPKD cysts, ADPKD cysts appear ovoid or spherical. The number of cysts increases with the age of the patient.[45] Despite the large number of cysts, the pelvicaliceal system is not obstructed.

MICROSCOPIC FEATURES

The cysts, derived from the tubules, are lined by a cuboidal epithelium that becomes progressively flattened as the cysts enlarge (see **Fig. 5**A). Both proximal and distal tubular markers have been demonstrated in ADPKD cysts.[51] The cysts begin as outpouchings from the tubular epithelium. As the cysts enlarge, they lose their connections with the tubules and continue to grow. Visualized under the microscope, the cysts appear as solitary structures, unconnected to the surrounding nephrons. Some cysts may show papillary growth of the epithelial lining or micropolyp formation, even in the absence of dialysis therapy (see **Fig. 5**B). This hyperproliferative phenotype of the cyst epithelia is thought to predispose ADPKD patients to renal cell carcinomas. The residual renal parenchyma shows varying degrees of global glomerulosclerosis, interstitial fibrosis, tubular atrophy, and chronic inflammation. The extent of renal parenchymal disease correlates with the severity of renal insufficiency. Glomerular cysts are frequently identified, particularly in the pediatric population.[31] A variant of ADPKD presents early in childhood and even before birth. Such cases may present predominantly with glomerular cysts and be diagnosed as glomerulocystic kidney disease (GCKD). GCKD is defined as glomerular cysts involving greater than 5% of glomeruli. A glomerular cyst is characterized by dilatation of the Bowman space greater than 2 times normal. In addition to ADPKD, ARPKD and other entities cause GCKD, for example, patients with mutations in $HNF1\beta$ may present with GCKD.[33]

MEDULLARY CYSTIC KIDNEY DISEASE/ NEPHRONOPHTHISIS

Medullary cystic kidney disease (MCKD) and NPHP represent a group of related inherited cystic kidney diseases with similar causes.[52] MCKD and NPHP are inherited in autosomal dominant and autosomal recessive fashion, respectively. Collectively, NPHP-MCKD are termed, *ciliopathies*, because they are secondary to a variety of defects in the renal tubular cilia proteins. The clinical presentation is initially mild with polyuria, polydipsia, and anemia. The kidneys inevitably fail at a young age in patients with NPHP and as adults in patients with MCKD.[53] Juvenile NPHP represents the most frequent genetic cause of end-stage renal disease in the first 3 decades of life, with renal loss occurring at a median age of 13 years.[53] The less common infantile and adolescent forms of NPHP have median ages of end-stage renal disease (ESRD) of 1 and 19 years of age, respectively. Other organs may be affected, with the retina the most common in addition to the kidney. MCKD has 2 forms, termed *MCKD1* and *MCKD2*, both of which are associated with hyperuricemia and gout. In contrast to NPHP, patients with MCKD1 and MCKD2 develop ESRD as adults at median ages of 62 and 32 years, respectively. A multitude of genetic mutations have been identified (see **Table 2**).[52]

GROSS FEATURES

In contrast to ADPKD, kidneys from patients with NPHP-MCKD are normal or somewhat reduced in size.[52] Sectioning the kidneys shows corticomedullary cysts as opposed to the more uniform distribution of cysts seen in patients with ADPKD and ARPKD. Gross examination does not distinguish NPHP from MCKD.

MICROSCOPIC FEATURES

Microscopic examination shows corticomedullary cysts that are lined by a simple, flattened low-cuboidal epithelium. The tubule basement membranes appear disrupted and atrophic. There is interstitial chronic inflammation and fibrosis. The glomeruli are unremarkable appearing, with some nonspecific periglomerular fibrosis.[53] There are no specific microscopic findings that distinguish MCKD from NPHP.

REFERENCES

1. Adamson AS, Nadjmaldin AS, Atwell JD. Total nephrectomy in children: a clinicopathological review. Br J Urol 1992;70(5):550–3.
2. Sammon J, Zhu G, Sood A, et al. Pediatric nephrectomy: incidence, indications and use of minimally invasive techniques. J Urol 2014;191(3):764–70.
3. Tada M, Jimi S, Hisano S, et al. Histopathological evidence of poor prognosis in patients with vesicoureteral reflux. Pediatr Nephrol 2001;16(6):482–7.
4. Mattoo TK. Vesicoureteral reflux and reflux nephropathy. Adv Chronic Kidney Dis 2011;18(5):348–54.
5. Williams G, Fletcher JT, Alexander SI, et al. Vesicoureteral reflux. J Am Soc Nephrol 2008;19(5):847–62.

6. Lebowitz RL, Olbing H, Parkkulainen KV, et al. International system of radiographic grading of vesicoureteric reflux. International Reflux Study in Children. Pediatr Radiol 1985;15(2):105–9.

7. Chantler C, Carter JE, Bewick M, et al. 10 years' experience with regular haemodialysis and renal transplantation. Arch Dis Child 1980;55(6):435–45.

8. Deleau J, Andre JL, Briancon S, et al. Chronic renal failure in children: an epidemiological survey in Lorraine (France) 1975-1990. Pediatr Nephrol 1994; 8(4):472–6.

9. Weiss M, Liapis H, Tomaszewski JE, et al. Pyelonephritis and other infections, reflux nephropathy, hydronephrosis, and nephrolithiasis. In: Jennette JC, Olson JL, Schwartz MM, et al, editors. Heptinstall's pathology of the kidney, vol. 2, 6th edition. Philadelphia: Lippincott Williams & Wilkins; 2007. p. 992–1081.

10. Arant BS Jr, Sotelo-Avila C, Bernstein J. Segmental "hypoplasia" of the kidney (Ask-Upmark). J Pediatr 1979;95(6):931–9.

11. Ingraham SE, McHugh KM. Current perspectives on congenital obstructive nephropathy. Pediatr Nephrol 2011;26(9):1453–61.

12. Woodward M, Frank D. Postnatal management of antenatal hydronephrosis. BJU Int 2002;89(2): 149–56.

13. Liapis H. Biology of congenital obstructive nephropathy. Nephron Exp Nephrol 2003;93(3):e87–91.

14. Malek RS, Greene LF, DeWeerd JH, et al. Xanthogranulomatous pyelonephritis. Br J Urol 1972;44(3): 296–308.

15. Li L, Parwani AV. Xanthogranulomatous pyelonephritis. Arch Pathol Lab Med 2011;135(5):671–4.

16. Loffroy R, Guiu B, Watfa J, et al. Xanthogranulomatous pyelonephritis in adults: clinical and radiological findings in diffuse and focal forms. Clin Radiol 2007;62(9):884–90.

17. Malek RS, Elder JS. Xanthogranulomatous pyelonephritis: a critical analysis of 26 cases and of the literature. J Urol 1978;119(5):589–93.

18. Inouye BM, Chiang G, Newbury RO, et al. Adolescent xanthogranulomatous pyelonephritis mimicking renal cell carcinoma on urine cytology: an atypical presentation. Urology 2013;81(4):885–7.

19. Winyard P, Chitty LS. Dysplastic kidneys. Semin Fetal Neonatal Med 2008;13(3):142–51.

20. Gordon AC, Thomas DF, Arthur RJ, et al. Multicystic dysplastic kidney: is nephrectomy still appropriate? J Urol 1988;140(5 Pt 2):1231–4.

21. Fugelseth D, Lindemann R, Sande HA, et al. Prenatal diagnosis of urinary tract anomalies. The value of two ultrasound examinations. Acta Obstet Gynecol Scand 1994;73(4):290–3.

22. Eckoldt F, Woderich R, Smith RD, et al. Antenatal diagnostic aspects of unilateral multicystic kidney dysplasia–sensitivity, specificity, predictive values, differential diagnoses, associated malformations and consequences. Fetal Diagn Ther 2004;19(2): 163–9.

23. Al Naimi A, Baumuller JC, Spahn S, et al. Prenatal diagnosis of multicystic dysplastic kidney disease in the second trimester screening. Prenat Diagn 2013;33(8):726–31.

24. Pruthi R, O'Brien C, Casula A, et al. UK Renal Registry 15th annual report: chapter 4 demography of the UK paediatric renal replacement therapy population in 2011. Nephron Clin Pract 2013; 123(Suppl 1):81–92.

25. Aslam M, Watson AR. Unilateral multicystic dysplastic kidney: long term outcomes. Arch Dis Child 2006;91(10):820–3.

26. Damen-Elias HA, Stoutenbeek PH, Visser GH, et al. Concomitant anomalies in 100 children with unilateral multicystic kidney. Ultrasound Obstet Gynecol 2005;25(4):384–8.

27. Cambio AJ, Evans CP, Kurzrock EA. Non-surgical management of multicystic dysplastic kidney. BJU Int 2008;101(7):804–8.

28. McPherson E, Carey J, Kramer A, et al. Dominantly inherited renal adysplasia. Am J Med Genet 1987; 26(4):863–72.

29. McPherson E. Renal anomalies in families of individuals with congenital solitary kidney. Genet Med 2007;9(5):298–302.

30. Jain S, Suarez AA, McGuire J, et al. Expression profiles of congenital renal dysplasia reveal new insights into renal development and disease. Pediatr Nephrol 2007;22(7):962–74.

31. Liapis H, Winyard P. Cystic diseases and developmental defects. In: Jennette JC, Olson JL, Schwartz MM, et al, editors. Heptinstall's pathology of the kidney, vol. 2, 6th edition. Philadelphia: Lippincott Williams & Wilkins; 2007. p. 1257–306.

32. Bonsib SM. The classification of renal cystic diseases and other congenital malformations of the kidney and urinary tract. Arch Pathol Lab Med 2010;134(4):554–68.

33. Lennerz JK, Spence DC, Iskandar SS, et al. Glomerulocystic kidney: one hundred-year perspective. Arch Pathol Lab Med 2010;134(4): 583–605.

34. Narchi H. Risk of Wilms' tumour with multicystic kidney disease: a systematic review. Arch Dis Child 2005;90(2):147–9.

35. Igarashi P, Somlo S. Genetics and pathogenesis of polycystic kidney disease. J Am Soc Nephrol 2002; 13(9):2384–98.

36. Dell KM. The spectrum of polycystic kidney disease in children. Adv Chronic Kidney Dis 2011; 18(5):339–47.

37. Sweeney WE Jr, Avner ED. Diagnosis and management of childhood polycystic kidney disease. Pediatr Nephrol 2011;26(5):675–92.

38. Buscher R, Buscher AK, Weber S, et al. Clinical manifestations of autosomal recessive polycystic kidney disease (ARPKD): kidney-related and non-kidney-related phenotypes. Pediatr Nephrol 2013. [Epub ahead of print].
39. Gunay-Aygun M, Font-Montgomery E, Lukose L, et al. Correlation of kidney function, volume and imaging findings, and PKHD1 mutations in 73 patients with autosomal recessive polycystic kidney disease. Clin J Am Soc Nephrol 2010;5(6):972–84.
40. Guay-Woodford LM, Desmond RA. Autosomal recessive polycystic kidney disease: the clinical experience in North America. Pediatrics 2003;111(5 Pt 1):1072–80.
41. Wolf MT, Hildebrandt F. Nephronophthisis. Pediatr Nephrol 2011;26(2):181–94.
42. Hildebrandt F, Attanasio M, Otto E. Nephronophthisis: disease mechanisms of a ciliopathy. J Am Soc Nephrol 2009;20(1):23–35.
43. Bergmann C, Senderek J, Kupper F, et al. PKHD1 mutations in autosomal recessive polycystic kidney disease (ARPKD). Hum Mutat 2004;23(5):453–63.
44. Blickman JG, Bramson RT, Herrin JT. Autosomal recessive polycystic kidney disease: long-term sonographic findings in patients surviving the neonatal period. AJR Am J Roentgenol 1995;164(5):1247–50.
45. Grantham JJ. Clinical practice. Autosomal dominant polycystic kidney disease. N Engl J Med 2008;359(14):1477–85.
46. Torres VE, Wilson DM, Hattery RR, et al. Renal stone disease in autosomal dominant polycystic kidney disease. Am J Kidney Dis 1993;22(4):513–9.
47. Harris PC, Torres VE. Polycystic kidney disease. Annu Rev Med 2009;60:321–37.
48. Sklar AH, Caruana RJ, Lammers JE, et al. Renal infections in autosomal dominant polycystic kidney disease. Am J Kidney Dis 1987;10(2):81–8.
49. Bonsib SM. Renal cystic diseases and renal neoplasms: a mini-review. Clin J Am Soc Nephrol 2009;4(12):1998–2007.
50. Harris PC. 2008 Homer W. Smith Award: insights into the pathogenesis of polycystic kidney disease from gene discovery. J Am Soc Nephrol 2009;20(6):1188–98.
51. Faraggiana T, Bernstein J, Strauss L, et al. Use of lectins in the study of histogenesis of renal cysts. Lab Invest 1985;53(5):575–9.
52. Hurd TW, Hildebrandt F. Mechanisms of nephronophthisis and related ciliopathies. Nephron Exp Nephrol 2011;118(1):e9–14.
53. Hildebrandt F, Otto E. Molecular genetics of nephronophthisis and medullary cystic kidney disease. J Am Soc Nephrol 2000;11(9):1753–61.

Autopsy Renal Pathology

Paisit Paueksakon, MD*, Agnes B. Fogo

KEYWORDS

- Gross examination • Glomeruli • Tubules • Interstitium • Light microscopy
- Immunofluorescence microscopy • Electron microscopy • Congenital abnormalities

ABSTRACT

We provide an overview of assessment of the kidneys at autopsy, with special considerations for pediatric versus adult kidneys. We describe the approach to gross examination, tissue allocation when needed for additional studies of potential medical renal disease, the spectrum of congenital abnormalities of the kidneys and urinary tract, and approach to cystic diseases of the kidney. We also discuss common lesions seen at autopsy, including acute tubular injury, ischemic versus toxic contributions to this injury, interstitial nephritis, and common vascular diseases. Infections commonly involve the kidney at autopsy, and the key features and differential diagnoses are also discussed.

APPROACH TO GROSS DISSECTION

TISSUE ALLOCATION

In any patient with renal functional abnormalities premortem, or with clinical suspicion of medical renal disease, tissue should be saved and allocated for potential immunofluorescence and electron microscopy (EM) studies. Tissue for immunofluorescence should be taken from the cortex. Pieces should be 2 to 3 mm thick, and approximately 5 × 2 to 3 mm and either directly snap-frozen or placed in Michel transport media. This tissue can then be stored for several days, before freezing for potential immunofluorescence studies. Immunofluorescence microscopy is much less sensitive on tissue that has already been fixed, and therefore it is imperative that fresh tissue is preserved for these studies. In contrast, EM can be done from tissue that has been fixed in any non–mercury-based fixative. For ease of maintaining optimal tissue allocation, we recommend that small rectangular pieces of tissue 2 to 3 mm × 2 to 3 mm be quickly place in glutaraldehyde. It is important that this tissue is cut with a fresh sharp blade on a clean surface, to avoid crushing and contamination of the tissue. The tissue allocated for these EM studies should come from the cortex. In cases in which regional abnormalities are present, the nonscarred and non-necrotic areas should be designated for immunofluorescence and EM studies.

In special circumstances, molecular studies may be indicated. Although DNA mutation analysis is better done from peripheral blood leukocytes or fibroblast-rich tissue sources, additional stains or assessment of specific markers may occasionally be necessary to reach a specific diagnosis. Allocation of tissue depends on the specific test needed, and a specialized reference laboratory should be consulted.

POSTMORTEM ALTERATIONS

The autopsy kidney will always show variable postmortem changes of autolysis. These changes may be minimal in infants, or patients with low body mass with a short postmortem interval, or when the body was quickly cooled. In contrast, even with a relatively short postmortem interval, patients with a high body mass may have kidneys that show extensive postmortem autolysis, due to maintenance of a higher inner core temperature for a longer period of time, as the body does not cool as quickly in this setting. The changes of autolysis consist of pyknosis of tubular epithelial nuclei, retraction and loss of continuity between the tubular epithelium and basement membrane, and degeneration of the tubular epithelium (**Fig. 1**). Although these findings overlap somewhat with those of acute tubular injury (ATI) (see later in this

Department of Pathology, Microbiology, and Immunology, Vanderbilt University Medical Center, MCN C3310, 1161 21st Avenue South, Nashville, TN 37232-2561, USA
* Corresponding author.
E-mail address: paisit.paueksakon@vanderbilt.edu

Surgical Pathology 7 (2014) 321–355
http://dx.doi.org/10.1016/j.path.2014.04.008

surgpath.theclinics.com

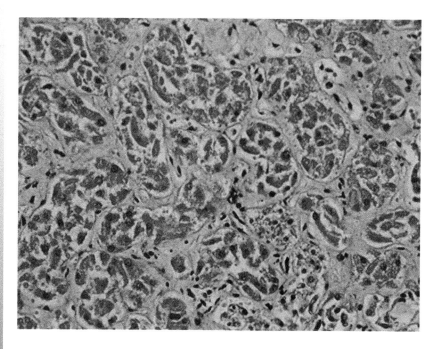

Fig. 1. Autolysis. There is pyknosis of tubular epithelial nuclei, retraction and loss of continuity between the tubular epithelial basement membranes and cells and degeneration of the tubular epithelium (H&E stain, original magnification ×200).

article), they may be distinguished from ATI by the uniform extent of these findings and the similar appearance of pyknotic changes of nuclei in other anatomic compartments of the kidney. Thus, in ATI, the proximal tubules are preferentially affected, whereas in postmortem injury, all of the nuclei have a similar pyknotic appearance and all of the tubules show similar degenerative changes. Regenerating changes of flattened epithelium (**Fig. 2**) and mitotic figures also distinguish ATI from autolysis.

MEDICAL RENAL DISEASES

A variety of medical renal diseases may be present in the autopsy kidney, most often clinically known before death. Comparison with any renal biopsies done antemortem is useful in determining

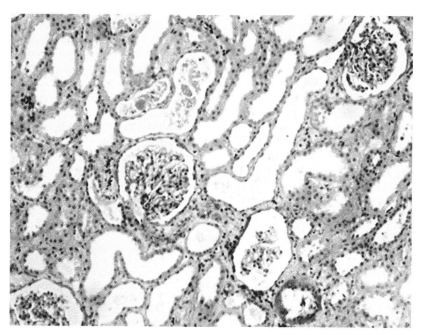

Fig. 2. Regenerative acute tubular injury. The proximal tubules are preferentially affected. Regenerating changes of flattened epithelium also distinguish ATI from autolysis (PAS stain, original magnification ×200).

progression of disease. Therefore, in any patient with a history of medical renal disease, or with significant proteinuria in which undiagnosed medical renal disease may be present, tissue should be saved for possible immunofluorescence and EM (see earlier in this article).

The kidney should be carefully examined grossly at autopsy, as detailed previously, and sections to illustrate any lesional areas and also nonlesional areas taken, to include cortex and medulla. In patients with history of proteinuria or medical renal disease, we recommend that additional special stains, in particular Jones and/or periodic acid-Schiff (PAS) or trichrome stains be done, as indicated by the initial light microscopic findings from hematoxylin-eosin (H&E) sections. Depending on abnormalities found by these stains, immunofluorescence may then be done as indicated. Depending on the clinical setting, immunofluorescence may be done for the usual panel of immunoglobulin (Ig)G, IgA, IgM, C3, C1q, kappa, and lambda. In the transplant, C4d studies may be done, depending on findings in premortem kidney biopsies. In patients with a history of polyomavirus nephropathy, an SV40 stain may be useful at autopsy to determine any change in extent of viral cytopathic lesions. It should be recognized that in patients who have received a transplant, it is necessary to examine both the transplanted kidney (or kidneys in case of recipients of multiple grafts) and the native kidney. In patients with cessation or decrease of immunosuppression due to complicated clinical course premortem, fulminant rejection, including antibody-mediated rejection, may be uncovered at autopsy.

If the previously mentioned special stains or immunofluorescence or clinical history indicate suspicion of medical renal disease, workup should proceed as is standard for assessment of medical renal disease, including EM as necessary. Immune complex deposits may robustly still be detected in autopsy specimens. Tissue fixed in formalin is still suitable for EM. Although fixation may be less than optimal, the autolysis present at autopsy makes the minor difference seen between glutaraldehyde-fixed and formalin-fixed tissues a moot point. Even deposits of, for instance light chain deposition disease, are robustly maintained and can be detected postmortem.

DISSECTION AND EXAMINATION OF THE KIDNEYS

Adults

At autopsy, the kidneys are taken out with their ureters and the urinary bladder. The simplest way is to grasp the kidney in situ through fat after making sweeping cuts just outside the lateral borders, through the peritoneum and fat. Blunt dissection with fingers then identify the organs by palpation. The ureter is then located and freed down to its entry to the bladder. The kidneys are then removed by blunt dissection in the plane between the renal capsule and the perinephric fat. Adherent fat should be removed to obtain accurate weight of the kidneys and a detailed external gross assessment. In most cases, the kidneys may be separated from the urinary bladder. It is then key to identify laterality by, for example, a tie, dye mark, or other means. When hydronephrosis is suspected, the organs should not be separated. The kidney is then bisected and the average thickness of the cortex and medulla is assessed. The cortex, medullary pyramids, and pelvis are examined, opening individual major and minor calyces as needed. Any calculi present should be preserved for possible biochemical analysis. The renal capsule should be completely stripped to allow examination of the cortical surfaces for any lesions or irregularities. Small cysts may not be detected if the capsules are left intact. The ease of capsular adherence and its appearance, whether fibrotic and thickened, or thin and translucent, should be noted. Fetal lobulations (see later in this article) may persist into adulthood and should be noted when present.

Children

Pediatric and fetal kidneys consist of small lobes (reniculi), each with a papilla. The kidney grows in development by progressively adding nephrons in a centrifugal pattern; therefore, assessment of the capsular and subcapsular regions has much greater importance in the developing kidneys. In contrast to the adult kidney, the pediatric kidney capsule should not initially be stripped. First assess for any variability in the appearance of the lobes before the kidneys are separated from the inferior vena cava. Abnormal blood supply, either arterial or venous, may sometimes occur in abnormal or dysplastic lobes. Inject the renal tract with saline if there is suspicion of obstruction, and observe if fluid passes through from the ureter into the bladder and from the bladder to the urethra. The kidney is then bisected. The renal capsule is then stripped as for adult kidneys. A list of abnormalities to note as present or absent for both pediatric and adult kidneys is given in **Box 1**

The kidneys are then dissected by making thin (3–5 mm) bread-loaf slices. Features of dysplasia should be assessed, as indicated in **Box 2**.[1,2]

Box 1
Abnormalities to assess on gross examination

1. Regularity of the renal lobes
2. Shape of the papillae
3. Thickness of cortex and medulla
4. Presence of cortical necrosis or papillary necrosis
5. Presence of cysts
6. Presence of fetal lobulations

COMMON PATHOLOGIC CHANGES OF KIDNEYS AT AUTOPSY

CONGENITAL ANOMALIES OF THE KIDNEY AND URINARY TRACT

Introduction

Defective development of kidney and urinary tract is referred to collectively as congenital anomalies of the kidney and urinary tract (CAKUT). CAKUT constitutes approximately 20% to 30% of all anomalies identified in the prenatal period. Incidence varies by type of malformation. Approximately 25% of patients with end-stage renal disease have CAKUT as the underlying disease. Defects can be bilateral or unilateral.

Categories of CAKUT

CAKUT can occur in isolation or as part of systemic clinical syndromes. In this article, only the

---

Box 2
Features of dysplasia

1. Smaller or larger kidneys than normal
2. Irregular, small or large lobes with rough edges or abnormal number of lobes
3. Indistinct line between cortex and medulla
4. Small or large cysts present; specify whether uniformly or in patchy distribution, whether cortical or medullary, whether round or saccular, give range of size, and contents of cysts
5. Irregular or firmer texture of kidneys than normal
6. Irregularities in coloration (eg, congested or pale areas)
7. Abnormality in thickness and form of renal pelvis

---

more important categories (listed as follows) are discussed:

- Renal agenesis
- Renal hypoplasia
- Renal dysplasia
- Ectopic and fused kidneys

RENAL AGENESIS

Introduction

Renal agenesis (RA) is defined as the complete absence of renal tissue, and may be bilateral or unilateral. The incidence of RA is 1 in 500 to 3200 births and males are more commonly affected than females, with a male-to-female ratio of 1.7:1.0. Bilateral RA is incompatible with life. Most infants with this anomaly are stillborn due to resulting oligohydramnios and hypoplastic lungs. Patients with unilateral RA have a higher risk of hypertension and albuminuria as adults. Unilateral RA is thus compatible with normal life and is often identified only as an incidental finding during imaging, surgery, or at postmortem examination.

Gross Features

At autopsy, RA is characterized by complete absence of one or both kidneys, with associated complete absence of the ureters and urinary bladder trigone. With unilateral RA, the remaining kidney usually shows hypertrophy.

Microscopic Features

The diagnosis of RA is made when no renal tissue is present either grossly or microscopically. With unilateral RA, the remaining contralateral kidney undergoes compensatory hypertrophy with glomerulomegaly and enlargement of tubules. Patients with unilateral agenesis are at increased risk for developing secondary focal segmental glomerulosclerosis (FSGS), likely as an adaptive response to loss of renal mass, both due to absence of one kidney and a reduced number of functioning nephrons in the single remaining kidney. When this happens, microscopic examination of the single remaining kidney shows FSGS characterized by perihilar sclerosis, and hyalinosis and glomerulomegaly.

Differential Diagnosis

The major differential diagnosis is renal aplastic dysplasia, which may result in a very small amount of malformed renal tissue that is difficult to identify by gross examination. The dysplastic tissue, such as bone or cartilage, is found by microscopic examination of tissue at the site where the kidney should be.

Clinical Correlation and Prognosis

Bilateral RA results in stillbirth in approximately 40% of affected infants. Most who are born alive are premature and die shortly after birth because of respiratory failure secondary to pulmonary hypoplasia. Unilateral RA is usually asymptomatic, but there is increase risk of hypertension and albuminuria, and later secondary FSGS.

Key Points: Renal Agenesis

- Complete absence of renal tissue

- Bilateral or unilateral

- Bilateral agenesis is incompatible with life

- Unilateral agenesis is compatible with normal life if no other abnormalities exist

- Enlarged remaining kidney as a result of compensatory hypertrophy in unilateral agenesis

- Increased risk for developing secondary focal segmental glomerulosclerosis

---

RENAL HYPOPLASIA

Introduction

Renal hypoplasia is defined as a reduction in renal mass due to inadequate genesis of normal renal tissue. Simple renal hypoplasia has no other pathologic alternations. Oligomeganephronic hypoplasia is characterized by marked compensatory growth of the reduced number of nephrons.

Gross Features

At autopsy, hypoplastic kidneys are small with weight less than 50% of age-matched normal kidneys. Oligomeganephronic hypoplasia is usually bilateral, whereas simple hypoplasia is usually unilateral. Hypoplastic kidneys may be rounder than normal or reniform. The kidney shows reduced number of renal lobes and pyramids, usually 6 or fewer on cut surface.

Microscopic Features

Unilateral simple hypoplasia shows no discernible histologic abnormalities or only mild glomerular hypertrophy. Bilateral simple hypoplasia is likely to manifest findings of oligomeganephronic hypoplasia. Microscopically, oligomeganephronic

hypoplasia displays glomerular hypertrophy and tubular enlargement. Oligomeganephronic hypoplasia predisposes to the development of FSGS mediated by adaptive responses to a reduced number of functioning nephrons.

Differential Diagnosis

The major differential diagnostic consideration is reduced renal size caused by other congenital or acquired pathologic processes and aplastic dysplasia, which can be readily distinguished microscopically.

Clinical Correlation

Bilateral renal hypoplasia is an important cause of end-stage renal disease in children and causes renal insufficiency from birth. Delayed-onset kidney failure may be caused by the development of secondary FSGS, which clinically manifests as proteinuria.[3,4]

Key Points: Renal Hypoplasia

- Reduction in renal mass caused by inadequate genesis of normal renal tissue

- Unilateral simple hypoplasia shows no discernible histologic abnormalities

- Bilateral simple hypoplasia is likely to manifest findings of oligomeganephronic hypoplasia

---

Key Points: Oligomeganephronic Hypoplasia

- Marked compensatory growth and glomerulomegaly of the remaining reduced number of nephrons

- Glomerular and tubular hypertrophy

- Hypoplasia predisposes to the development of focal segmental glomerulosclerosis

---

ECTOPIC AND FUSED KIDNEYS

Introduction

Ectopic kidneys are sited in an abdominal or pelvic location, rather than the normal retroperitoneal location. The ectopy may involve only one kidney or it may be bilateral. Fused kidneys are ectopic, nearer the midline than normal, or in the pelvis. Fusion of the upper or lower poles of the kidneys produces a horseshoe-shaped structure that is continuous across the midline anterior to the great vessels, so-called "horseshoe kidneys." This anomaly is common and is found in approximately 1 in 400 autopsies.

Gross Features

At autopsy, ectopic kidneys that are not fused typically have reniform shape and are often abnormally rotated. The ureters of ectopic kidneys may be more tortuous than normal, especially in the proximal portion, causing obstruction and hydronephrosis.

Horseshoe kidneys are usually fused at the lower pole. Complete fusion of the kidneys (**Fig. 3**) most often produces a formless mass in the pelvis that gives rise to 2 or more ureters.

Microscopic Features

The ectopic and fused kidney is usually normal microscopically unless there are acquired related diseases, such as chronic pyelonephritis and obstructive nephropathy.

Differential Diagnosis

The major differential diagnoses are clinical rather than pathologic. An ectopic or fused kidney may be palpated during physical examination or seen by imaging studies and misinterpreted as tumor. This has resulted in unnecessary surgery. With modern imaging techniques, such as magnetic resonance imaging, such a misdiagnosis is extremely rare.

Clinical Correlation

In the absence of secondary complications, such as infection and/or obstruction, prognosis is excellent and no treatment is necessary.[3,5]

Key Points: Ectopic Kidneys

- Abdominal location, usually in the pelvis
- Reniform shape
- Tortuous ureter may cause obstruction
- Normal microscopic findings

Key Points: Fused Kidneys

- Ectopic, nearer the midline or in the pelvis
- Fusion of the upper or lower poles of the kidneys produces a horseshoe-shaped structure that is continuous across the midline anterior to the great vessels
- Normal microscopic findings

CYSTIC DISEASES OF THE KIDNEY

Introduction

Cystic diseases of kidney comprise hereditary, developmental, and acquired disorders. A useful classification of cystic diseases of the kidney is shown in **Box 3**.

Only the more important categories in **Box 3** are discussed in this article.

AUTOSOMAL DOMINANT (ADULT) POLYCYSTIC KIDNEY DISEASE

Introduction

Autosomal dominant (adult) polycystic kidney disease (ADPKD) is the most common cystic and genetic kidney disease, occurring in 1:500 to 1:1000 births. It is a major cause of end-stage kidney disease. It is inherited in an autosomal dominant fashion. Although the disease has complete penetrance and all individuals with the genetic defect develop cysts, not all patients develop renal failure, and, thus, not all are diagnosed. Spontaneous mutations also occur. Thus, not all affected patients have a positive family history. ADPKD is associated with defects in 2 genes: polycystin 1 (PKD1), coded on chromosome 16p 13.3 (the underlying defect in 90% of patients) and polycystin 2 (PKD2), coded on chromosome 4q21 (10% of patients). Polycystin-1 is localized to tubular epithelial cells, particularly those of the distal nephron, and consists of a large, receptorlike integral membrane glycoprotein involved in cell-cell and cell-matrix interactions. Polycystin-1 also activates polycystin-2, another transmembrane protein, which acts as a calcium channel at the plasma membrane after translocation from the endoplasmic reticulum. Patients with mutations in PKD2 have a slower rate of progression of disease than those with PKD1 mutations. A 2-hit theory is proposed, with a second injury and loss of heterozygosity leading to cyst development in early adulthood and progression at age 40 to 50 years. Many of these patients remain

Fig. 3. Horseshoe kidneys. Horseshoe kidneys are usually fused at the lower pole and have 2 separate collecting systems.

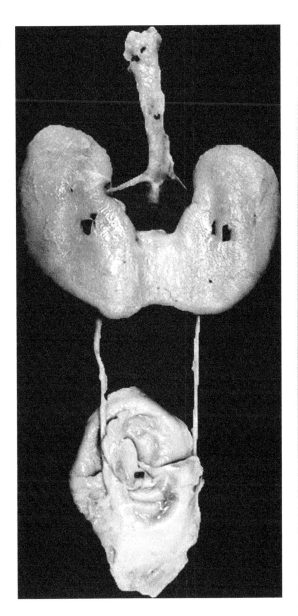

asymptomatic until renal insufficiency pronounces the presence of disease. Other patients may present with hematuria, hypertension, flank pain, urinary tract infection, or nephrolithiasis. They also can develop cysts in other organs, including the liver, pancreas, and spleen. About 5% to 15% will develop a berry aneurysm in the Circle of Willis in the brain.

Gross Features

Once cysts are fully developed, the kidneys become markedly enlarged bilaterally. Both kidneys are similarly affected in most patients. At autopsy, each kidney weighs approximately 6 lb in severely affected adults, with a range from 4.5 to 10.0 lb (**Fig. 4**). The external contour of the kidney is cobbled by numerous cysts filled with clear fluid, most of which range from 0.5 cm to 5.0 cm, without intervening parenchyma by gross examination.

Microscopic Features

In the early stages of the disease, the intervening renal parenchyma is normal, but as the cysts enlarge, the intervening tissue becomes fibrotic and atrophic and glomeruli also become sclerosed. The cysts are lined by a single layer of benign flattened epithelial cells. Cystic dilatation

---

Box 3
Cystic diseases of the kidney

1. Polycystic kidney disease
   a. Autosomal-dominant (adult) polycystic kidney disease (ADPKD)
   b. Autosomal-recessive (childhood) polycystic disease (ARPKD)
2. Multicystic renal dysplasia
3. Medullary cystic disease
   a. Medullary sponge kidney
   b. Nephronophthisis/Medullary cystic kidney disease
4. Acquired (dialysis-associated) cystic disease
5. Localized (simple) renal cyst
6. Renal cysts in hereditary malformation syndromes (eg, tuberous sclerosis)
7. Glomerulocystic disease
8. Extraparenchymal renal cysts (pyelocalyceal cysts, hilar lymphangitic cysts)

---

of Bowman space around glomeruli (glomerular cyst) may occur.

Differential Diagnosis

Simple renal cysts (see later in this article) may rarely be so numerous to raise the possibility of adult polycystic kidney disease. However, kidneys are typically not markedly enlarged, as in ADPKD. Simple renal cysts usually occur in the outer cortex, bulging the capsule and also are typically lined by flat epithelium. Associated glomerular cysts are not present in simple renal cysts. Multicystic renal dysplasia is readily distinguished microscopically by the presence of dysplastic mesenchyme, such as cartilage or bone and primitive tubules and ducts.

Clinical Correlation and Prognosis

Once renal function begins to deteriorate, the rate of deterioration accelerates with progressive increase in renal cyst volume and overall renal size, with concomitant reduction in renal parenchyma and glomerular filtration rate. Patients with ADPKD also are predisposed to develop renal carcinomas, which occur in 1% to 5% of cases.

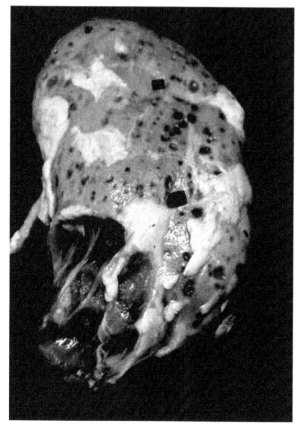

Fig. 4. ADPKD. Both kidneys are enlarged. The external contour of the kidney is cobbled by numerous cysts filled with clear fluid.

These renal carcinomas more often are papillary rather than clear-cell type.

Key Points: ADPKD

- Most common cystic and genetic kidney disease

- Incidence 1:500 to 1:1000

- Autosomal dominant

- Defects in 2 genes: Polycystin 1 (PKD1) or Polycystin 2 (PKD2); second hit leads to disease phenotype in adulthood

- Cysts in other organs, including the pancreas, liver, and spleen

- 5% to 15% develop berry aneurysm in the Circle of Willis in the brain

---

**Key Features
ADPKD**

- Cysts vary in size and shape

- Cysts are widespread throughout the renal parenchyma and replace the entire kidney

- The cysts are lined by a single layer of benign flattened epithelial cells

- Glomerular cysts also may occur

AUTOSOMAL RECESSIVE (CHILDHOOD) POLYCYSTIC KIDNEY DISEASE

Introduction

Autosomal recessive (childhood) polycystic kidney disease (ARPKD) is a rare autosomal recessive condition with an incidence of between 1:6000 to 14,000 births. There is often bilateral kidney involvement. In most cases, the disease is associated with a defect on PKHD1 on chromosome 6p21-p23, which codes for fibrocystin, a component of the cilia of the collecting ducts. The function of fibrocystin is still poorly understood, but it is thought to modulate cell differentiation and proliferation in response to flow. ARPKD often leads to stillbirth or death within days after birth due to oligohydramnios and resulting pulmonary hypoplasia (Potter sequence). There is also a strong association with congenital hepatic fibrosis. Some patients have survived into adolescence, but they usually suffer respiratory failure or portal hypertension and esophageal varice, due to hepatic fibrosis.

Gross Features

At autopsy, both kidneys are markedly symmetrically enlarged with preservation of the reniform shape and often accentuated fetal lobation (**Fig. 5**). The kidney resembles a sponge, with numerous radially oriented, fusiform cysts (1–2 mm), which represent dilated collecting ducts, replacing the entire kidney. Cut surfaces reveal elongated, fusiform cysts in the cortex that are arranged perpendicularly to the capsule, thus producing a radial pattern.

Microscopic Features

There are conspicuous elongated cortical cysts with the long axis perpendicular to the renal capsule. The cysts arise predominantly from the collecting ducts. Medullary cysts are usually round or oval rather than elongated.

Differential Diagnosis

ARPKD must be distinguished from multicystic renal dysplasia and early-onset autosomal dominant polycystic kidney disease. Multicystic renal dysplasia is readily distinguished microscopically by the presence of dysplastic mesenchyme and primitive tubules and ducts. Early-onset autosomal dominant polycystic kidney disease often has glomerular cysts, which do not occur in ARPKD. ADPKD does not show the distinct elongated, radial cysts of ARPKD.

Clinical Correlation

If patients survive past the perinatal period, they are at high risk for developing progressive renal failure, systemic hypertension, respiratory failure, and portal hypertension. Renal transplantation in the infant or child can improve prognosis and extend life. However, many still die from complications of congenital hepatic fibrosis.

Key Points: ARPKD

- Autosomal recessive condition

- Incidence of between 1:6000 and 14,000 births

- Defect in PKHD1 on chromosome 6p21-p23, which codes for fibrocystin

- Bilateral kidney involvement

- Leads to stillbirth or death within days after birth due to oligohydramnios and resulting pulmonary hypoplasia (Potter sequence)

- Association with congenital hepatic fibrosis

Key Features
ARPKD

- Sponge appearance with numerous radially oriented, fusiform cysts
- Cysts are perpendicular to the capsule, thus producing a radial pattern
- Cysts arise predominantly from the collecting ducts

MULTICYSTIC RENAL DYSPLASIA

Introduction

Renal dysplasia is characterized by the presence of malformed kidney tissue elements. Characteristic microscopic abnormalities include geographic disorganization of nephron elements, maldifferentiation of mesenchymal and epithelial elements, decreased number of nephrons, and metaplastic transformation of metanephric mesenchyme to cartilage and bone. Renal dysplasia may be unilateral or bilateral and occurs in 2 to 4 per 1000 births. The male-to-female ratio for bilateral renal dysplasia is 1.3:1.0, and for unilateral dysplasia 1.9:1.0. Renal dysplasia may also have cysts, so-called multicystic renal dysplasia, which is usually unilateral.

Gross Features

At autopsy, the kidney is usually enlarged, extremely irregular, and often multicystic. The kidney does not have the usual beanlike shape, but rather resembles an irregular mass of grapes. The cysts vary in size from microscopic structures to several centimeters in diameter.

Microscopic Features

The histologic hallmarks of renal dysplasia are primitive tubules and ducts lined by cuboidal epithelium and surrounded by poorly differentiated mesenchymal tissue. There are islands of undifferentiated mesenchyme, often with cartilage, smooth muscle, adipose tissue, and immature collecting ducts (**Table 1**). The cysts are lined by flattened epithelium.

Differential Diagnosis

The clinical differential diagnosis for a large, unilateral, multicystic dysplastic kidney is an abdominal neoplasm, especially neuroblastoma or Wilms' tumor. The diagnosis usually can be resolved by imaging studies. Multicystic renal dysplasia must be distinguished from autosomal recessive polycystic kidney disease and early-onset autosomal dominant polycystic kidney disease. The presence of primitive mesenchyme and undifferentiated tubules between the cysts indicates dysplasia.

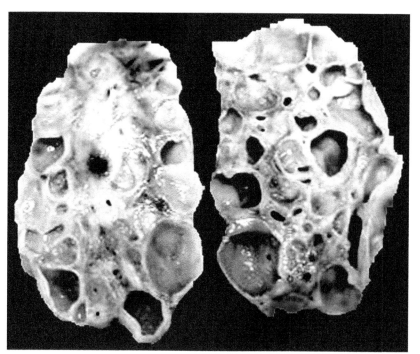

Fig. 5. ARPKD. There are round cysts in the cortex and medulla in a patient with ARPKD who survived beyond the perinatal period, and thus gross pathologic differentiation between ADPKD and ARPKD become more challenging. Microscopic examination can help to distinguish these entities.

Table 1
Dysplasia/Hypoplasia/Agenesis

	Dysplasia	Hypoplasia	Agenesis
Definition	Disorganized architecture, undifferentiated mesenchyme and stroma	Small, architecturally normal kidney, reduced nephron number	Absent kidney
Gross features	Nonreniform irregular mass of multiple, variably sized cysts	Small, normally shaped kidneys, reduced number of pyramids	No kidney
Microscopic features	Primitive ducts and mesenchyme, cartilage	Normal organization; large nephrons in oligomeganephronia	Normal or compensatory hypertrophy in unilateral renal agenesis

Clinical Correlation

A patient with large unilateral, multicystic renal dysplasia may have discomfort because of hemorrhage, infarction, or inflammation. The prognosis for patients with multicystic renal dysplasia often is influenced as much or more by concomitant abnormalities in other organs.[6–8]

Key Points: Multicystic Renal Dysplasia

- Presence of malformed kidney tissue elements, including mesenchymal and epithelial elements
- Decreased number of nephrons
- Usually unilateral

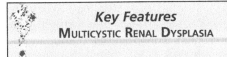

Key Features
MULTICYSTIC RENAL DYSPLASIA

- Multicystic, nonreniform
- Irregular mass of multiple, variably sized cysts from microscopic to several centimeters
- Primitive tubules and ducts, undifferentiated mesenchyme, often with cartilage and immature collecting ducts

---

CYSTIC DISEASE OF THE RENAL MEDULLA

The 3 major types of medullary cystic disease are medullary sponge kidney, nephronophthisis (NPHP), and adult-onset medullary cystic disease.

MEDULLARY SPONGE KIDNEY

Introduction

Medullary sponge kidney is defined by congenital cystic dilatation of the terminal collecting ducts (ducts of Bellini), and occurs in 1 in 5000 to 20,000. Patients are asymptomatic unless the disease is complicated by infection, stones, obstruction or hematuria, which typically manifest by age 30 to 40 years.

Gross Features

Kidneys are usually of normal size, but about 30% of patients have slight renal enlargement. The cut surfaces reveal cysts in the medullary pyramid, most numerous at the papillary tips. These cysts may reach 8 to 10 mm and in at least 50% of patients contain intense calcium deposits or stones.

Microscopic Features

Cysts arise from distal collecting ducts, including ducts of Bellini. The cysts are usually lined by cuboidal epithelium or occasionally by transitional epithelium.

Cyst lumens may contain calcium deposits, clotted blood, or leukocytes.

Differential Diagnosis

Medullary sponge kidney must be distinguished from NPHP. The former essentially always involves the papillary tips, whereas papillary tip involvement is rare with NPHP. In addition, calcification is common in the cysts of medullary sponge kidney but does not occur in the cysts of NPHP.

Clinical Correlation

Medullary sponge kidney usually does not cause renal failure. Although the defect of tubular development is present at birth, the etiology is unknown and it does not appear to be inherited. Hemorrhage may occur in the absence of stones or infection but resolves spontaneously.

Key Points: Medullary Sponge Kidney

- Congenital cystic dilatation of ducts of Bellini
- Asymptomatic unless the disease is complicated by infection, stones, obstruction, or hematuria
- Cysts in medullary pyramid, most numerous at the papillary tips
- The cysts are lined by cuboidal epithelium or occasionally by transitional epithelium
- Calcium deposits, clotted blood, or leukocytes in cyst lumina

---

NEPHRONOPHTHISIS AND ADULT-ONSET MEDULLARY CYSTIC DISEASE

Introduction

This is a group of progressive renal disorders. The common characteristic is the presence of variable numbers of cysts in the medulla, usually concentrated in the corticomedullary junction. Initially, injury probably involves the distal tubules with tubular basement membrane disruption, followed by chronic and progressive tubular atrophy involving both medulla and cortex, and ultimately interstitial fibrosis. Although the presence of medullary cysts is important, the cortical tubulointerstitial damage is the cause of eventual renal insufficiency.

Gross Features

At autopsy, in NPHP and adult-onset medullary cystic disease, kidney size is normal or slightly decreased, depending on the extent of chronic tubulointerstitial injury. The external surface is variably granular. With advanced disease, the kidneys are fibrotic and shrunken. The cut surfaces of the kidney show multiple 1-mm to 15-mm cysts, predominantly at the corticomedullary junction. Not all patients have identifiable cysts; therefore, cysts are not required for a pathologic diagnosis of NPHP and adult-onset medullary cystic disease.

Microscopic Features

Microscopically, cysts and diverticula are lined by flattened or detached epithelial cells and are usually surrounded by either inflammatory cells or fibrous tissue. There is widespread atrophy and thickening of tubular basement membranes of proximal and distal tubules in the cortex together with interstitial fibrosis. The thickened tubular basement membranes may have a very frilly, lamellated or loosely woven appearance by EM.

Nephronophthisis

NPHP is a group of autosomal recessive cystic kidney diseases and is the most common cause of inheritable end-stage renal diseases (ESRD) in the first 3 decades of life, with the median onset of ESRD 13 years. The disease can be subdivided clinically based on the age of onset of ESRD into infantile, juvenile, and adolescent categories with the mean age at onset 1, 13, and 19 years of age, respectively. The juvenile form is the most frequent. Affected children present first with polyuria and polydipsia, which reflect a marked defect in the renal concentrating ability. Sodium wasting and tubular acidosis also are prominent. Renal ultrasound reveals normal kidney size, increased echogenicity, and corticomedullary cysts. Some variants of juvenile NPHP can have extrarenal associations, including oculomotor abnormalities, retinal dystrophy, liver fibrosis, and cerebellar abnormalities.

At least 11 responsible gene loci have been identified. NPH1, which is mutated in approximately 20% of all cases of NPHP, encodes the protein nephrocystin 1, a protein that interacts with components of cell-cell and cell-matrix signaling and is involved in motility of primary cilia of renal epithelial cells. The NPHP2 gene, which is mutated in infantile NPHP, encodes the inversin protein, which mediates left-right patterning during embryogenesis. Mutation of the NPHP3 gene, which encodes nephrocystin 3, has been found in patients with adolescent NPHP.

Medullary Cystic Kidney Disease

Medullary cystic kidney disease (MCKD) has an autosomal dominant inheritance and is relatively rare. MCKD and NPHP share symptoms including decreased urine-concentrating capacity, polydipsia, polyuria, and renal cyst formation in the corticomedullary junction. Two genes (MCKD1 and MCKD2) have been identified as causing MCKD.

Differential Diagnosis

When medullary cysts are prominent, the gross pathologic differential includes medullary sponge kidney (see earlier in this article). The cysts in medullary sponge kidneys essentially always involve the papillary tips, whereas papillary tip involvement is rare with NPHP and adult-onset medullary cystic disease. In addition, calcification is common in the cysts of medullary sponge kidney, but does not occur in the cysts of NPHP and adult-onset medullary cystic disease.

Clinical Correlation

There is no specific treatment for NPHP and adult-onset medullary cystic disease. Therapy is thus directed at managing the consequences of the injury, including correction of electrolyte disturbance, acid-base balance, and water balance. Patients often eventually require kidney transplantation.[9,10]

Key Points: Nephronophthisis

- Autosomal recessive cystic kidney diseases
- The most common cause of inheritable end-stage renal diseases in the first 3 decades of life
- At least 11 responsible gene loci have been identified:
  - NPH1; nephrocystin 1
  - NPH2; inversin
  - NPH3; nephrocystin 3

Key Findings: Medullary Cystic Kidney Disease

- Autosomal dominant
- Decreased urine concentrating capacity, polydipsia, polyuria, and renal cyst formation in the corticomedullary junction
- Two gene loci identified:
  - MCKD1
  - MCKD2

Key Findings: Nephronophthisis and Medullary Cystic Disease

- Identical histologic findings
- Cysts and diverticula lined by flattened or detached epithelial cells and surrounded by either inflammatory cells or fibrous tissue, particularly at corticomedullary junction
- Widespread atrophy and thickening of tubular basement membranes of proximal and distal tubules in the cortex together with interstitial fibrosis
- Thickened tubular basement membranes with very frilly, lamellated, or loosely woven appearance

---

ACQUIRED RENAL CYSTIC DISEASE

Introduction

The kidneys from patients with end stage renal disease who have undergone prolonged dialysis sometimes show numerous cortical and medullary cysts. About 8% of patients have cysts at time of initiation of dialysis, about 50% after 3–5 years of dialysis, and about 90% after 10 years of dialysis.

Gross Features

At autopsy, the gross appearance of kidneys with acquired cystic disease can resemble autosomal dominant polycystic kidney disease. Cysts typically present bilaterally. The cysts are irregular in shape and distributed through the cortex and medulla. The cysts measure from 0.5 to 2.0 cm in diameter and contain clear fluid. However, the size and weight of the kidneys in acquired cystic disease are much less than in autosomal dominant polycystic kidney disease. The underlying scarred parenchyma typical of the end-stage kidney is usually apparent.

Microscopic Features

The cysts are lined by either hyperplastic or flattened tubular epithelium. The cysts probably form as a result of obstruction of tubules by interstitial fibrosis or by oxalate crystals. Most patients are asymptomatic, but sometimes the cysts bleed, causing hematuria.

Differential Diagnosis

Acquired renal cystic disease must be distinguished from autosomal dominant polycystic kidney disease. The history of dialysis and the presence of calcium oxalate crystals indicate acquired renal cystic disease.

Clinical Correlation

The most ominous complication is the development of papillary renal cell carcinoma arising from these cysts, occurring in 7% of dialyzed patients, and papillary adenoma, occurring in 10% to 20% of patients observed for at least 10 years.

Key Points: Acquired Renal Cystic Disease

- Seen in patients with end-stage renal disease who have undergone prolonged dialysis
- Cortical and medullary cysts are lined by either hyperplastic or flattened tubular epithelium
- Cysts often contain calcium oxalate crystals

SIMPLE CYSTS

Introduction

Simple cysts are common postmortem findings without clinical significance.

Gross Features

Simple renal cysts usually occur in the outer cortex, bulging the capsule (**Fig. 6**). These may be multiple or single, and usually are cortical and vary widely in diameter, from 1 to 5 cm up to 10 cm or more. They are translucent, lined by a gray glistening, smooth membrane, and filled with clear fluid.

Microscopic Findings

These cyst membranes are composed of a single layer of cuboidal or flattened cuboidal epithelial cells, which in many instances may be completely atrophic.

Differential Diagnosis

Multiple simple renal cysts may be so numerous to raise the possibility of adult polycystic kidney disease. Simple renal cysts usually occur in the outer cortex, bulging the capsule, in contrast to the cysts in autosomal dominant polycystic kidney disease, which occur in the cortex and medulla, and cause a uniform cobblestone appearance of the surface.

Clinical Correlation

No treatment is required and there is no significant health consequence in most cases.[8,11]

Key Points: Simple Cysts

- Common postmortem finding without clinical significance
- Occur in the outer cortex, bulging the capsule
- Multiple or single
- Single layer of cuboidal or flattened cuboidal epithelial cells

---

TUBULAR DISEASES

ACUTE TUBULAR NECROSIS

Introduction

Acute tubular necrosis (ATN), now often called ATI, is characterized by primary destruction or alteration of the renal tubular epithelium. Clinically, it is the most common cause of acute kidney injury, resulting in elevation of serum creatinine and blood urea nitrogen, and often causing oliguria or anuria. There are 2 major forms of ATN: ischemic and toxic.

Gross Findings

At autopsy, the kidneys are enlarged and pale. On cross section, the renal parenchyma is swollen and bulges from the capsule. The cortex is widened and there is accentuation of the corticomedullary junction, with the medulla appearing dark in contrast to the paler cortex and papillary tips (**Fig. 7**). This darkening of the medulla is caused by congestion of the vasa recta.

Microscopic Findings

There are many changes in the early phase of ATN that may be evident by microscopic examination (**Box 4**).

Ischemic ATN/ATI is characterized by tubular epithelial cell damage along multiple patchy segments of the nephrons, especially proximal segments, with associated tubular basement membrane breaks (tubulorrhexis) and tubular luminal casts (**Table 2**). The necrosis is quite subtle and easily missed by microscopic examination. Toxic ATN/ATI often shows more obvious

Fig. 6. Simple cyst. The simple cyst occurs in the outer cortex, bulging the capsule. It is translucent, lined by a gray glistening and smooth epithelium.

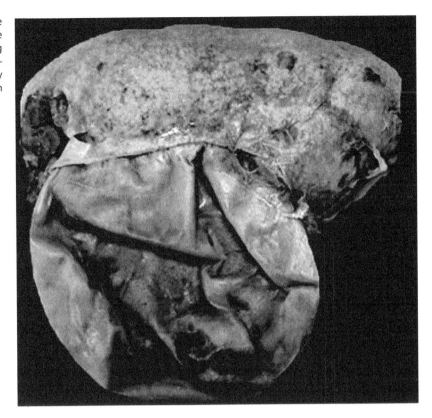

and extensive tubular epithelial cell necrosis because the proximal tubular segment of the nephron is the most common site responsible for the excretion of organic acids, drugs, toxins, and ions. Heavy metals and organic toxins usually lead to extensive destruction of all nephron segments, with greater involvement of cortical nephrons. Ethylene glycol causes marked ballooning and hydropic vacuolar changes in the proximal tubular cells with intraluminal calcium

Fig. 7. Acute tubular injury/necrosis. Cross sections of the kidneys show deep red medulla with paler cortex and papillary tips.

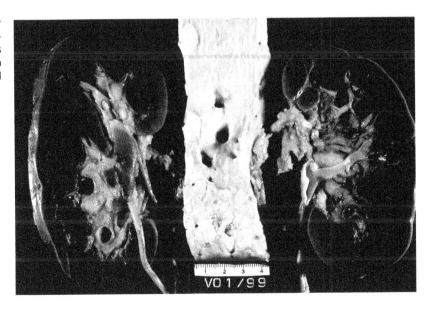

Box 4
Characteristics of acute tubular necrosis

Acute injury stage:

1. Injury with degeneration and necrosis of tubular epithelial cells with coagulative necrosis characterized by loss of cell nuclei with karyorrhexis, and pyknosis but partial preservation of cell outlines

2. Apical blebs of proximal tubular epithelial cells with shedding of cells into the tubular lumens and denuded areas of underlying basement membranes

3. Swelling of tubular epithelium with ballooning of cytoplasm

4. Loss or attenuation of brush border of the proximal tubular epithelial cells

5. Tubular dilatation

6. Presence of hyaline, pigmented, eosinophilic, or granular casts, especially in distal tubules

7. Numerous nucleated cells (myeloid precursors) in the vasa recta of the outer medulla

8. Scant, if any, peritubular capillaritis (peritubular capillary dilatation containing mononuclear cells and neutrophils)

Reparative/Regenerative stage findings:

1. Basophilic staining of the cytoplasm of tubular epithelial cells

2. Large hyperchromatic nuclei with prominent nucleoli

3. Mitotic figures in tubular epithelial cells

4. Simplification and flattening of tubular epithelial cell lining

oxalate crystals, which are fan-shaped, clear on H&E stain, and polarizable. Enteric hyperoxaluria or other causes of increased oxaluria also cause calcium oxalate crystals. Severe crush injuries can cause extensive muscle damage and rhabdomyolysis, causing pigmented globular myoglobin casts in tubular lumina. In patients with severe liver failure with high serum bilirubin level, greenish-brown pigmented casts of bilirubin in tubules may be identified by H&E stain and are highlighted by bilirubin special stain (Hall stain). In aminoglyocide nephrotoxicity, myeloid bodies in lysosomes in proximal tubules can be identified by EM. In 2,8-dihydroxyadeninuria, a rare autosomal recessive disorder caused by complete adenine phosphoribosyltransferase deficiency, there is diffuse acute tubular injury with globular and rod-shaped brownish-green intratubular crystals on H&E stain, which are birefringent under polarized light. These should not be confused with the clear calcium oxalate crystals. Occasional calcium phosphate crystals are common in scarred kidneys. Numerous calcium phosphate crystals, which are purplish on H&E stain, may be seen with any hypercalcemic/calciuric condition, such as hyperparathyroidism, or with excess phosphate load, as seen with oral sodium phosphate solution for colonoscopy preparation.

Differential Diagnosis

The most important morphologic differential diagnosis is between primary acute interstitial nephritis with secondary involvement of the nearby tubules, and primary severe ATN. The presence of focal or diffuse interstitial inflammation with or without eosinophils and associated tubulitis favors primary acute interstitial nephritis. The presence of increased interstitial eosinophils and eosinophilic tubulitis suggests a hypersensitivity reaction. ATN/ATI due to ischemia has minimal inflammation.

At autopsy, it might not be easy to distinguish ATN from autolysis of tubular epithelial cells. Autolysis usually shows detached tubular epithelial cells of the whole tubular cross section in the lumina (see earlier in this article). However, brush borders are intact, as best seen by PAS stain. Autolysis does not show nucleated cells (myeloid precursors) in the vasa recta of the outer medulla, in contrast to ATN. Autolysis also tends to be widespread, whereas ATN is more regional and patchy in distribution.

Table 2
Ischemic and toxic acute tubular necrosis

ATN	Ischemic	Toxic
Microscopic findings	Tubular epithelial cell damage along multiple patchy segments, subtle coagulative necrosis	More obvious and extensive frank tubular epithelial cell necrosis

Clinical Correlation and Prognosis

Patients with oliguria and ATN have a worse prognosis than patients with normal urine output. Patient survival is more often a function of other organ system involvement and complications, such as accompanying sepsis or multiorgan failure.

Key Points: Acute Tubular Necrosis

- Primary destruction or alteration of renal tubular epithelium
- The most common cause of acute kidney injury
- Two major forms: ischemic and toxic

Key Gross Findings: Acute Tubular Necrosis

- Widened cortex
- Accentuation of the corticomedullary junction
- Dark medulla and pale cortex and papillary tip

Key Microscopic Findings: Acute Tubular Necrosis

- Coagulative necrosis (in severe ischemic form)
- Apical blebs of proximal tubular epithelial cells
- Swelling of tubular epithelium with ballooning of cytoplasm
- Sloughing off of tubular epithelial cells from underlying tubular basement membranes
- Loss or attenuation of brush border of the proximal tubular epithelial cells

---

RENAL CORTICAL NECROSIS

Introduction

Renal cortical necrosis is defined as multifocal or diffuse coagulative necrosis of the renal cortex, thus including necrosis of glomeruli and tubules; 50% to 60% of cases are associated with obstetric complications, including abruptio placenta with hemorrhage, placenta previa with hemorrhage, septic abortion, and puerperal sepsis with placental retention. Additional causes include shock associated with acute pancreatitis, diabetic ketoacidosis, postoperative gastrointestinal hemorrhage, transfusion reactions, burns, thrombotic microangiopathy, and antibody-mediated renal allograft rejection.

Gross Findings

At autopsy, in the acute phase, the kidneys show yellow cortex with subcapsular and juxtamedullary congestion. In the later phase, the kidneys reveal irregular scarring with thin cortex and calcification.

Microscopic Features

There is multifocal or diffuse coagulative necrosis of cortex, characterized by acute tubular necrosis and glomerular necrosis. The subcapsular cortex, juxtamedullary cortex, and medulla are spared.

Differential Diagnosis

The most important morphologic differential diagnosis is between renal cortical necrosis and autolysis (see earlier in this article).

Clinical Correlation and Prognosis

Duration of oliguria is proportional to the extent of renal cortical necrosis. Renal survival correlates with the extent of necrosis.[12–14]

Key Points: Renal Cortical Necrosis

- Multifocal or diffuse coagulative necrosis of renal cortex, characterized by acute tubular necrosis and glomerular necrosis
- Associated with obstetric complications, sepsis, shock, severe thrombotic microangiopathy, and so forth
- Glomerular and acute tubular necrosis

BILE (BILIRUBIN) CAST NEPHROPATHY

Introduction

Renal dysfunction is a common and important complication in patients with hepatic failure. Hepatorenal syndrome (HRS) is defined by the presence of acute or chronic liver diseases with advanced hepatic failure, and renal dysfunction. HRS is thought to be due to marked intrarenal vasoconstriction resulting in functional impairment of the kidneys, and thus, pathologic changes of ATI would be anticipated. However, several historical articles have described intrarenal bile casts (cholemic nephrosis) as a mechanism for renal dysfunction in the setting of hepatic failure. Cholemic nephrosis or bile cast nephropathy can occur in adults and children with a wide spectrum of liver disorders, as well as in patients with or without cirrhosis, but generally these casts are only observed with severe hyperbilirubinemia.

Gross Findings

At autopsy, there is green discoloration of the surface of the kidneys. On cross sections, the renal pyramids usually show a darker green color, as the concentration of bilirubin is higher in these regions compared with the cortex. Bile casts also can be seen as linear green streaks throughout the cortex and medulla.

Microscopic Findings

Bile casts are present by light microscopy, and are mainly limited to distal nephrons. These casts appear acellular and greenish-tinged brown on H&E and distinctly green on Hall special stain (**Figs. 8** and **9**). There is variable ATI with attenuated tubular epithelium and loss of brush borders.

Differential Diagnosis

The top differential diagnoses include myoglobin cast nephropathy, and hemoglobin casts. Myoglobin cast nephropathy shows brown pigmented casts in distal tubules that stain for myoglobin, and are seen with rhabdomyolysis. Reddish brown casts also occur with hemolysis, and stain with an iron stain. In contrast, light-chain cast nephropathy shows pale pink metachromatic fractured-appearing casts with giant cell reaction. Monoclonal staining for kappa or lambda light chains helps to confirm diagnosis. However, the absence of monoclonal staining of the casts cannot rule out light-chain cast nephropathy in that only approximately 50% of cases with light-chain cast nephropathy show monoclonal staining.

Pathogenesis and Clinical Correlations

In the clinical setting of liver failure, serum bile and bilirubin levels increase and can impair proximal tubular function (proximal tubulopathy). Bile cast formation increases with prolonged exposure to

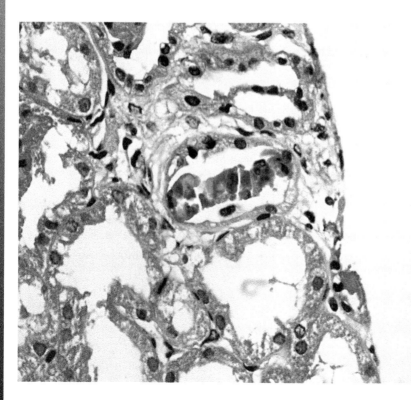

Fig. 8. Bile (bilirubin) casts. Bile casts are seen as brownish casts with slight green tinge with associated tubular injury with attenuated tubular epithelium (H&E stain, original magnification ×200).

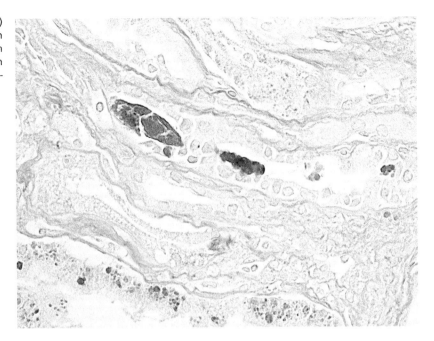

Fig. 9. Bile (bilirubin) casts. Bile casts are seen as distinctly green with special stain for bilirubin (Hall stain, original magnification ×200).

high bilirubin levels. van Slambrouck and colleagues[15] purposed that bile casts may contribute to kidney injury in severely jaundiced patients by direct bile and bilirubin toxicity, and tubular obstruction. Both mechanisms are analogous to the tubular injury caused by light-chain cast nephropathy, or hemoglobin, or myoglobin casts. However, Heyman and colleagues[16] suggested that bile casts might be merely an epiphenomenon, reflecting reduced glomerular filtration rate and diminished washout of casts, rather than playing a role in the pathogenesis of renal dysfunction in the setting of severe hepatic disease.[17,18]

Key Points: Bile (Bilirubin) Cast Nephropathy

- Described in patients with severe hepatic disease, regardless of cause

- Acellular and yellowish-green granular/globular casts on H&E and Hall special stain

- Top differential diagnoses of pigmented casts are hemoglobin, and myoglobin cast nephropathy

- Light-chain cast nephropathy has pale pink metachromatic fractured-appearing casts

---

TUBULOINTERSTITIAL NEPHRITIS

Introduction

Tubulointerstitial nephritis (TIN) refers to acute or chronic inflammation of tubules and interstitium. The diagnosis often requires renal biopsy, as clinical features are usually nonspecific. TIN is a relatively common cause of unexplained (nonischemic) acute kidney injury. There are many causes of TIN. In this article, we discuss only the common causes of TIN.

Infection

Organisms can directly infect the kidney, or can cause acute pyelonephritis (see later in this article) or interstitial nephritis, discussed here.

Polyomavirus

The BK virus was originally isolated from a patient named B.K., a Sudanese patient who had distal donor ureteral stenosis, 3 months after a living related kidney transplant. BK virus is related to JC virus and to simian kidney virus (SV40). These polyomaviruses are double-stranded nonencapsulated DNA viruses, and are in the family of Polyomaviridae, which also include the papilloma viruses. The BK virus commonly infects the urothelium but does not cause morbidity in immunocompetent individuals. However, in patients who have received a renal transplant, 3 lesions have been contributed to by BK virus: hemorrhagic cystitis, stenosis of the ureter, and acute interstitial nephritis.

Emphysematous Pyelonephritis

This reaction to gas-forming bacteria results in necrosis with areas of gas formation. At autopsy, this may be demonstrated by sectioning the kidney and removing its capsule while immersed in water or saline, allowing detection of the gases leaking out. Microscopically, large saccular dilated spaces are present around the necrotic areas.

Drug-Induced Interstitial Nephritis

Drug-induced interstitial nephritis is an allergic reaction triggered by drugs or other substances (eg, antibiotics, nonsteroidal anti-inflammatory drugs [NSAIDs], diuretics, and antiviral drugs, or herbal or other supplements).

Autoimmune TIN

The group of TIN with autoimmune pathogenesis includes TIN with uveitis, lupus nephritis, Sjögren's syndrome, antitubular basement membrane disease, tubular basement membrane immune complex disease (with or without membranous glomerulopathy), and IgG4-associated autoimmune pancreatitis and interstitial nephritis.

TIN Associated with IgG4 Deposits and Autoimmune Pancreatitis

A new form of tubulointerstitial disease has recently been recognized, which is part of a systemic syndrome with tumorlike inflammatory lesions in the pancreas (autoimmune pancreatitis), lung, salivary glands, kidney, and other organs. In the kidney, the disease is manifested by immune complex deposits along the tubular basement membranes in about 80% of cases, which stain dominantly for IgG4, but also for other IgG subclasses. The affected organs, including the kidney, demonstrate aggregates of polyclonal plasma cells expressing IgG4, and a whorling, storiform pattern of interstitial fibrosis.

Pathology

Gross findings

At autopsy, the kidneys may be slightly enlarged due to interstitial inflammation and edema. In IgG4-related disease, masses may be present.

Light microscopy, immunofluorescence, and EM

In polyomavirus-induced interstitial nephritis, the tubular epithelium shows viral cytopathic changes with nucleoli and viral inclusions. Cells may be enlarged. Polyomavirus is diagnosed specifically by immunostaining for the large T antigen of the polyoma species. Characteristic intranuclear paracrystalline arrays of virus particles of 40 to 50 nm are present by EM. Urine cytology usually shows decoy cells with inclusions of so-called "Haufen" cells, and may be more sensitive for diagnosis in urine (ie, 3-dimensional aggregates of infected cells).

In drug-induced interstitial nephritis, there is interstitial infiltrate with mononuclear cells accompanied by interstitial edema with a variable number of eosinophils. The infiltrate is usually focal and particularly predominant at the corticomedullary junction. The medulla is rarely affected. The number of plasma cells is quite variable. Eosinophils may comprise approximately 20% to 25% of the infiltrating leukocytes. The eosinophils tend to be concentrated in small foci and may even form abscesses. Eosinophilic tubulitis may be seen. However, the absence of significant eosinophils does not rule out a hypersensitivity reaction; nor is their presence pathognomonic of this etiology. Multinucleated giant cells may be present. A granulomatous reaction is not uncommon. Granulomas are non-necrotizing and not well-formed.

In TIN associated with IgG4 deposits and autoimmune pancreatitis, there is dense lymphoplasmacytic infiltrate. The interstitial fibrosis is patchy, expansile, and destructive, with a whorling pattern. It usually shows accompanying interstitial eosinophils. IgG4 subclass staining shows dominance of IgG4-positive plasma cells in the most affected dense areas with more than 10 plasma cells per high-power field. Most cases show granular tubular basement membrane deposits by immunofluorescence and by EM. These deposits stain dominantly but not exclusively for IgG4. Glomeruli usually show no deposits, although rarely membranous glomerulopathy is present. The disease is often responsive to steroids.[19–22]

Key Points: Tubulointerstitial Nephritis

- Characterized by acute and chronic inflammation of tubules and interstitium, with numerous causes

- Infection

- Reactive interstitial nephritis

- Drug-induced interstitial nephritis

- Autoimmune (eg, tubulointerstitial nephritis associated with IgG4 deposits and autoimmune pancreatitis)

VASCULAR DISEASES

Thrombosis and Embolic Disease

Renal vein thrombosis

Introduction There are many risk factors for renal vein thrombosis, including nephrotic syndrome; antiphospholipid antibody syndrome; neoplasms, such as renal cell carcinoma and urothelial carcinoma; infections; trauma; surgical procedure; immobilization; dehydration; and diuretics, such as furosemide.

Gross findings At autopsy, the kidney is enlarged with vascular congestion and thrombus is identified in a renal vein.

Microscopic findings Thrombus is present in the renal vein and renal venules. There is glomerular capillary and peritubular capillary dilatation containing red blood cells, neutrophils, and mononuclear cells. Interstitial edema is present. There may be concurrent glomerular disease, such as membranous glomerulopathy or FSGS.

Differential diagnosis Thrombotic microangiopathy and renal artery thrombosis are the main differential diagnoses. Thrombotic microangiopathy shows fibrin thrombi in glomerular capillaries, arterioles, or arteries, but not veins or venules. Renal artery thrombosis shows hemorrhage, necrosis, infarct, and thrombi in renal artery and branches, but not in renal vein or venules.

Clinical correlation The prognosis for recovery of renal function depends on the cause of renal vein thrombosis. Treatment with anticoagulation and fibrinolytic therapy or the underlying cause (ie, nephrotic syndrome) is helpful.[23,24]

Key Points: Renal Vein Thrombosis

- Thrombus involving renal vein
- Risk factors: nephrotic syndrome, antiphospholipid antibody syndrome, neoplasms, infections, trauma, surgical procedure, immobilization, dehydration, and diuretics, such as furosemide

---

Renal artery thrombosis

Introduction Renal artery thrombosis is characterized by thrombus in the main renal artery. Renal artery thrombosis is associated with many conditions, including renal artery stenosis, fibromuscular dysplasia, renal or abdominal aortic aneurysm, trauma, hypercoagulable states, vasculitis, infections, and cocaine use.

Gross findings At autopsy, the kidneys show hemorrhagic necrosis or wedge infarcts. There is thrombus in the main renal artery or branches of the renal artery (**Fig. 10**).

Microscopic findings Arterial thrombi show lines of Zahn, that is, layers of platelets/fibrin alternating with red blood cells. There is associated interstitial hemorrhage and acute tubular injury, and often cortical necrosis (see previously in this article).

Differential diagnosis The main differential diagnoses include thrombotic microangiopathy, renal vein thrombosis, and atheromatous emboli. Thrombotic microangiopathy shows fibrin thrombi in glomerular capillaries, arterioles, or arteries, not in the main renal artery or branches. Renal vein thrombosis shows thrombi in the renal artery and branches, but not in the renal vein or venules. Atheromatous emboli show cholesterol clefts within the occluded artery.

Clinical correlation The prognosis for recovery of renal function depends on the cause of renal artery thrombosis. Treatment with anticoagulation and fibrinolytic therapy may be helpful, depending on the underlying cause.[25,26]

Key Points: Renal Artery Thrombosis

- Thrombus of the main renal artery
- Associated with renal artery stenosis, fibromuscular dysplasia, renal or abdominal aortic aneurysm, trauma, hypercoagulable state, vasculitis, infections, or cocaine use

---

Renal atheroembolization

Introduction Renal atheroembolization is defined as embolization of athermatous debris, mostly composed of cholesterol crystals, into the renal vasculature, including arteries, arterioles, and glomerular capillaries. It occurs most often in elderly patients with severe atherosclerotic vascular disease. The distribution is downstream from the most severely affected arteries, and thus typically involves many organs, including skin of flanks and lower extremities, kidneys,

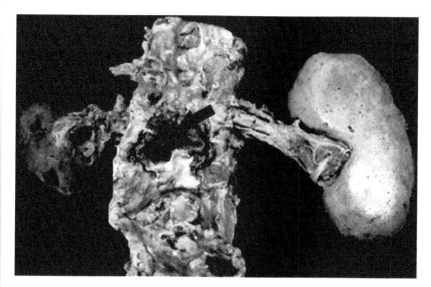

Fig. 10. Renal artery thrombosis. There is thrombus in the right renal artery (*arrow*). The affected right kidney is atrophic. There is severe atherosclerosis of aorta and both renal arteries.

gastrointestinal tract, spleen, and adrenals. Eyes, brain, and thoracic organs are rarely affected. About 50% of patients with atheroembolization have renal involvement. It can cause acute or subacute kidney injury that develops immediately after an inciting event, such as angiography or aortic surgery, often with new-onset or worsened hypertension, livedo reticularis, and eosinophilia. Atheroemboli may also occur spontaneously.

Gross findings At autopsy, cholesterol emboli usually do not produce specific gross lesions. In rare patients, acute or larger arteries may be occluded, resulting in wedge-shaped cortical infarcts with red borders and pale centers.

Microscopic findings Atheroembolization is characterized by the presence of elongated clefts in the lumen of small arteries (100–200 μm in diameter) resulting from the cholesterol being dissolved by standard processing of tissue for light microscopy. Occasionally, the cholesterol crystals extend into glomeruli. In the acute phase, the cholesterol crystals are surrounded by atheromatous debris or thrombus. The crystals induce a leukocyte response and become surrounded by leukocytes, especially macrophages, including multinucleated giant cells. Later, there is intimal proliferation that encloses the crystals within a thickened intima.

Differential diagnosis The clinical differential diagnosis includes antineutrophil cytoplasmic antibody (ANCA)-associated vasculitis and cryoglobulinemic vasculitis. ANCA-associated vasculitis usually shows fibrinoid necrosis of small arteries and capillaries and glomerular crescents. The presence of strong PAS-positive material in arterial walls with associated inflammatory reaction and in the lumen of glomeruli (cryo plugs) is characteristic of cryoglobulinemic glomerulonephritis with vasculitis. Cholesterol clefts are very focal and are easily overlooked, unless specifically sought.

Clinical correlation The prognosis for recovery of renal function in atheroembolization is poor. Only rare patients who develop severe acute kidney injury that requires dialysis recover enough renal function to come off dialysis. Anticoagulation treatment may further destabilize atherosclerotic plaque and promote additional showering of emboli.[27–29]

Key Points: Atheroembolization

- Atheromatous debris, mostly composed of cholesterol crystals, into the renal vasculature, including small arteries (100–200 μm), arterioles, and glomerular capillaries
- Cholesterol clefts in the lumen of arteries

Arterionephrosclerosis

Introduction Arterionephrosclerosis is a term that encompasses the vascular and parenchymal damages observed associated with hypertension and aging. The renal injury is clinically characterized by varying degrees of proteinuria and renal insufficiency. Proteinuria occasionally can be nephrotic range, especially if hypertension is severe.

Gross findings So called "benign" nephrosclerosis is associated with hypertension below the "malignant range," and results in small kidneys with finely granular surface and thinned cortex in the late stage. Arcuate and interlobular arteries usually have thickened pale walls with a "pipe stem" appearance due to sclerosis.

Microscopic findings Interlobular and larger arteries show varying degree of tunica media hyperplasia and intimal fibrosis with reduplication of the internal elastic lamina and there is hyalinosis of afferent arterioles. There are associated glomerular ischemic changes with variable corrugation and thickening of the glomerular basement membranes, global sclerosis, tubular atrophy, and interstitial fibrosis. Global sclerosis can be either obsolescent type, which shows fibrous material filling the Bowman space, or the solidified type, which is characterized by contracted and corrugated glomerular basement membranes of the entire glomerular tuft without collagenous material within the Bowman space. Secondary FSGS also may be present, often with associated corrugation and reduplication of the glomerular basement membranes, periglomerular fibrosis, and subtotal foot process effacement. Immunofluorescence may show entrapment of IgM and C3 in glomeruli, but there are no immune complexes.

Differential diagnosis Arterionephrosclerosis must be distinguished from other forms of chronic renal disease, such as chronic ischemic nephropathy secondary to renal artery stenosis, chronic thrombotic microangiopathy, and chronic interstitial nephritis. As is discussed in detail later in this article, chronic ischemic nephropathy secondary to renal artery stenosis is characterized by a distinctive pattern of proximal tubular injury with very small tubules and inapparent lumina and mild to moderate interstitial fibrosis. The reduced tubular volume brings the glomeruli closer together, in contrast to arterionephrosclerosis, which shows zones of global sclerosis and atrophic tubules surrounded by interstitial fibrosis and interstitial inflammation. Chronic thrombotic microangiopathy shows prominent replication of the glomerular basement membranes, and often intimal proliferation of arterioles. Chronic TIN shows excess tubulointerstitial fibrosis and interstitial inflammation in comparison

with the severity of glomerular and vascular damages, in contrast to arterionephrosclerosis, where vascular lesions and global sclerosis dominate. In end-stage kidneys, distinctions may not be possible.

Clinical correlation Angiotensin-converting enzyme inhibitors and angiotensin receptor antagonists may slow the progression of renal failure.

Key Features
ARTERIONEPHROSCLEROSIS

- Hyalinosis of afferent arterioles
- Tunica media hyperplasia and intimal fibrosis with reduplication of internal elastic lamina of arteries
- Wrinkling and thickening of the glomerular basement membranes
- Obsolescent and solidified global glomerulosclerosis
- Secondary focal segmental glomerulosclerosis
- Nonspecific IgM and C3 trapping by immunofluorescence periglomerular fibrosis and subtotal foot process effacement. Immunofluorescence may show entrapment of IgM and C3 in glomeruli.

Malignant hypertensive nephropathy

Introduction Malignant hypertension is defined by severe hypertension that causes acute tissue injury in multiple organs. About 50% of the patients with malignant hypertensive nephropathy have a history of arterionephrosclerosis.

Gross findings Malignant hypertensive nephropathy is often superimposed on usual findings of arterionephrosclerosis; therefore, the pathologic features of arterionephrosclerosis may dominate the gross findings. At autopsy, the acute gross appearance of malignant hypertensive nephropathy includes renal swelling and scattered irregular red specks caused by hemorrhage from foci of fibrinoid necrosis of arterioles and glomeruli. This so-called "flea-bitten" kidney appearance is similar to the gross findings in severe crescentic glomerulonephritis, or other conditions with necrosis of small arteries.

Microscopic findings The characteristic findings of acute phase of malignant hypertensive nephropathy are mucoid change and fibrinoid necrosis of arteries. Glomeruli also may show fibrin thrombi; however, glomeruli are not the dominant site of injury. The late phase of injury is characterized by corrugation and reduplication of the glomerular basement membranes as a result of cellular interposition. Arterioles show intimal proliferation of myofibroblasts and lamination of internal elastic lamina forming an "onion-skin" appearance. By EM, glomeruli show expansion of lamina rara interna with flocculent material of the glomerular basement membranes. There is extension of infiltrating monocytes or mesangial cell cytoplasm into the expanded lamina rara interna and underlying deposition of new basement membrane material.

Differential diagnosis The gross and histologic features of malignant hypertensive nephropathy cannot be distinguished definitely from those caused by any other forms of thrombotic microangiopathy, such as hemolytic uremic syndrome, thrombotic thrombocytopenic purpura, scleroderma renal crisis, and antiphospholipid antibody syndrome. As discussed previously, glomeruli are not the dominant site of injury in malignant hypertensive nephropathy. In contrast, hemolytic uremic syndrome and thrombotic thrombocytopenic purpura involve glomeruli more than arteries.

Pathogenesis Malignant hypertension alone can cause renal vascular fibrinoid necrosis. The extremely high blood pressure in patients directly injures endothelial cells of arteries, causing insudation of plasma proteins into the arterial walls, including fibrin at sites of fibrinoid necrosis.[30,31]

Key Findings: Malignant Hypertensive Nephropathy

- "Flea-bitten" gross appearance
- Mucoid change with fibrinoid necrosis of arteries in acute phase
- Intimal proliferation with luminal narrowing in chronic phase
- May have fibrin thrombi in glomeruli
- Severe glomerular basement membrane corrugation and reduplication
- Expansion of lamina rara interna with cellular interposition

---

Renal artery stenosis

Introduction Renal artery stenosis is defined by luminal narrowing of the main renal artery, which can be asymptomatic or can cause renovascular hypertension and may result in chronic ischemic nephropathy characterized by severe atrophy of cortical tubules. There are many causes of renal artery stenosis, such as atherosclerosis, fibromuscular dysplasia, dissecting aneurysm, vasculitis, retroperitoneal fibrosis, neurofibromatosis, and compression by intra-abdominal neoplasm. It is present in approximately 1% to 5% of patients with hypertension and is more frequent in older adults and children. Atherosclerosis is a significant cause of renal artery stenosis (10%–40% in elderly). In children, fibromuscular dysplasia is the most common case of renal artery stenosis. Renal artery stenosis due to fibromuscular dysplasia is much more common in women than men.

Gross findings At autopsy, there is narrowing of the renal artery. A combination of friable lipid debris, calcification, and dense fibrosis implicates atherosclerosis as the cause. In fibromuscular dysplasia, there are multiple ridges of hyperplastic tissue alternating with a thinned wall of aneurysms. An elastin stain can demonstrate the abnormal elastic lamina.

Microscopic findings The characteristic finding of long-standing renal artery stenosis is a distinctive pattern of tubular injury resulting in the appearance of crowding of glomeruli. Glomeruli are crowded together due to reduction in size of tubules, especially proximal tubules. Glomeruli are smaller than normal with mild Bowman space dilatation. There is mild to moderate hyperplasia of the juxtaglomerular apparatuses.

Fibromuscular dysplasia usually involves the distal two-thirds of the main renal artery. There are 3 major types of fibromuscular dysplasia: intimal fibroplasia, medial fibromuscular dysplasia, and periarterial dysplasia. Approximately 95% of fibromuscular dysplasia cases are caused by medial fibromuscular dysplasia.

Differential diagnosis Chronic ischemic nephropathy in renal artery stenosis must be distinguished from hypertension-associated arterionephrosclerosis. As detailed previously, chronic ischemic nephropathy secondary to renal artery stenosis is characterized by a distinctive pattern of proximal tubular injury with very small tubules and inapparent lumina and mild to moderate interstitial fibrosis. The reduced tubular volume brings the glomeruli closer together. In contrast, in hypertension-associated nephrosclerosis, there is patchy interstitial fibrosis and tubular atrophy with chronic inflammation, and varying degrees of glomerular sclerosis, including globally sclerotic glomeruli mostly clustered beneath the capsule.

Pathogenesis The tubular injury in chronic ischemic nephropathy due to renal artery stenosis is because of the high energy requirement of the tubules for mitochondrial respiration to support their high rate of solute support. Sublethal ischemia induces atrophy, whereas lethal ischemia induces cell death, probably primarily through apoptosis. Segmental proximal tubular cell loss through apoptosis or necrosis induces atubular glomeruli. The etiology and pathogenesis of the various types of fibromuscular dysplasia are unknown, but probably secondary to congenital abnormalities in composition or structure that manifest only later in life.[32,33]

Key Points: Renal Artery Stenosis

- Most common causes: atherosclerosis and fibromuscular dysplasia
- Fibromuscular dysplasia is more common in women than in men

---

Thrombotic microangiopathy

Introduction Thrombotic microangiopathy (TMA) is a pathologic term describing a lesion characterized by endothelial cell injury and thrombosis in glomeruli and arterioles, occasionally extending to interlobular arteries. This lesion often manifests clinically as hemolytic uremic syndrome (HUS), characterized by thrombocytopenia, microangiopathic hemolytic anemia, and variable organ involvement. Renal involvement with TMA occurs with multiple etiologies, including HUS, malignant hypertension, scleroderma, and antiphospholipid antibody syndrome, and in disseminated intravascular coagulation, preeclampsia, eclampsia, and drug toxicities, such as anti–vascular endothelial growth factor (VEGF) antibody bevacizumab, or with inherited or acquired complement dysregulation. Thrombotic thrombocytopenic purpura (TTP) is characterized by fever, hemolytic anemia, thrombocytopenia, fluctuating neurologic symptoms, and variable, but typically mild, renal involvement.

Gross findings Regardless of cause of TMA, kidneys are enlarged at autopsy. There may be petechial and purpuric hemorrhages on the external and cut surfaces in the acute phase. In severe cases, where arteries are involved, focal or widespread cortical necrosis appears as bulging pale zones. The zones of necrosis usually are not wedge-shaped, which differs from the typical wedge-shaped infarcts due to occlusion of large arteries. In the chronic phase, the kidneys are small and may have scattered depressed scars and calcifications at sites of early cortical necrosis.

Light microscopic findings In the earliest phase of TMA, glomeruli may appear bloodless due to obliteration of the glomerular capillary lumina by swollen endothelial cells and products of coagulation, preventing perfusion. Glomerular capillary lumina are occluded by fibrin thrombi, which have a characteristic bright eosinophilic chunky appearance on H&E, or pale pink on Jones stain (**Fig. 11**). Glomerular capillaries may be congested with erythrocytes and neutrophils. Mesangiolysis, defined as dissolution of the mesangial matrix and injury of mesangial cells, occurs in the acute phase. Because the glomerular basement membranes are normally anchored to the mesangial cells, loss of these attachments due to mesangiolysis can result in aneurysmal dilatation of the glomerular capillaries. In the more chronic phase of TMA, glomeruli show double contours of glomerular basement membranes, with increased lamina rara interna with cellular interposition without immune complexes, culminating in varying degrees of glomerulosclerosis, including both segmental or global glomerulosclerosis. Vascular lesions of TMA may involve small arteries and/or arterioles. Acute lesions typically show intravascular fibrin thrombi with endothelial swelling and necrosis and red blood cell fragments within the wall. Subacute lesions show a pale edematous intimal mucopolysaccharide ground substance, referred to as "mucoid changes," culminating in the classic onion-skin proliferation of the intima.

Immunofluorescence findings Lesions with thrombi show intense staining for fibrin-related antigen. IgM and C3 may be positive in glomeruli with thrombi or sclerosis, likely representing nonspecific trapped immune reactants due to increase in permeability of damaged endothelial cells.

Electron microscopic findings There is swelling of endothelial cells. Intraluminal fibrin tactoids and platelet aggregates are present in affected glomeruli. There is increase in lucency of the lamina rara interna with electron flocculent

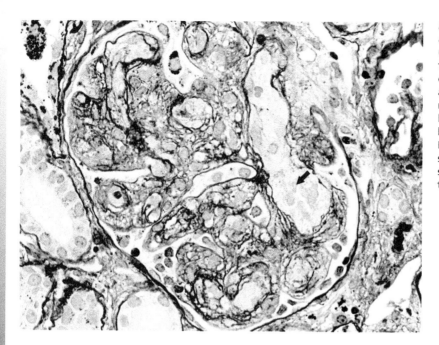

Fig. 11. Thrombotic microangiopathy. The glomerulus shows thickening of the capillary wall due to endothelial cell swelling and accumulation of material between the endothelial cells and glomerular basement membranes. Fibrin thrombi also are present (*arrow*) (Jones silver stain, original magnification ×400).

materials with cellular interposition, with new basement membrane formation. Mesangiolysis may be present.

Clinical correlation and pathogenesis There are many causes of TMA.

- Classical diarrhea (D+) HUS is caused by shiga-like exotoxin or verotoxin (VT), most commonly produced by *Escherichia coli* O157:H7, but occasionally caused by other *E coli* serotypes and non–*E coli* organisms, such as *Shigella dysenteriae*. VT causes proteolytic cellular injury to intestinal epithelial cells, producing colitis and bloody diarrhea. Hematogenous dissemination of the VT from the intestinal tract causes vascular endothelial cell injury in distant organs, such as kidneys.
- Atypical diarrhea (D−) HUS lacks a diarrheal prodrome and may result from infectious and noninfectious agents. Approximately 30% to 50% of patients with D− HUS have genetic defects in key component regulatory molecules, such as complement factor H, I, B, or membrane cofactor protein, resulting in continuous complement C3 activation at the endothelial cell surface, and ensuing injury and thrombosis.
- TTP endothelial cell perturbation leads to the release of unusually large von Willebrand factor aggregates (UlvWF) that promote platelet adhesion to endothelium. The persistence of UlvWF molecules on the surface of endothelium

leads to platelet binding and thrombosis. Most patients with hereditary/familial TTP have severe deficiency (<3%–5% normal activity) of vWF cleaving proteinase (ADAMTS13), a serum metalloprotease that normally cleaves UlvWF. Acquired TTP often is due to an autoantibody that decreases ADAMTS activity.

Other causes:

Antiphospholipid antibody (APLA) syndrome: APLA may be primary or arise in the clinical setting of autoimmune connective tissue disease, such as systemic lupus erythematosus, hepatitis C infection, Lyme disease, or lymphoproliferative disease. How APLA promotes thrombosis is unclear; possible mechanisms may include binding to apoptotic cells, dysregulation of coagulation, platelet activation, and direct endothelial injury. Clinical manifestations of APLA syndrome include arterial and venous thromboses, thrombocytopenia, and recurrent abortion. Renal manifestations vary depending on the size of vessel involvement and may include hypertension, proteinuria, acute kidney injury, renal cortical necrosis, and progressive chronic kidney injury.

Scleroderma and malignant hypertension tend to dominantly involve arterioles and interlobular arteries, whereas HUS is glomerular dominant. Disseminated intravascular coagulation (DIC) tends to be more diffuse and uniform in involvement and also affects glomeruli predominantly.

TMA may occur as a complication of treatment, including cytotoxic drugs, such as mitomycin, calcineurin inhibitor, anti-VEGF agents, mammalian target of rapamycin inhibitors, radiation, and stem cell transplantation.

Differential diagnosis TMA of different causes has pathologic changes that are indistinguishable from each other. A common cause of TMA at autopsy is DIC. This condition is characterized by activation of both coagulation and fibrinolytic systems, with formation of platelet and fibrin thrombi in multiple organs and depletion of coagulation factors and platelets, leading to paradoxic concomitant hemorrhage.

DIC is characterized by prolonged prothrombin time, partial thromboplastin time, decreased platelets and fibrinogen, and increased fibrin degradation products. Precipitating causes include sepsis, head trauma, and neoplasia, and may follow the introduction of brain, fat, amniotic fluid, or other strong thromboplastins into the circulation. The pathomechanisms involve increased release of tissue factor from stimulated endothelium, leading to activation of coagulation via the extrinsic pathway. The simultaneous development of a consumption coagulopathy leads to extensive hemorrhage. The glomerular lesions in DIC are usually more widespread and severe than HUS or other causes of TMA discussed previously.[34,35]

Key Points: Thrombotic Microangiopathy

- Endothelial cell injury with thrombosis and fibrin thrombi in small vessels/glomeruli

- Numerous causes
  - Hemolytic uremic syndrome
  - Scleroderma
  - Malignant hypertension
  - Antiphospholipid antibody syndrome
  - Disseminated intravascular coagulation

Diabetic nephropathy

Introduction Diabetic nephropathy (DN) is the most common cause of ESRD in the United States. Approximately 30% to 40% of patients with either diabetes type 1 (insulin dependent) or diabetes type 2 (non–insulin dependent) develop severe or ESRD. There are no differences in the pathology of DN per se in patients with either type 1 or type 2 diabetes.

Gross findings At autopsy, the kidneys are diffusely and symmetrically enlarged in the early stage of disease. However, in the late stage, kidney size may be small when scarring is extensive, or normal. Papillary necrosis with loss of pyramids may be present.

Microscopic findings In the earliest phase, glomeruli may be enlarged. The earliest detectable morphologic changes are thickening of the glomerular basement membranes, seen by EM, and widening of the mesangium, due to increased accumulation of matrix more than cells, seen by light microscopy. In the advanced phase of DN, the mesangial matrix expansion often forms nodules known as Kimmelstiel-Wilson nodules. There is hyaline deposition (insudation of plasma protein) in afferent and efferent arterioles. By immunofluorescence, there is linear accentuation along glomerular basement membranes for IgG and albumin (**Table 3**). Granular patterns of immunofluorescence staining for immunoglobulin and complement in autopsies indicate alternate or superimposed immune complex–mediated forms of glomerulonephritis.

Differential diagnosis A number of glomerular lesions resemble nodular sclerosis in DN by light microscopy (eg, light-chain deposition disease [LCDD], amyloidosis, and idiopathic nodular sclerosis). The Jones silver stain reveals less argyrophilia in the nodules of LCDD than in DN. In LCDD, there is monoclonal kappa or lambda ribbonlike staining by immunofluorescence along tubular and glomerular basement membranes with chunky or granular deposits in the mesangium. There are corresponding punctate, amorphous deposits by EM. Amyloidosis involving glomeruli may have a nodular appearance, resembling DN. The amyloid nodules are usually acellular and negative on Jones and PAS stains, but stain with Congo red with apple green birefringence under polarized light. By EM, randomly arranged fibrils (8–10 nm in diameter) are present in amyloidosis. Idiopathic nodular glomerulosclerosis shows identical morphologic findings, as seen in DN. This morphologic lesion is diagnosed by exclusion of diabetes clinically and is associated with history of smoking hypertension, and occurs more commonly in middle-aged or older white men.

Key Findings: Diabetic Nephropathy

- Mesangial matrix expansion with or without nodular sclerosis
- Hyalinosis of afferent and efferent arterioles
- Diffusely thickened glomerular basement membranes by electron microscopy

⚠⚠ Differential Diagnosis
NODULAR GLOMERULOSCLEROSIS

- Diabetic nephropathy
- Light chain deposition disease
- Amyloidosis
- Idiopathic nodular sclerosis
- Other

Clinical correlation Patients with DN but without unusual clinical features rarely undergo renal biopsy in the United States. Patients with atypical clinical features, such as acute kidney injury or sudden onset of massive proteinuria, often are biopsied in efforts to identify a superimposed, treatable form of renal disease. All of the common glomerular and tubulointerstitial lesions have been documented to occur in patients with diabetes.[36–38]

RENAL INFECTION

ACUTE PYELONEPHRITIS

Introduction

Acute pyelonephritis is defined as acute inflammation of the kidney parenchyma caused by bacterial infection. Acute pyelonephritis is secondary to ascending infections in 95% of patients, with the bacteria gaining access to the kidney via retrograde urine flow from the ureters. The remaining cases are caused by hematogenous spreading of the bacteria from an infected source outside of the kidney.

Gross Findings

At autopsy, the kidneys are enlarged and swollen with yellow or white microabscesses, usually confined to the cortex with pale streaks extending from medulla to cortex, representing collecting ducts filled with pus. The distribution of these lesions is random and patchy. The mucosa of renal calyces is edematous and red and covered by a purulent exudate. The pelvis is dilated and the papillae are flattened and blunted or may be necrotic. Papillary necrosis can occur with severe infection and may be unilateral or bilateral, and can involve few or all of the papillae. The papillary tips of the distal two-thirds of the papillae have

---

Table 3
Summary of pathologic findings in diabetic nephropathy

Light Microscopy	Immunofluorescence	Electron Microscopy
Glomeruli		
Glomerular hypertrophy Prominent glomerular basement membranes Diffuse mesangial expansion Nodular sclerosis Capillary microaneurysm, mesangiolysis Capsular drops	Linear accentuation of glomerular basement membranes for IgG and albumin	Thickened glomerular basement membranes Increase in mesangial matrix Fibrillosis (nonamyloidotic) fibrils in mesangial matrix
Tubules and interstitium		
Atrophy Prominent tubular basement membranes Interstitial fibrosis	Linear accentuation along tubular basement membranes for IgG (polyclonal) and albumin	Thickened tubular basement membranes Increase in interstitial collagen
Blood vessels		
Hyalinosis of afferent and efferent arterioles Intimal fibrosis of arteries	No characteristic alterations	Subendothelial and transmural hyaline deposits in arterioles and small arteries

gray-white to yellow discoloration, representing necrosis (**Fig. 12**). Long-term use of NSAIDs also can cause papillary necrosis. Papillary necrosis has been reported in association with phenacetin, indomethacin, phenylbutazone, ibuprofen, and fenoprofen.

Microscopic Findings

The characteristic findings of acute pyelonephritis are polymorphonuclear leukocytes present in tubular lumina forming neutrophilic plugs, as well as invading tubular epithelium and interstitium. Interstitial lymphocytes, plasma cells, and eosinophils may be present, with areas of necrosis and microabscesses. Hematogenous infection of the kidneys results in small cortical abscess formation with medullary involvement. In papillary necrosis, there is coagulative necrosis with retention of medulla outlines but little cellular detail.

Differential Diagnosis

The differential diagnosis of the accompanying interstitial inflammation includes drug-induced hypersensitivity reaction and viral renal infection, such as adenovirus or Hanta virus, in which the infiltrate is often hemorrhagic and mononuclear cells predominate. However, the presence of tubular neutrophilic plugs is quite characteristic of acute pyelonephritis.

Clinical Correlation

Acute uncomplicated pyelonephritis usually occurs in young healthy women. It must be distinguished from acute complicated pyelonephritis that is associated with urinary tract obstruction or reflux nephropathy. *E coli* is the major causative pathogen in acute uncomplicated pyelonephritis in young women in approximately 70% to 95% of the cases. In the older age group, there is increase in infections due to *Klebsiella* sp. Hematogenous infections are most commonly caused by *Staphylococcus aureus* or atypical bacteria (*Mycobacterium avium intracellulare*) or fungi, including *Candida* and *Aspergillus*. The renal biopsy rarely samples the renal papillae and pelvis, but at autopsy, careful examination of these areas can detect these infections.

Key Points: Acute Pyelonephritis

- Acute inflammation of renal parenchyma due to bacterial infection

- Ascending infection (95%)

- Retrograde infection via urethra, urinary bladder, and ureters

- *E coli*, most common organism

- With hematogenous infection, *S aureus* most common organism

- Tubular neutrophilic plugs by light microscopy

- Microabscesses and papillary necrosis may arise

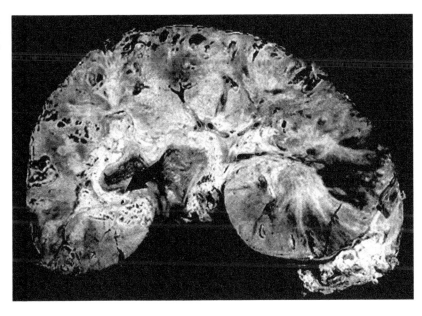

Fig. 12. Acute pyelonephritis with papillary necrosis. The papillary tips of the papillae (*arrow*) have yellow discoloration, representing necrosis.

CHRONIC PYELONEPHRITIS

Introduction

Chronic pyelonephritis is defined as a chronic tubulointerstitial disease characterized by renal damage caused by repeat bacterial infection and scarring. Chronic pyelonephritis affects more women than men. A history of urinary tract anomalies, nephrolithiasis, obstruction, or urologic surgical repair is common.

Gross Findings

The characteristic gross finding is irregular scarred renal cortices. The cortical scars are single, or multiple, large broad-based (**Fig. 13**), or U-shaped. Cortical scars are more common in the upper and lower poles of the kidney, rather than in the mid section.

Microscopic Findings

There is patchy chronic tubulointerstitial inflammation containing lymphocytes, plasma cells, and mononuclear cells, with associated geographic/jigsaw pattern of interstitial fibrosis and tubular atrophy. There is sharp demarcation between areas of inflammation and preserved parenchyma. Tubular thyroidization is present, characterized by atrophic tubules with attenuated epithelium and luminal colloidlike hyaline casts. A definite

diagnosis of chronic pyelonephritis requires that the pyelocalyceal regions be sampled and that they show evidence of chronic inflammation. Periglomerular fibrosis is noted, but glomeruli are usually spared. However, with progression, secondary FSGS may develop.

Differential Diagnosis

The differential diagnosis includes chronic tubulointerstitial nephritis and arterionephrosclerosis. Pericalyceal inflammation and tubular thyroidization are more prominent in chronic pyelonephritis than in chronic tubulointerstitial nephritis. Arterionephrosclerosis can lead to wedge-shaped or U-shaped cortical scars resembling those of chronic pyelonephritis; however, the underlying medulla and calyceal areas are usually normal in arterionephrosclerosis, in contrast to the striking changes in chronic pyelonephritis.

Clinical Correlation

Chronic pyelonephritis is the consequence of persistent untreated and incompletely resolved acute pyelonephritis, and, therefore, has many of the same risk factors and pathogenesis as these acute illnesses. In addition, structural abnormalities promoting reflux of urine contribute to the lesions of chronic pyelonephritis and reflux nephropathy.[39,40]

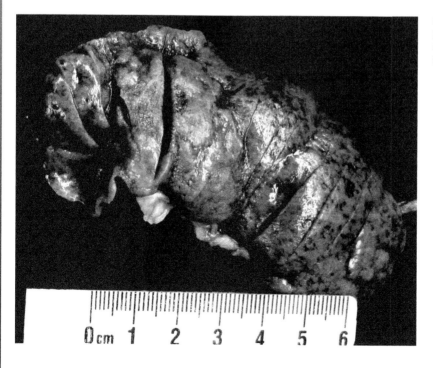

Fig. 13. Chronic pyelonephritis. Deep broad-based cortical scars (*arrow*) are seen in the kidney.

Key Points: Chronic Pyelonephritis

- Renal damage caused by repeated bacterial infection and scarring
- Urinary tract infection and reflux nephropathy
- Large irregular scars on the surface of cortex; inflammation and scarring involves pelvis and calyces
- Dilated calyces
- Jigsaw/geographic pattern of interstitial fibrosis with associated chronic inflammatory cell infiltrates
- Tubular thyroidization
- Periglomerular fibrosis
- Secondary focal segmental glomerulosclerosis may be present

XANTHOGRANULOMATOUS PYELONEPHRITIS

Introduction

Xanthogranulomatous pyelonephritis (XPN) is a variant of chronic pyelonephritis characterized by mass lesions with numerous foamy macrophages. XPN occurs most often in middle-aged women with history of recurrent urinary tract infection. *Proteus mirabilis* is the most common causative agent (>50%) followed by *E coli, Pseudomonas* sp, and *Klebsiella* sp. Nephrolithiasis, urinary tract obstruction, and diabetes mellitus are predisposing factors. XPN is usually unilateral and occurs predominantly in the pelvicalyceal regions.

Gross Findings

At autopsy, the kidneys are enlarged with perirenal adhesions. The pericalyceal system is dilated with deformed papillae and yellow necrotic materials in calyces. Large yellow nodules may mimic renal cell carcinoma. Staghorn calculi are commonly present.

Extrarenal extension to the perinephric soft tissue is present in approximately 30% and may also mimic renal cell carcinoma.

Microscopic Findings

There is diffuse granulomatous inflammatory tubulointerstitial infiltrate, which includes numerous foamy, lipid-laden macrophages and occasional multinucleated giant cells in addition to lymphocytes, plasma cells, and neutrophils. The lesion is very destructive and recognizable renal parenchyma may be ablated.

Differential Diagnosis

Top differential diagnoses are clear-cell renal cell carcinoma and renal medullary tuberculosis. Clear cells of renal cell carcinoma may mimic foamy, lipid-laden macrophages in XPN. Macrophage immunohistochemical markers, such as CD163 and CD68 are negative in clear cells in renal cell carcinoma, but epithelial cell markers, such as CKAE1/CAM5.2 and epithelial membrane antigen, are positive. Renal medullary tuberculosis shows necrotizing granulomatous inflammation with epithelioid histiocytes and multinucleated giant cells. Acid-fast mycobacteria usually can be demonstrated by special stain.

Clinical Correlation

XPN is caused by a defect in macrophage processing of bacteria. Renal cell carcinoma may coexist with XPN.[41,42]

Key Points: Xanthogranulomatous Pyelonephritis

- Variant of chronic pyelonephritis
- Numerous foamy, lipid-laden macrophages
- *Proteus* sp, *E coli, Klebsiella* sp
- Urinary tract obstruction, nephrolithiasis, and diabetes
- Dilated pelvicalyceal system and deformed papillae with yellow necrotic material in calyces
- Sheets of foamy, lipid-laden macrophages admixed with mononuclear cells, lymphocytes, and plasma cells

MALAKOPLAKIA

Introduction

Malakoplakia is caused by chronic bacterial infection with numerous macrophages containing Michaelis-Gutmann bodies. Malakoplakia is an uncommon consequence of inflammatory reaction, most commonly secondary to infection by *E coli*, and is thought to be initiated by defective intracytoplasmic macrophage bactericidal function.

It is thought to be a chronic sequela of xanthogranulomatous pyelonephritis.

Gross Findings

At autopsy, the kidneys are enlarged with raised, yellow nodules. These may be multiple and occur on the pelvic lining, on the capsular surface, or extend into the parenchyma.

Microscopic Findings

There are clusters of macrophages with foamy eosinophilic cytoplasm (von Hanseman cells) in the mass lesions. There are scattered lymphocytes and plasma cells. Diagnostic Michaelis-Gutmann bodies are inclusions (4–10 μm) present in cytoplasm or extracellularly. They stain positively with von Kossa (phosphate), Prussian blue, and PAS. They are thought to represent an aggregation of calcium phosphate–containing crystals, and are induced by a central nidus of bacterial breakdown products.

Differential Diagnosis

The lesions are easily misdiagnosed radiographically as a cancer because of their nodular appearance. In renal cell carcinoma, immunohistochemistry for CKAE1/CAM5.2 (epithelial cells) is positive, whereas CD163 and CD68 (macrophage marker) are negative.

Clinical Correlation

Mass lesion is detected on ultrasound or computed tomography scan and high level of suspicion is needed for definite diagnosis.[43,44]

Key Points: Malakoplakia

- Chronic bacterial infection with numerous macrophages containing foamy eosinophilic cytoplasm
- *E coli* most common pathogen
- Defective intracytoplasmic macrophage bactericidal activity
- Michaelis-Gutmann bodies stain for
  - Calcium phosphate (positive Von Kossa)
  - Iron (Prussian blue)
  - PAS

RENAL TUBERCULOSIS

Introduction

Renal tuberculosis is a renal infection caused by *Mycobacterium* sp. The kidney is affected in approximately 10% of extrapulmonary tuberculosis cases. *Mycobacterium tuberculosis* is the most common organism. *Mycobacterium bovis* can rarely cause renal tuberculosis. *Mycobacterium avium-intracellulare* occurs in immunosuppressed patients. Renal tuberculosis may occur in acute infection, hematogenous dissemination of active pulmonary tuberculosis, or reactivation of latent infection. Higher frequency of renal tuberculosis is present in immunosuppressed individuals (AIDS, transplantation, and dialysis), endemic areas, and in drug-resistant tuberculosis.

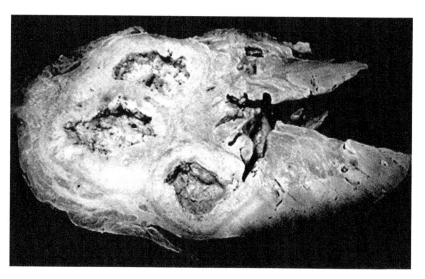

Fig. 14. Renal tuberculosis. The cross section of the kidney shows destruction and dilatation of the renal pelvic system, with caseous cheesy material.

Fig. 15. Miliary tuberculosis of the kidney. There are numerous small foci of cheesy caseous necrosis in the cortex and medulla.

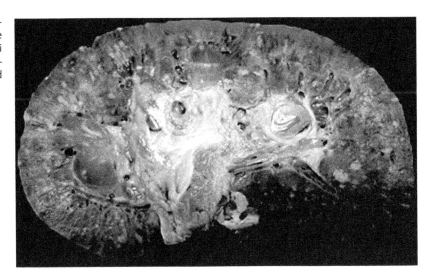

Gross Findings

The initial lesions occur in the renal pelvic calyces and papillae, with ulceration of the epithelium with caseous cheesy materials. The ureteropelvic junction can become obstructed by caseous cheesy materials producing hydronephrosis (**Fig. 14**). The renal cortex can become atrophic with extensive destruction of renal parenchyma. Renal miliary tuberculosis (**Fig. 15**) is difficult to distinguish from xanthogranulomatous pyelonephritis on gross examination.

Microscopic Findings

The earliest findings are neutrophils and macrophages in the renal medulla. This is followed by production of granulomas, often with caseous necrosis. There is usually interstitial fibrosis and tubular atrophy in the renal cortex with associated interstitial lymphoplasmacytic infiltrate. Persistent infection of the medulla may form large tumorlike masses (tuberculomas). The mycobacterial organisms can usually be identified with acid-fast stains, such as Ziehl-Neelsen or Fite. Fluorochromes, such as auramine rhodamine, are helpful to demonstrate the organisms.

Differential Diagnosis

XPN and sarcoidosis are the top differential diagnoses. The presence of caseating granulomas leads to the diagnosis of renal tuberculosis. Renal sarcoidosis shows confluent noncaseating granulomas. Multinucleated giant cells may be found in XPN. However, foamy, lipid-laden macrophages are predominant in XPN.

Clinical Correlation

Spread to the kidney probably occurs hematogenously during the primary tuberculosis infection, before cell-mediated immunity develops against the organism. In most cases, the organism is confined and the lesions heal. In a small number of cases, infection persists in the medulla, resulting in caseating granulomas.[45,46]

Key Points: Renal Tuberculosis

- Infection by *Mycobacterium* sp
- Hematogenous dissemination of active primary infection or reactivated latent infection
- Destruction of pelvic calyces and papillae with caseous necrosis
- Caseating granulomas with acid fast bacilli

ACKNOWLEDGMENTS

We thank Colonel Sureeporn Poungphong and Colonel Pipat Sritanabutr from the Department of Pathology, Phramongkutklao College of Medicine, in retrieving gross images.

REFERENCES

1. Gilbert-Barness E, Lacson A. A urinary tract and male genital system. In: Sternberg SS, editor. Diagnostic surgical pathology. 4th edition. Philadelphia: Lippincott Williams and Wilkins; 2003. p. 1845–62.

2. Gilbert-Barness E, Debich-Spicer DE. Renal system. In: Opitz JM, editor. Handbook of pediatric autopsy pathology. Totowa (NJ): Human Press Inc; 2004. p. 301–36.

3. Song R, Yosypiv IV. Genetics of congenital anomalies of the kidney and urinary tract. Pediatr Nephrol 2011;26:353–64.

4. Hiraoka M, Tsukahara H, Ohshima Y, et al. Renal aplasia is the predominant cause of congenital solitary kidneys. Kidney Int 2002;61:1840–4.

5. van den Bosch CM, van Wijk JA, Beckers GM, et al. Urological and nephrological findings in renal ectopia. J Urol 2010;183:1574–8.

6. Bonsib SM. The classification of renal cystic disease and other congenital malformations of the kidney and urinary tract. Arch Pathol Lab Med 2010;134: 554–68.

7. Wilson PD, Goilav B. Cystic disease of the kidney. Annu Rev Pathol 2007;2:341–68.

8. Bisceglia M, Galliani CA, Senger C, et al. Renal cystic disease; a review. Adv Anat Pathol 2006;13: 25–56.

9. Hurd TW, Hildebrandt F. Mechanisms of nephronophthisis and related ciliopathies. Nephron Exp Nephro 2011;118:9–14.

10. Hildebrandt F, Attanasio M, Otto E. Nephronophthisis: disease mechanisms of a ciliopathy. J Am Soc Nephrol 2009;20:23–35.

11. Caglioti A, Esposito C, Fuiano G, et al. Prevalence of symptoms in patients with simple renal cysts. BMJ 1993;306:430–1.

12. Solez K, Morel-Maroger L, Sraer JD. The morphology of "acute tubular necrosis" in man: analysis of 57 renal biopsies and a comparison with the glycerol model. Medicine (Baltimore) 1979;58:362–76.

13. Chugh KS, Jha V, Sakhuja V, et al. Acute renal cortical necrosis—a study of 113 patients. Ren Fail 1994;16:37–47.

14. Rosen S, Heyman SN. Difficulties in understanding human "acute tubular necrosis": limited data and flawed animal models. Kidney Int 2001;60:1220–4.

15. van Slambrouck CM, Salem F, Meehan SM, et al. Bile cast nephropathy is a common pathologic finding for kidney injury associated with severe liver dysfunction. Kidney Int 2013;84:192–7.

16. Heyman SN, Darmon D, Ackerman Z, et al. Bile cast nephropathy. Kidney Int 2014;85:479.

17. Betjes MG, Bajema I. The pathology of jaundice-related renal insufficiency: cholemic nephrosis revisited. J Nephrol 2006;19:229–33.

18. Najafian B, Franklin DB, Fogo AB. Acute renal failure and myalgia in a transplant patient. J Am Soc Nephrol 2007;18:2870–4.

19. Colvin RB, Fang LS. Interstitial nephritis. In: Tisher C, Brenner BM, editors. Renal pathology. Philadelphia: JB Lippincott; 1994. p. 723–68.

20. Randhawa PS, Finkelstein S, Scantlebury V, et al. Human polyoma virus-associated interstitial nephritis in the allograft kidney. Transplantation 1999;67:103–9.

21. Magil AB. Drug-induced acute interstitial nephritis with granulomas. Hum Pathol 1983;14:36–41.

22. Cornell LD. IgG4-related kidney disease. Curr Opin Nephrol Hypertens 2012;21:279–88.

23. Arneil GC, MacDonald AM, Sweet EM. Renal venous thrombosis. Clin Nephrol 1973;1:119–31.

24. Rosenmann E, Pollak VE, Pirani CL. Renal vein thrombosis in the adult: a clinical and pathologic study based on renal biopsies. Medicine (Baltimore) 1968;47:269–335.

25. Tektonidou MG. Renal involvement in the antiphospholipid syndrome (APS)-APS nephropathy. Clin Rev Allergy Immunol 2009;36:131–40.

26. Farkas JC, Tabet G, Marzelle J, et al. Arterial thrombosis: a rare complication of the nephrotic syndrome. Cardiovasc Surg 1993;1:265–9.

27. Mittal BV, Alexander MP, Rennke HG, et al. Atheroembolic renal disease: a silent masquerader. Kidney Int 2008;73:126–30.

28. Modi KS, Rao VK. Atheroembolic renal disease. J Am Soc Nephrol 2001;12:1781–7.

29. Fogo A, Stone WJ. Atheroembolic renal disease. In: Martinez-Maldonado M, editor. Hypertension and renal disease in the elderly. Cambridge (MA): Blackwell Scientific; 1992. p. 261–71.

30. Hill GS. Hypertensive nephrosclerosis. Curr Opin Nephrol Hypertens 2008;17:266–70.

31. Marcantoni C, Fogo AB. A perspective on arterionephrosclerosis: from pathology to potential pathogenesis. J Nephrol 2007;20:518–24.

32. Shanley PF. The pathology of chronic renal ischemia. Semin Nephrol 1996;16:21–32.

33. Textor SC, Wilcox CS. Renal artery stenosis: a common, treatable, cause of renal failure? Annu Rev Med 2001;52:421–42.

34. Moake JL. Thrombotic microangiopathies. N Engl J Med 2002;347:589–600.

35. Noris M, Remuzzi G. Hemolytic uremic syndrome. J Am Soc Nephrol 2005;16:1035–50.

36. Kimmelstiel P, Wilson C. Intracapillary lesions in glomeruli of the kidney. Am J Pathol 1936;12: 83–98.7.

37. Gambara V, Mecca G, Remuzzi G, et al. Heterogeneous nature of renal lesions in type II diabetes. J Am Soc Nephrol 1993;3:1458–66.

38. Fioretto P, Mauer SM, Bilous RW, et al. Effects of pancreas transplantation on glomerular structure in insulin-dependent diabetic patients with their own kidneys. Lancet 1993;342:1193–6.

39. Craig WD, Wagner BJ, Travis MD. Pyelonephritis: radiologic-pathologic review. Radiographics 2008; 28:255–77.

40. Cotran RS. The renal lesion in chronic pyelonephritis: immunofluorescent and ultrastructural studies. J Infect Dis 1969;120:109–18.

41. Zugor V, Schott GE, Labanaris AP. Xanthogranulomatous pyelonephritis in childhood: a critical analysis of 10 cases and of the literature. Urology 2007;70:157–60.

42. Antonakopoulos GN, Chapple CR, Newman J, et al. Xanthogranulomatous pyelonephritis. A reappraisal and immunohistochemical study. Arch Pathol Lab Med 1988;112:275–81.

43. Kobayashi A, Utsunomiya Y, Kono M, et al. Malakoplakia of the kidney. Am J Kidney Dis 2008;5:326–30.

44. Tam VK, Kung WH, Li R, et al. Renal parenchymal malacoplakia: a rare cause of ARF with a review of recent literature. Am J Kidney Dis 2003;41:E13–7.

45. Wise GJ, Marella VK. Genitourinary manifestations of tuberculosis. Urol Clin North Am 2003;30:111–21.

46. Eastwood JB, Corbishley CM, Grange JM. Tuberculosis and the kidney. J Am Soc Nephrol 2001;12:1307–14.

Donor Kidney Evaluation

Nasreen Mohamed, MD, FRCPA[a], Lynn D. Cornell, MD[b],*

KEYWORDS

- Kidney transplant • Donor biopsy • Expanded criteria donor • Zero time biopsy

ABSTRACT

In patients with end-stage renal disease, kidney transplantation is the best means to extend survival and offer a better quality of life. The current shortage of organs available for transplantation has led to an effort to expand the kidney donor pool, including the use of nonideal donor kidneys. Assessment of the quality of the donated kidney is essential, and would facilitate the decision to transplant a potential organ or discard it. Multiple clinical and histologic parameters have been examined to evaluate the donor kidney and relate the findings to the graft outcome, but clear-cut criteria are yet to be defined.

OVERVIEW

Kidney transplantation is the best choice of treatment for most patients with end-stage renal disease. Patients who do not have an acceptable living kidney donor may turn to the deceased donor waiting list. The shortage of organs available for donation with the growing waiting list has been a major challenge in the field. Clinicians started to turn their focus toward expanding the kidney donor pool by using nonideal kidneys, and in recent years, there has been an increasing use of kidneys from older donors and from donors with comorbidities, such as hypertension.[1,2]

Expanded criteria donor (ECD) kidneys are generally defined as those from patients 60 years or older, or age 50 to 59 with 2 of 3 of the following factors: death due to cerebrovascular cause, history of hypertension, or serum creatinine greater than 1.5 mg/dL (or creatinine clearance<60 mL/min).[3] Kidneys retrieved from ECDs are at higher risk of delayed graft function and primary nonfunction, and have decreased graft survival compared with kidneys from standard criteria donors (SCDs).[4] ECD kidneys are typified by having reduced creatinine clearance with a higher percentage of sclerotic glomeruli as a sequel to aging or other coexisting diseases. The remaining viable nephrons might not have the capacity to withstand additional stress during the transplantation procedure, nephrotoxic immunosuppression, and requirement to function instead of 2 kidneys. Thus, the quality of the donor organ is a critically important matter, that is, the number of surviving nephrons having the ability to withstand the injury will determine the long-term function and survival. One study found that donor factors accounted for 64% of the variability in allograft function at 6 months posttransplant.[5,6] The greater risk of delayed graft function and poor long-term function might compel the surgeon to err to the side of discarding the organ.

The increasing evidence of reduced graft survival rate from deceased donors necessitates assessment of the quality of the donated kidney before transplantation. Many institutes have acquired the practice of biopsy evaluation before transplantation. Evaluation of the donor biopsy can help determine the functional reserve of a donor kidney under consideration for transplantation and to improve both short-term and long-term graft function. In the United States, approximately 75% of kidneys from ECDs are biopsied and 41% of those are discarded because of the histopathologic characteristics.[7] Azancot and colleagues showed poor reproducibility of donor biopsy evaluation between on-call (non-renal) pathologists and renal pathologists.[8] Recipient outcomes (one-year eGFR and death censored graft survival) correlated with scores by the renal pathologists but not by the on-call

Disclosure and Conflict of Interest: None.
[a] Department of Pathology and Laboratory Medicine, King Fahad Specialist Hospital-Dammam, Amer Bin Thabet Street-mbc035, PO Box 15215, Dammam 31444, Kingdom of Saudi Arabia; [b] Division of Anatomic Pathology, Department of Laboratory Medicine and Pathology, Mayo Clinic, 200 First Street Southwest, Rochester, MN 55905, USA
* Corresponding author.
E-mail address: Cornell.Lynn@mayo.edu

Surgical Pathology 7 (2014) 357–365
http://dx.doi.org/10.1016/j.path.2014.04.002
1875-9181/14/$ – see front matter

pathologists. In addition, a subset of discarded kidneys deemed unsuitable by the on-call pathologist was considered by the renal pathologist to be adequate for transplantation. These results suggest that donor biopsies be evaluated by a renal pathologist. One possibility to consider is whole-slide imaging and evaluation by a renal pathologist on-call at a distant site, if a local renal pathologist is not available, particularly as these biopsies are not used for primary patient diagnosis.[9] Although ECD kidneys are not ideal, they can be used for elderly recipients to offer a better quality of life and survival. Surgeons might also consider using dual kidney transplantation to improve the nephron mass and increase the GFR in the recipient.

CLASSIFICATION OF DONORS

The deceased donor kidneys are classified into 2 broad groups, reflecting the quality of the organ and driven by the risk of graft loss: SCDs and ECDs.[4,10]

ECD

A donor at the time of death is 60 years or older or a donor aged 50 to 59 years and has any of the following 3 criteria: (1) cause of death is cerebrovascular accident, (2) history of hypertension, (3) terminal serum creatinine greater than 1.5 mg/dL.[3,10,11] Other categories of deceased donor kidneys are donation after cardiac death (DCD) and donation after brain death (DBD).

SCD

Any donor who does not fulfill the criteria of ECD.[10]

DBD

A donor who has primarily brain death with maintained cardiac and respiratory circulation by medical measures. The donor can be SCD or ECD.[10]

DCD

DCD includes donors who do not fit the brain death category but who have cardiac standstill or cessation of cardiac function before organ procurement. They can be divided into controlled DCD and uncontrolled DCD. Controlled DCD includes donors whose life support will be withdrawn in the controlled environment of the operating room. The donor hemodynamic and respiratory functions are maintained. Uncontrolled DCD includes candidates who die in the emergency room before consent is obtained for organ donation and a catheter is placed in the femoral vessels and peritoneum to cool the organs. It also includes candidates who consented for organ donation, but suffer a cardiac arrest requiring cardiopulmonary resuscitation during procurement of organs.[10]

CLINICAL AND LABORATORY EVALUATION OF DONORS

Clinical history and laboratory results of the potential donor should be reviewed before considering that patient's organs for donation. Patients with a history of diabetes, hypertension, and other conditions are considered as potential donors, as well as patients with perimortal disseminated intravascular coagulation and acute tubular injury.[1,12] In patients with traumatic death, a complete clinical history may not be available, and so some centers have used donor age as a surrogate marker for renal function and a guide to suitability of the organ for transplantation. We know that global glomerulosclerosis and other chronic histopathologic changes increase with age on the whole in normal-functioning kidneys,[13,14] but there is considerable variability among individual kidneys, and so age alone is not a satisfactory factor. Even among healthy living donors, glomerulosclerosis occurs with increasing age that is not explained by chronic kidney disease risk factors.[13] The calculated donor glomerular filtration rate (GFR) may be a better clinical indicator of quality of a kidney for transplantation than age alone; one study suggested a calculated donor GFR of less than 85 mL per minute as an indicator of poor donor kidney quality.[15] Some clinicians have used a creatinine clearance of greater than 60 to 70 mL per minute as the acceptable cutoff value for accepting organs for single kidney donation, whereas others recommend dual kidney transplantation with a lower creatinine clearance.[16–18] Rao and colleagues[19] put forth the Kidney Donor Profile Index (KDPI), which is a score that estimates the risk of graft failure and takes into account donor age, race/ethnicity, height and weight, history of hypertension and diabetes, serum creatinine, cerebrovascular cause of death, DCD, and hepatitis C status. KDRI values can help allocate kidneys and determine whether to transplant a single kidney or 2 kidneys.[20,21]

DONOR BIOPSY ASSESSMENT

Renal biopsy is performed after procurement and before kidney transplantation, and serves as an important tool for evaluation of the kidney, particularly with ECD. In approximately 85% of potential donors older than 65, the organ undergoes histologic assessment pretransplantation.[11] Approximately 40% of ECD kidneys are discarded. The main reason for kidneys to be discarded in the United States was the biopsy findings, as reported to the United Network for Organ Sharing.[11] Donor biopsies may also be performed to evaluate for a suspected neoplasm. The donor biopsy, performed before transplantation for rapid evaluation of suitability of an organ for transplantation, is to be distinguished from the implantation or "time-zero" biopsy. The time-zero biopsy is generally performed after perfusion of the transplanted graft and is done for the purpose of evaluating baseline chronic changes in a graft that is already deemed acceptable for transplantation.

The preimplantation biopsy may be a wedge biopsy or a needle-core biopsy. Most surgeons prefer wedge biopsies to reduce the risk of damaging large arteries and result in uncontrolled bleeding.[22] The wedge biopsy, however, may overrepresent the degree of global glomerulosclerosis, which tends to affect disproportionally the subcapsular glomeruli in patients with vascular disease. Wedge biopsies also may be superficial and not sample arteries, compared with needle-core biopsies, which are more likely to contain arteries.[23]

Urgent assessment of the donor biopsy is essential when the decision to transplant a kidney is contingent with the extent of the chronic changes, and so rapid evaluation is important. The biopsy tissue can undergo rapid processing, with a permanent section available within 2 to 3 hours; the other most widely used alternative is frozen section. The frozen section will provide morphology to identify sclerotic glomeruli, interstitial fibrosis, and arteriosclerosis (**Fig. 1**). The drawback to the frozen section is freezing artifact, or simply the "normal" physiologic appearance of the kidney that has not gone through dehydration steps of routine tissue processing. Frozen sections typically show interstitial edema, which can be misinterpreted as fibrosis. Assessment of mesangial cellularity or mesangial matrix expansion and glomerular capillary loop thickening or duplication is often not reliable on frozen sections, which is particularly important to consider in a donor with a history of diabetes (**Fig. 2**). There is consistent agreement among pathologists that formalin-fixed, paraffin-embedded tissue is superior to frozen sections for more detailed evaluation.

DONOR BIOPSY PATHOLOGY EVALUATION AND REPORT

On biopsy, the pathologist should assess the different renal "compartments": glomeruli, tubules and interstitium, and vessels. For glomeruli, the total number of glomeruli and percentage of global glomerulosclerosis are reported (**Box 1**). An adequate sample contains at least 25 glomeruli, including those from the deep cortex. Sometimes the surgeon will sample a distinct subcapsular scar in a wedge biopsy, sometimes due to targeted sampling of a firm or white area seen grossly on the kidney surface. Globally sclerotic glomeruli are clustered in a subcapsular scar and these should not be included in the overall percentage of global glomerulosclerosis. Any other glomerular abnormality, such as thrombi or segmental

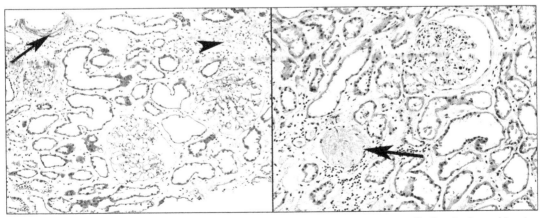

Fig. 1. Mild fibrous intimal thickening (*arrow, left panel*) in an artery is a common finding in donor biopsies, particularly in older donors. There is focal interstitial fibrosis (*arrowhead*). This section also shows significant tubular epithelial flattening, a feature of acute tubular injury commonly seen in donor biopsies. Interstitial edema, shown here, is typically seen on frozen sections. A globally sclerotic glomerulus is identified on this frozen section (*arrow, right panel*) (Hematoxylin and eosin stains, original magnification ×100, *left*; original magnification ×200, *right*).

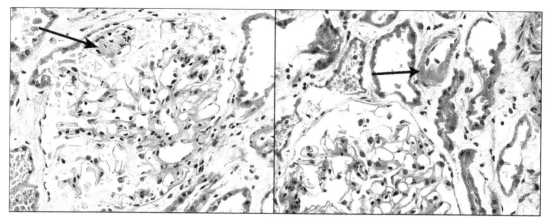

Fig. 2. Assessment of mesangial cellularity or mesangial matrix expansion and glomerular capillary loop thickening or duplication is often not reliable on frozen sections, which is particularly important to consider in a donor with a history of diabetes, although mesangial expansion can occasionally be seen, as shown here (*arrow, left panel*). Arteriolar hyalinosis (*right panel, arrow*) also sometimes can be seen, especially in patients with a history of diabetes or hypertension (Hematoxylin and eosin stains, original magnification ×400, *left and right*).

glomerulosclerosis, should also be sought and reported if present. The pathologist must recognize that normal glomeruli often appear hypercellular in frozen sections. In the tubulointerstitial compartment, the degree of interstitial fibrosis and tubular atrophy is reported. Another possible tubulointerstitial finding is interstitial inflammation. Acute tubular injury may be present, although frozen artifact precludes optimal evaluation for acute tubular injury. The presence or absence of arteries should be reported; at least 2 arteries are present in an adequate sample. The degree (none, mild, moderate, or severe) of fibrous intimal thickening in arteries should be reported. Arterioles, best seen near glomeruli, may show hyalinosis, most commonly in the intimal location but occasionally arterioles show peripheral hyalinosis. Fibrin thrombi in vessels should be reported (**Fig. 3**). Another point to highlight in the donor kidney

biopsy report is evidence of chronic diseases, such as diabetic nephropathy, although as mentioned previously, these features may not be evaluable on frozen section.

GLOMERULAR CHANGES

The extent of acceptable chronic changes within donor kidney is not absolute, but the most widely accepted guideline is that a donor kidney with more than 20% glomerulosclerosis should not be used for transplantation.[24] This guideline was based on the findings presented by Gaber and colleagues,[24] who showed that more than 20% of glomerulosclerosis is associated with delayed graft function in 88% of cases and graft loss in 38% of cases.[24] Escofet and colleagues[15] and Bajwa and colleagues[25] found that greater than 10% and greater than 5% glomerulosclerosis is a better predictor for reduction of graft survival, respectively. The incidence of graft dysfunction at 12 months posttransplantation for kidney biopsies with 0% glomerulosclerosis, 1% to 10% glomerulosclerosis, and 11% to 20% glomerulosclerosis was 25%, 46%, and 60%, respectively.[1] Pokorna and colleagues[26] showed that the 3-year graft survival is 75% when 20% to 48% of the glomeruli show global sclerosis, whereas 11% of cases show primary graft nonfunction. In contrast, a few investigators found no predictive value for glomerulosclerosis.[27,28] Despite significant glomerulosclerosis (approximately 15%–50%) that might represent a higher-risk graft, these kidneys could still be used for particular patients, such as for highly sensitized patients with an acceptable match or for older patients.

Box 1
Reporting donor biopsy (frozen or permanent)

Type of the biopsy (wedge, needle)

Total number of glomeruli and number of globally sclerosed glomeruli

Number of arteries

Arterial intimal fibrosis and arteriolar hyalinosis

Percentage of interstitial fibrosis/tubular atrophy in cortex

Presence of thrombi within glomeruli or vessels

Any other notable features

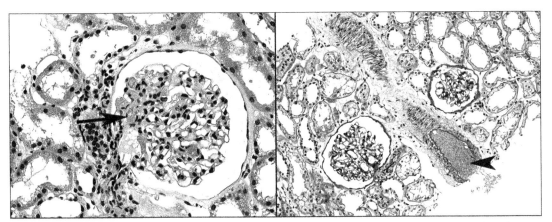

Fig. 3. Thrombi are seen in a glomerulus (*arrow, left panel*) or in an artery (*arrowhead, right panel*) in these examples (Hematoxylin and eosin, original magnification ×400, *left*; periodic acid-Schiff, original magnification ×200, *right*).

The presence of scattered fibrin thrombi in a few glomeruli does not contraindicate transplantation; these thrombi will likely dissolve by an intact fibrinolytic system.[29] Gaber and colleagues[30] found no effect on graft outcome in donor biopsies that showed thrombi in fewer than 50% of glomeruli. In another study, Pokorna and colleagues[26] documented fibrin thrombi within glomerular capillaries in 5 donor kidneys, which were transplanted into 10 patients. In 33% there was a nonfunctioning graft, 56% had delayed graft function, and 11% had immediate graft function. Although the glomerular thrombi did not affect graft survival, 63% of recipients had delayed graft function.[31]

Occasionally, pretransplant or posttransplant biopsies show donor-derived glomerulonephritis. The most frequent of these is immunoglobulin (Ig) A nephropathy or mesangial IgA-dominant deposits, which tends to have no impact on graft function and usually resolves with time.[32] Indeed, IgA-dominant immune complex deposits have been reported in approximately 10% of normal donor kidneys,[33,34] and so IgA deposits in the absence of clinically apparent disease or mesangial hypercellularity may not represent the disease of IgA nephropathy. A recent study concluded that even donor biopsies that showed mesangial expansion with IgA deposits did not affect the transplant prognosis.[35] Subsequent biopsies of grafts with donor-derived IgA deposits show progressive lessening and eventual disappearance of the deposits.[36] Other documented glomerular lesions in donor kidneys include membranous glomerulonephritis and focal segmental glomerulosclerosis.

VASCULAR CHANGES

Besides glomerulosclerosis, at least moderate arteriosclerosis (>25% luminal narrowing) is another predictor of worse graft outcome and is a common reason for discarding organs.[2,12] Generally, significant vascular changes have been associated with delayed graft function and the graft outcome,[27,28,37–39] although scoring arteries in donor biopsies might not be possible because of limited sample size in most cases.[40] Vascular pathology was independently associated with risk of graft failure in the Maryland Aggregate Pathology Index (MAPI) study (see later in this article).

TUBULOINTERSTITIAL CHANGES

Acute tubular injury is often present in donor biopsies; studies have shown that histologic scoring of acute tubular necrosis[26,41] and apoptosis[29] predicts delayed graft function. The value of interstitial fibrosis and tubular atrophy has not been examined extensively, some suggested its adverse effect on graft outcome,[1] whereas others found little value of scoring them.[26]

LIVING DONOR BIOPSIES

The presence of microscopic hematuria and/or mild proteinuria in a potential living donor warrants further investigation, including consideration of a renal biopsy. Biopsy assessment, including use of immunofluorescence and electron microscopy, will aid in the decision to proceed with organ donation or not. Relevant pathology is generally considered a contraindication for donation to protect the donor from developing progressive kidney disease aggravated further by reduced nephron mass. Kidneys with thin glomerular basement membrane nephropathy may be considered for transplantation, however, so long as Alport syndrome, including carrier status of Alport syndrome and Alport syndrome with a thin basement membrane phenotype, can be excluded. In this case, relevant personal and family history, and ancillary genetic tests if available, also should be considered.

CLINICAL AND HISTOPATHOLOGIC SCORING SYSTEMS FOR DONOR BIOPSIES

A study by Munivenkatappa and colleagues[42] examined a combination of donor clinical and histopathologic variables to come up with an aggregate score that would help predict allograft outcome. This group showed that donor age and terminal creatinine were by themselves statistically significant clinical factors affecting graft loss. The independently significant histopathological features were percentage of glomerulosclerosis, presence of periglomerular fibrosis, wall-to-lumen ratio of interlobular arteries, presence of arteriolar hyalinosis, and the presence of tubulointerstitial scarring involving an area including at least 10 atrophic tubules. From these data, the group proposed the MAPI, where scores between 7 and 11 were threshold cutoffs for grouping MAPI scores into 3 groups designated as low, intermediate, and high risk for graft failure (Table 1). The 5-year graft survival with MAPI scores from 0 to 7 (low risk) was 90%, with scores from 8 to 11 (intermediate risk) 5-year graft survival was 63%, and with scores from 12 to 15 (high risk) 5-year graft survival was 53%. This scoring system has predicted graft outcome independent of the other donor characteristics.[42] The 5-year graft survival for glomerulosclerosis greater than 15%, wall-to-lumen ratio of 0.5 or higher (equivalent to cv3 in the Banff score), presence of arteriolar hyalinosis, localized fibrosis, and periglomerular fibrosis is 46%, 52%, 48%, 54%, and 54%, respectively.[42]

Another scoring system developed by Nyberg and colleagues[43] is based purely on 7 clinical parameters of the donor. The total final score ranged from 0 to 32 points, and a grade was assigned to the kidney based on the total score: A (0–5), B (6–10), C (11–15), or D (≥16). In this scoring system, the renal biopsy findings, including glomerulosclerosis, did not predict the early renal function.[43]

Another group investigated the significance of clinical donor characteristics and the histopathologic features at the biopsy. The group was able to conclude that donor history of hypertension, serum creatinine before organ recovery, and the presence of 10% or more glomerulosclerosis had a significant impact on graft survival (Table 2).[44] The composite scoring system that included donor serum creatinine levels (<150 μmol/L or ≥150 μmol/L), donor hypertension, and glomerulosclerosis (≥10% or <10%) showed the highest predictive value for low GFR at 1 year posttransplantation. The vascular and tubulointerstitial changes of the donor kidneys had no significant impact on graft survival.[44]

Surprisingly, a few studies have failed to identify a correlation between donor biopsy findings and later posttransplant graft function.[45–49] These studies included small sample size with mainly mild changes.[2]

Table 1 Maryland aggregate pathology index	
Variables	Points
Periglomerular fibrosis (present or absent)	4
Arteriolar hyalinosis (present/absent)	4
Scar (focus of scar or IF/TA >10 tubules) (present/absent)	3
Global glomerulosclerosis ≥15%	2
Wall-to-lumen ratio of interlobular arteries ≥0.5	2
5-y graft survival	
Low risk (0–7)	90%
Intermediate risk (8–11)	63%
High risk (12–15)	53%

Abbreviations: IF, interstitial fibrosis; TA, tubular atrophy.

Table 2 French clinico-pathological composite score	
Variables	Points
Glomerulosclerosis >10% (absent/ present)	0/1
Donor hypertension and/or donor serum creatinine ≥150 μmol/L (absent/present)	0/1
eGFR <25 mL/min at 1 y	
GS = 0 and DHC = 0	5.2%
GS = 1 and DHC = 0	12.5%
GS = 0 and DHC = 1	13.5%
GS = 1 and DHC = 1	35.1%

Abbreviations: DHC, donor hypertension or serum creatinine ≥150 μmol/L; eGFR, estimated glomerular filtration rate; GS, glomerulosclerosis.

MOLECULAR EVALUATION OF DONOR BIOPSIES

As molecular studies have been proposed or used in other areas of renal transplant pathology, so have they in the evaluation of donor biopsies. Molecular studies might detect changes associated with tissue injury and repair, and give additional predictive information about the suitability of an organ for transplantation.

In one study, using a cDNA microarray technique, deceased donor kidneys showed high expression of genes related to signal transduction pathways, cell-cycle regulation, and cell growth/metabolism, and these were related to development of acute renal failure in recipients.[50] In addition, microarray analyses have shown that inflammation-associated transcriptome profile differentiates living donor from deceased donor kidneys.[50,51] Naesens and colleagues[52] showed that the complement gene expression is higher in deceased donor kidneys in comparison with living donor kidneys.[50] Gene expression of implantation biopsies was able to identify kidneys at risk of delayed graft function better than clinical and histologic parameters.[53] Kainz and colleagues[51] showed that gene sets of the tubulointerstitial compartments is abundantly expressed in deceased donor kidneys in comparison with the living donor kidney, whereas the gene expression of the glomerular compartment did not show a difference.

The changes in gene expression are more sensitive than clinical and histologic markers in identifying acute tissue injury, but it is not likely to reflect the degree of glomerulosclerosis, the reserve capacity, or the presence of hypertensive or diabetic changes.[54] Transcriptome and gene expression evaluation may emerge as a complementary method to clinical history and renal biopsy findings to optimize the interpretation of the quality of the donated organ.

REFERENCES

1. Randhawa PS, Minervini MI, Lombardero M, et al. Biopsy of marginal donor kidneys: correlation of histologic findings with graft dysfunction. Transplantation 2000;69(7):1352–7.
2. Randhawa P. Role of donor kidney biopsies in renal transplantation. Transplantation 2001;71(10):1361–5.
3. Port FK, Bragg-Gresham JL, Metzger RA, et al. Donor characteristics associated with reduced graft survival: an approach to expanding the pool of kidney donors. Transplantation 2002;74(9): 1281–6.
4. Metzger RA, Delmonico FL, Feng S, et al. Expanded criteria donors for kidney transplantation. Am J Transplant 2003;3(Suppl 4):114–25.
5. Cosio FG, Qiu W, Henry ML, et al. Factors related to the donor organ are major determinants of renal allograft function and survival. Transplantation 1996;62(11):1571–6.
6. Suri D, Meyer TW. Influence of donor factors on early function of graft kidneys. J Am Soc Nephrol 1999;10(6):1317–23.
7. Sung RS, Christensen LL, Leichtman AB, et al. Determinants of discard of expanded criteria donor kidneys: impact of biopsy and machine perfusion. Am J Transplant 2008;8(4):783–92.
8. Azancot MA, Moreso F, Salcedo M, et al. The reproducibility and predictive value on outcome of renal biopsies from expanded criteria donors. Kidney Int 2014 May;85(5):1161–8.
9. Haas M. Donor kidney biopsies: pathology matters, and so does the pathologist. Kidney Int 2014 May; 85(5):1016–9.
10. Rao PS, Ojo A. The alphabet soup of kidney transplantation: SCD, DCD, ECD—fundamentals for the practicing nephrologist. Clin J Am Soc Nephrol 2009;4(11):1827–31.
11. Cecka JM, Cohen B, Rosendale J, et al. Could more effective use of kidneys recovered from older deceased donors result in more kidney transplants for older patients? Transplantation 2006;81(7): 966–70.
12. Verran D, Sheridan A, Barnwell A, et al. Biopsy of potential cadaveric renal allografts at the time of retrieval. Nephrology (Carlton) 2005;10(4):414–7.
13. Rule AD, Amer H, Cornell LD, et al. The association between age and nephrosclerosis on renal biopsy among healthy adults. Ann Intern Med 2010; 152(9):561–7.
14. Kaplan C, Pasternack B, Shah H, et al. Age-related incidence of sclerotic glomeruli in human kidneys. Am J Pathol 1975;80(2):227–34.
15. Escofet X, Osman H, Griffiths DF, et al. The presence of glomerular sclerosis at time zero has a significant impact on function after cadaveric renal transplantation. Transplantation 2003;75(3): 344–6.
16. Sola R, Guirado L, Lopez Navidad A, et al. Renal transplantation with limit donors: to what should the good results obtained be attributed? Transplantation 1998;66(9):1159–63.
17. Velosa JA, Offord KP, Schroeder DR. Effect of age, sex, and glomerular filtration rate on renal function outcome of living kidney donors. Transplantation 1995;60(12):1618–21.
18. Lee CM, Scandling JD, Shen GK, et al. The kidneys that nobody wanted: support for the utilization of expanded criteria donors. Transplantation 1996; 62(12):1832–41.

19. Rao PS, Schaubel DE, Guidinger MK, et al. A comprehensive risk quantification score for deceased donor kidneys: the kidney donor risk index. Transplantation 2009;88(2):231–6.

20. Klair T, Gregg A, Phair J, et al. Outcomes of adult dual kidney transplants by KDRI in the United States. Am J Transplant 2013;13(9):2433–40.

21. Bennett WM, McEvoy KM. A new system for kidney allocation: the devil is in the details. Clin J Am Soc Nephrol 2011;6(9):2308–9.

22. Hopfer H, Kemeny E. Assessment of donor biopsies. Curr Opin Organ Transplant 2013;18(3):306–12.

23. Bago-Horvath Z, Kozakowski N, Soleiman A, et al. The cutting (w)edge—comparative evaluation of renal baseline biopsies obtained by two different methods. Nephrol Dial Transplant 2012;27(8):3241–8.

24. Gaber LW, Moore LW, Alloway RR, et al. Glomerulosclerosis as a determinant of posttransplant function of older donor renal allografts. Transplantation 1995;60(4):334–9.

25. Bajwa M, Cho YW, Pham PT, et al. Donor biopsy and kidney transplant outcomes: an analysis using the Organ Procurement and Transplantation Network/United Network for Organ Sharing (OPTN/UNOS) database. Transplantation 2007;84(11):1399–405.

26. Pokorna E, Vitko S, Chadimova M, et al. Proportion of glomerulosclerosis in procurement wedge renal biopsy cannot alone discriminate for acceptance of marginal donors. Transplantation 2000;69(1):36–43.

27. Karpinski J, Lajoie G, Cattran D, et al. Outcome of kidney transplantation from high-risk donors is determined by both structure and function. Transplantation 1999;67(8):1162–7.

28. Bosmans JL, Woestenburg A, Ysebaert DK, et al. Fibrous intimal thickening at implantation as a risk factor for the outcome of cadaveric renal allografts. Transplantation 2000;69(11):2388–94.

29. Oberbauer R, Rohrmoser M, Regele H, et al. Apoptosis of tubular epithelial cells in donor kidney biopsies predicts early renal allograft function. J Am Soc Nephrol 1999;10(9):2006–13.

30. Gaber LW, Gaber AO, Tolley EA, et al. Prediction by postrevascularization biopsies of cadaveric kidney allografts of rejection, graft loss, and preservation nephropathy. Transplantation 1992;53(6):1219–25.

31. McCall SJ, Tuttle-Newhall JE, Howell DN, et al. Prognostic significance of microvascular thrombosis in donor kidney allograft biopsies. Transplantation 2003;75(11):1847–52.

32. Silva FG, Chander P, Pirani CL, et al. Disappearance of glomerular mesangial IgA deposits after renal allograft transplantation. Transplantation 1982;33(2):241–6.

33. Cosyns JP, Malaise J, Hanique G, et al. Lesions in donor kidneys: nature, incidence, and influence on graft function. Transpl Int 1998;11(1):22–7.

34. Rosenberg HG, Martinez PS, Vaccarezza AS, et al. Morphological findings in 70 kidneys of living donors for renal transplant. Pathol Res Pract 1990;186(5):619–24.

35. Sofue T, Inui M, Hara T, et al. Latent IgA deposition from donor kidneys does not affect transplant prognosis, irrespective of mesangial expansion. Clin Transplant 2013;27(Suppl 26):14–21.

36. Ji S, Liu M, Chen J, et al. The fate of glomerular mesangial IgA deposition in the donated kidney after allograft transplantation. Clin Transplant 2004;18(5):536–40.

37. Minakawa R, Tyden G, Lindholm B, et al. Donor kidney vasculopathy: impact on outcome in kidney transplantation. Transpl Immunol 1996;4(4):309–12.

38. Cockfield SM, Moore RB, Todd G, et al. The prognostic utility of deceased donor implantation biopsy in determining function and graft survival after kidney transplantation. Transplantation 2010;89(5):559–66.

39. Wang HJ, Kjellstrand CM, Cockfield SM, et al. On the influence of sample size on the prognostic accuracy and reproducibility of renal transplant biopsy. Nephrol Dial Transplant 1998;13(1):165–72.

40. Pokorna E, Vitko S, Chadimova M, et al. Adverse effect of donor arteriolosclerosis on graft outcome after renal transplantation. Nephrol Dial Transplant 2000;15(5):705–10.

41. Kuypers DR, Chapman JR, O'Connell PJ, et al. Predictors of renal transplant histology at three months. Transplantation 1999;67(9):1222–30.

42. Munivenkatappa RB, Schweitzer EJ, Papadimitriou JC, et al. The Maryland aggregate pathology index: a deceased donor kidney biopsy scoring system for predicting graft failure. Am J Transplant 2008;8(11):2316–24.

43. Nyberg SL, Matas AJ, Rogers M, et al. Donor scoring system for cadaveric renal transplantation. Am J Transplant 2001;1(2):162–70.

44. Anglicheau D, Loupy A, Lefaucheur C, et al. A simple clinico-histopathological composite scoring system is highly predictive of graft outcomes in marginal donors. Am J Transplant 2008;8(11):2325–34.

45. Nyberg G, Hedman L, Blohme I, et al. Morphologic findings in baseline kidney biopsies from living related donors. Transplant Proc 1992;24(1):355–6.

46. Abdi R, Slakey D, Kittur D, et al. Baseline glomerular size as a predictor of function in human renal transplantation. Transplantation 1998;66(3):329–33.

47. Bosmans JL, Woestenburg AT, Helbert MJ, et al. Impact of donor-related vascular alterations in implantation biopsies on morphologic and functional outcome of cadaveric renal allografts. Transplant Proc 2000;32(2):379–80.

48. Curschellas E, Landmann J, Durig M, et al. Morphologic findings in "zero-hour" biopsies of renal transplants. Clin Nephrol 1991;36(5):215–22.

49. Sund S, Reisaeter AV, Fauchald P, et al. Living donor kidney transplants: a biopsy study 1 year after transplantation, compared with baseline changes and correlation to kidney function at 1 and 3 years. Nephrol Dial Transplant 1999;14(10):2445–54.

50. Hauser P, Schwarz C, Mitterbauer C, et al. Genome-wide gene-expression patterns of donor kidney biopsies distinguish primary allograft function. Lab Invest 2004;84(3):353–61.

51. Kainz A, Mitterbauer C, Hauser P, et al. Alterations in gene expression in cadaveric vs. live donor kidneys suggest impaired tubular counterbalance of oxidative stress at implantation. Am J Transplant 2004;4(10):1595–604.

52. Naesens M, Li L, Ying L, et al. Expression of complement components differs between kidney allografts from living and deceased donors. J Am Soc Nephrol 2009;20(8):1839–51.

53. Mueller TF, Reeve J, Jhangri GS, et al. The transcriptome of the implant biopsy identifies donor kidneys at increased risk of delayed graft function. Am J Transplant 2008;8(1):78–85.

54. Mueller TF, Solez K, Mas V. Assessment of kidney organ quality and prediction of outcome at time of transplantation. Semin Immunopathol 2011;33(2):185–99.

The Basics of Renal Allograft Pathology

Megan L. Troxell, MD, PhD[a],*, Donald C. Houghton, MD[b]

KEYWORDS

- Kidney • Transplant • T-cell–mediated rejection • Antibody-mediated rejection • C4d
- Polyomavirus

ABSTRACT

Renal allograft biopsy provides critical information in the management of renal transplant patients, and must be analyzed in close collaboration with the clinical team. The histologic correlates of acute T-cell mediated rejection are interstitial inflammation, tubulitis, and endothelialitis; polyomavirus nephropathy is a potential mimic. Evidence of antibody-mediated rejection includes C4d deposition; morphologic acute tissue injury; and donor specific antibodies. Acute tubular injury/necrosis is a reversible cause of impaired graft function, especially in the immediate post-transplant period. Drug toxicity, recurrent disease, chronic injury, and other entities affecting both native and transplant kidneys must also be evaluated.

OVERVIEW

Renal transplantation greatly enhances quality of life and survival of patients with end-stage renal failure, as compared with dialysis. Patients may receive a living donor kidney, or a deceased donor allograft through the United Network of Organ Sharing paradigm. ABO blood group compatibility is an important factor in kidney transplantation; however, a few centers perform ABO-incompatible transplants after desensitization protocols. Pretransplantation HLA crossmatching is a critical component of transplant evaluation, as preexisting antibodies to the kidney graft can result in immediate (hyperacute) rejection. Crossmatching technology has evolved considerably over the past 50 years; potential recipients are typed for HLA antigen expression, and have their serum tested for preformed anti-HLA antibodies as an important part of the pretransplant workup. Large studies have shown that the fewer the HLA mismatches between donor and recipient, the better the long-term allograft survival.[1] Once the HLA type of an available organ is characterized, a "virtual" crossmatch can be computed with potential recipients, usually but not always followed by tissue studies (such as cytotoxic, B-cell and T-cell crossmatches, **Table 1**).[1] Recipients also may develop antibodies to their kidney allograft after transplantation, which can be elucidated with so-called "donor-specific antibody" (DSA) testing: testing patient serum for HLA antibodies, and comparison with the donor HLA type or archived blood.[1]

Renal allograft biopsies are performed primarily for graft dysfunction, as measured by serum creatinine ("indication" or "for-cause" biopsies). In addition, many centers also perform so-called surveillance or protocol biopsies at defined post-transplantation intervals to assess for subclinical rejection and other pathology. Careful histopathologic evaluation of tissue sections, including special studies, is necessary to distinguish rejection from potential mimics; further, clinicopathologic correlation, including drug levels, medication compliance, clinical history, viral studies, DSAs, imaging, and so forth, is key to appropriate diagnosis and, thus, therapy.

[a] Department of Pathology, Oregon Health & Science University, 3181 Southwest Sam Jackson Park Road, Portland, OR 97239, USA; [b] Department of Pathology, Oregon Health & Science University, 3181 Southwest Sam Jackson Park Road, Portland, OR 97239, USA
* Corresponding author.
E-mail address: troxellm@ohsu.edu

Surgical Pathology 7 (2014) 367–387
http://dx.doi.org/10.1016/j.path.2014.04.009
1875-9181/14/$ – see front matter © 2014 Elsevier Inc. All rights reserved.

Table 1
HLA testing vocabulary

Cell based	
National Institutes of Health standard crossmatch	"Classic assay": most specific, least sensitive; complement-dependent cytotoxicity. Donor lymphocytes are incubated with dilutions of recipient serum in the presence of complement; cell death is assayed
Antiglobulin-enhanced cross match	Detects non–complement binding antibodies and lower-titer antibodies (more sensitive due to addition of antihuman globulin)
B-cell crossmatch	Detects both anti-Class I and II antibodies; detects anti-Class I even when standard crossmatch negative (tests lymphocyte population enriched for B cells)
T-cell crossmatch	Detects only anti-Class I antibodies (T cells do not express Class II HLA)
Flow crossmatch	Most sensitive current assay; does not require viable donor cells. Donor lymphocytes are mixed with recipient serum then with fluorochrome-tagged antihuman immunoglobulin; cells with bound antibody are detected by a flow cytometer
Bead based (Luminex)	
Flow panel reactive antibodies (PRA)	Detects HLA antigen (coated beads) that react with antibodies in patient serum (expressed as a % of antibodies in a pool)
Donor-specific antibody (DSA)	Detects HLA antigens that react with antibodies in patient serum (single antigen–coated beads)
Mean fluorescence intensity (MFI)	A measure of the strength/amount of antibody in a bead-based assay; thresholds are set by individual HLA laboratory tests.

Data from Delos Santos R, Langewisch E, Norman DJ. Immunologic assessment of the transplant patient. In: Kidney transplantation: a practical guide to medical management. Springer Science+Business Media, LLC; 2014.

ALLOGRAFT BIOPSY LABORATORY PREPARATION

Several excellent references outline methods for kidney biopsy tissue handling and reporting.[2–4] Briefly, for allograft biopsies, at least 2 cores of renal parenchyma containing generous proportions of kidney cortex (10 or preferably more glomeruli) for light microscopy are necessary to adequately assess allograft rejection, as inflammatory cell infiltrates and other abnormalities may be patchy. Depending on local practice, tissue also may be needed for immunofluorescence microscopy (IF; usually in Michels or Zeus solution, see C4d Staining in Antibody-Mediated Rejection section), or electron microscopy (EM; usually in glutaraldehyde). If there is proteinuria, hematuria, or any concern for glomerular disease, tissue containing glomeruli should be handled similarly to a native biopsy, and sent for all 3 studies (light microscopy, IF, EM).

For light microscopy, attention to handling and processing is necessary to prevent artifacts and tissue loss.[2,3] Renal biopsies require thin sections (2–3 μm), multiple levels, hematoxylin-eosin (H&E), and additional histochemical stains to fully assess various facets of allograft pathology. Periodic acid-Schiff (PAS) stains are particularly useful in

evaluating hyaline (as described in detail later in this article); PAS and other basement membrane stains (such as silver or Jones silver) help to reveal tubulitis.[2,3] As in native renal biopsies, trichrome staining is useful in assessing fibrosis.[2,3] Special immunostains, such as stains for C4d and polyomavirus, are essential in many scenarios, and are described in detail later in this article. Consensus guidelines for renal allograft reporting were recently published.[4]

ACUTE REJECTION: T-CELL MEDIATED

OVERVIEW

Acute T-cell–mediated rejection (acute cellular rejection) occurs most commonly within the first months after transplantation, but can arise at any time point. Interstitial inflammation, tubulitis, and endothelialitis are the hallmarks of acute T-cell–mediated rejection in the renal allograft, although these histopathologic findings are not entirely specific for rejection. Classification schemes have evolved for the assessment and grading of allograft rejection; the Banff classification system is used in many centers and is undergoing continual evaluation and revision as data emerge (**Box 1**).[5–8] Acute rejection is illustrated in the framework

Box 1
Diagnostic categories for renal allograft biopsies: Banff 2013 update

1. Normal

2. Antibody-mediated changes (may coincide with other categories below)

   Acute antibody-mediated rejection (all 3 of the following features must be present)

   1. Histologic evidence of tissue injury, including 1 or more of the following:
      - Microvascular inflammation (peritubular capillaritis and/or glomerulitis)
      - Acute thrombotic microangiopathy in the absence of other causes
      - Intimal (as type II) or transmural arteritis (as type III)
      - Acute tubular injury in the absence of other apparent causes

   2. Evidence of any antibody-endothelial interaction, including at least 1 of the following:
      - Linear C4d peritubular capillary deposition ($\geq$10% by immunofluorescence [IF] or any immunohistochemistry [IHC] staining)
      - At least moderate microvascular inflammation (peritubular capillaritis and/or glomerulitis)
      - Increased gene expression in biopsy tissue indicative of endothelial injury, if validated

   3. Serologic detection of circulating antidonor antibodies

   Chronic active antibody-mediated rejection (all 3 of the following features must be present)

   1. Morphologic evidence of chronic tissue injury, including 1 or more of the following:
      - Glomerular double contours (transplant glomerulopathy) without evidence of chronic thrombotic microangiopathy (TMA)
      - Severe peritubular capillary basement membrane multilayering (by electron microscopy)
      - Arterial intimal fibrosis of new onset, excluding other causes

   2. Evidence of any antibody-endothelial interaction, including at least 1 of the following:
      - Linear C4d peritubular capillary deposition ($\geq$10% by IF or any IHC staining)
      - At least moderate microvascular inflammation (peritubular capillaritis and/or glomerulitis)
      - Increased gene expression in biopsy tissue indicative of endothelial injury, if validated

   3. Serologic detection of circulating antidonor antibodies

   C4d deposition without evidence of active rejection (all 3 of the following features must be present)

   1. Linear C4d peritubular capillary deposition ($\geq$10% by IF or any IHC staining)
   2. No glomerulitis, no peritubular capillaritis, no intimal arteritis, no chronic glomerulopathy or ptc lamination, no TMA, no acute tubular injury
   3. No acute T-cell mediated rejection (TCMR) or borderline changes

3. Borderline changes: "suspicious" for acute T-cell–mediated rejection (may coincide with categories other than T-cell–mediated rejection)

   Focal tubulitis ($\geq$1 cell/tubular cross section) with minor interstitial infiltration (10%–25%) or

   Interstitial infiltration (>25%) with mild tubulitis (1–4 cells/tubular cross section)

4. T-cell–mediated rejection (may coincide with categories 2, 5, 6)

   Type IA: Significant interstitial infiltration (>25% of parenchyma affected) and foci of moderate tubulitis (5–10 cells/tubular cross section [or 10 tubular cells])

   Type IB: Significant interstitial infiltration (>25% of parenchyma affected) and foci of severe tubulitis (>10 cells/tubular cross section [or 10 tubular cells], or at least 2 areas of tubular basement membrane destruction and moderate tubulitis elsewhere)

   Type IIA: Mild-to-moderate intimal arteritis

Type IIB: Severe intimal arteritis comprising greater than 25% of the luminal area (25% luminal narrowing)

Type III: "Transmural" arteritis and/or arterial fibrinoid change and necrosis of medial smooth muscle cells with accompanying lymphocytic inflammation

Chronic active T-cell–mediated rejection

"Chronic allograft arteriopathy" (arterial intimal fibrosis with mononuclear cell infiltration in fibrosis, formation of neo-intima)

5. Interstitial fibrosis and tubular atrophy, *no evidence of any specific etiology* (severity graded by tubulointerstitial features, may include nonspecific vascular and glomerular sclerosis)

   I. Mild interstitial fibrosis and tubular atrophy (<25% of cortical area)

   II. Moderate interstitial fibrosis and tubular atrophy (26%–50% of cortical area)

   III. Severe interstitial fibrosis and tubular atrophy/loss (>50% of cortical area)

6. Other. Changes not considered to be due to rejection, and may coincide with categories above.

Note: The Banff schema provides criteria for (semi-)quantitative for assessment of each of tubulitis (t), interstitial inflammation (i), vasculitis (v), glomerulitis (g), vascular fibrous intimal thickening (cv), interstitial fibrosis (ci), tubular atrophy (ct), allograft glomerulopathy (cg), mesangial matrix increase (mm), arteriolar hyaline thickening (ah, aah), peritubular capillaritis (ptc), total inflammation (ti).
Adapted from Refs.[5–8,12]

---

of the Banff schema (see **Table 1**)[5–8]; however, some centers apply alternative classification schemes, such as the Comparative Clinical Trials in Transplantation (CCTT, **Box 2**, **Table 2**), or others.[9–11]

Pathologic Key Features
OF ACUTE REJECTION

T-cell–mediated rejection

  Mononuclear interstitial inflammation in nonatrophic cortex

  Tubulitis in nonatrophic cortex

  Endothelialitis

  Arterial fibrinoid necrosis, transmural arteritis

  Also: edema, activated lymphocytes

Antibody-mediated rejection

  Histologic changes

    Peritubular capillaritis

    Glomerular capillaritis (glomerulitis)

    Fibrin thrombi, arterial fibrinoid necrosis

  C4d staining in peritubular capillaries

  Correlate with donor-specific antibody studies

Note: See **Boxes 1** and **2** and **Table 2** for grading.

Box 2
Comparative Clinical Trials in Transplantation criteria for diagnosis of acute cellular rejection

Type I: At least 5% of the cortex must have interstitial mononuclear infiltration with at least 2 of the following 3 features:

- Edema

- Tubular degeneration/injury

- Activated lymphocytes

In addition, tubulitis must be present, with at least 3 tubules affected in 10 serial high-power fields (×40) from the areas with the most infiltrate.

Type II: Arterial or arteriolar mononuclear cell endothelial inflammation (endothelialitis or endarteritis) is present (with or without features of type I).

- A threshold of at least 1 cell under the endothelium is required

- A lymphocyte adherent to the luminal surface of an endothelial cell is not sufficient.

Type III: Arterial or arteriolar fibrinoid necrosis or transmural inflammation is present and may or may not be accompanied by thrombosis, parenchymal necrosis/recent infarction, or hemorrhage.

Adapted from Colvin RB, Cohen AH, Saiontz C, et al. Evaluation of pathologic criteria for acute renal allograft rejection: reproducibility, sensitivity and clinical correlation. J Am Soc Nephrol 1997;8:1931; with permission.

MICROSCOPIC DESCRIPTION

The histologic hallmarks of acute rejection include interstitial inflammation and tubulitis, often accompanied by interstitial edema, involving nonatrophic areas of renal parenchyma (**Fig. 1**). Tubulitis is characterized by mononuclear inflammatory cells (T or B lymphocytes, monocytes, rarely plasma cells) that have crossed the tubular basement membrane, and are thus admixed with tubular epithelial cells. Basement membrane stains, such as PAS, are helpful, if not crucial, in assessing tubulitis. Basement membrane stains also help define areas of tubular atrophy, characterized by smaller-diameter tubules, with thick wavy tubular basement membranes, usually separated by interstitial fibrosis. Lymphocyte nuclei must be distinguished from tubular epithelial cell nuclei in good-quality sections; on H&E-stained and PAS-stained sections, lymphocyte nuclei are smaller and darker as compared with larger, paler, and often rounder epithelial cell nuclei with nucleoli (see **Fig. 1**).

Endothelialitis (intimal arteritis or endarteritis) in the renal allograft, as in other settings, is defined as mononuclear inflammatory cells beneath the endothelium, and is most often associated with reactive or edematous changes in the endothelium, along with proliferation of intimal myofibroblasts (see **Fig. 1**). Even one lymphocyte under the endothelium is sufficient for a diagnosis of endothelialitis, and, thus, acute rejection. Neither marginating inflammatory cells on the endothelial surfaces nor venulitis meet criteria for endothelialitis in kidney allograft rejection.

Table 2
Simplified comparison of Banff and Comparative Clinical Trials in Transplantation (CCTT) classification schemes of acute cellular rejection

Histopathology	Banff	CCTT
Interstitial inflammation and tubulitis	Borderline Type I	Type I Type I
Endothelialitis	Type II	Type II
Arterial fibrinoid necrosis	Type III	Type III

Data from Refs.[5,9,10]

DIFFERENTIAL DIAGNOSIS

 Differential Diagnosis
OF KIDNEY ALLOGRAFT
INFLAMMATION

Acute rejection (T-cell mediated, antibody mediated)

Polyomavirus infection (BK), or postviral inflammation

Other viral infections (eg, cytomegalovirus, adenovirus)

Bacterial, fungal, or other infections

Reflux/obstruction

Acute interstitial nephritis

Posttransplant lymphoproliferative disorder

Chronic damage (especially in areas of tubular atrophy and interstitial fibrosis)

Borderline changes, suspicious for acute rejection, include interstitial inflammation and tubulitis that do not fully meet diagnostic criteria for acute T-cell–mediated rejection (in the Banff schema, 10%–25% interstitial inflammation, or <5 lymphocytes per tubule, see later in this article and **Box 1**).[5–8] Occasionally, delay in scheduling biopsy may lead to empiric (partial) treatment for rejection, resulting in borderline findings on biopsy. On the other hand, a follow-up biopsy too soon after treatment for rejection may retain enough inflammation to meet criteria for acute cellular rejection even though treatment will prove to be sufficient.

Several other entities, some rare, manifest as interstitial inflammation with tubulitis, and may overlap with acute rejection; clinicopathologic correlation is invaluable in these settings. Polyomavirus nephropathy is a notorious mimic of T-cell–mediated rejection, requiring markedly different therapy, and is discussed in detail later in this article. Acute interstitial nephritis (AIN) is rarely described in the renal allograft, no doubt in part because the histopathologic findings are quite similar to those of acute rejection.[10] Numerous eosinophils, together with an infiltrate that is more concentrated in the medulla, may suggest acute interstitial nephritis (see **Fig. 3**); nevertheless, eosinophils also may be seen in acute rejection. Review of new medications, or medications associated with AIN, with the nephrology team may provide relevant information. Allograft inflammation also may be due to pyelonephritis caused by urinary reflux or obstruction. Pyelonephritis

372

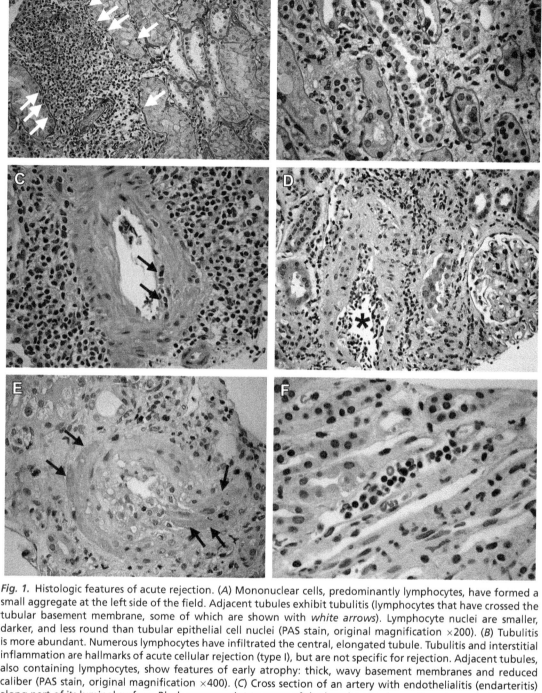

Fig. 1. Histologic features of acute rejection. (*A*) Mononuclear cells, predominantly lymphocytes, have formed a small aggregate at the left side of the field. Adjacent tubules exhibit tubulitis (lymphocytes that have crossed the tubular basement membrane, some of which are shown with *white arrows*). Lymphocyte nuclei are smaller, darker, and less round than tubular epithelial cell nuclei (PAS stain, original magnification ×200). (*B*) Tubulitis is more abundant. Numerous lymphocytes have infiltrated the central, elongated tubule. Tubulitis and interstitial inflammation are hallmarks of acute cellular rejection (type I), but are not specific for rejection. Adjacent tubules, also containing lymphocytes, show features of early atrophy: thick, wavy basement membranes and reduced caliber (PAS stain, original magnification ×400). (*C*) Cross section of an artery with endothelialitis (endarteritis) along part of its luminal surface. Black arrows point to some of the lymphocytes beneath and among the hyperplastic endothelium and myointimal cells. Even one lymphocyte under the endothelium is sufficient for a diagnosis of endothelialitis, and thus type II acute cellular rejection. The presence of perivascular inflammatory cells, as seen here, is not a criterion for rejection (H&E, original magnification ×400). (*D*) Severe endothelialitis in the artery marked by the asterisk, results in luminal narrowing (H&E, original magnification ×200). (*E*) Arteritis with fibrinoid necrosis is delineated (*black arrows*), accompanied by inflammatory cells and apoptotic bodies in the wall, and swollen intima. Fibrinoid necrosis is diagnostic of type III rejection, and may be seen in T-cell–mediated or AbMR. Fibrinoid necrosis is bright red and fibrillar on trichrome stain, although it is pale and often inconspicuous on PAS stain, not shown (H&E, original magnification ×400). (*F*) Peritubular capillaritis. The diagonal capillary in the center is filled with mononuclear inflammatory cells, one of the histologic features that may be seen in AbMR (H&E, original magnification ×400).

classically presents as exudative inflammation with neutrophilic casts, but focal changes may resemble acute cellular rejection. Correlation with clinical features indicative of urinary tract infection and/or obstruction are very helpful in making the distinction. Extensive dilation and disruption of tubules with accumulation of Tamm-Horsfall protein may suggest reflux nephropathy (see **Fig. 3**), although similar changes may be seen focally in acute cellular rejection.

DIAGNOSIS

The diagnosis and grading of acute T-cell–mediated rejection is based on the presence and degree of interstitial inflammation, tubulitis, and endothelialitis (see **Boxes 1** and **2, Table 2**).[5–11] Interstitial inflammation and tubulitis without endothelialitis indicate type I rejection ("tubulointerstitial") by the Banff schema; 25% parenchymal involvement by interstitial inflammation (plus sufficient tubulitis) is required for acute T-cell–mediated rejection type I, which is further subcategorized based on the extent of tubulitis (see **Box 1**, section 4).[5–8] Endothelialitis defines the more severe type II rejection ("vascular"); again this is subcategorized under the Banff schema based on degree of luminal narrowing (see **Box 1**).[5–8]

Transmural arteritis and/or arterial fibrinoid necrosis defines type III rejection in both classification systems (see **Fig. 1**).[5–11] This may be a manifestation of acute T-cell–mediated and/or acute antibody-mediated processes. Although it is rarely seen in the modern era, it requires prompt treatment and portends a poor outcome for the allograft. The finding of necrotic renal parenchyma on an allograft biopsy within a few days of transplantation is rare and is generally associated with graft loss. The differential diagnosis includes accelerated acute rejection (often antibody mediated and associated with low-titer or undetected preformed antibodies), or infarction due to thrombosis or surgical complication. These entities often cannot be distinguished on core biopsy, although antibody-mediated rejection (AbMR) may be associated with occlusion and thrombosis of numerous small vessel and other histologic clues, as described later in this article, whereas clinical vascular studies, second-look surgery, or examination of the eventual allograft nephrectomy specimen may elucidate infarction.

CLINICAL CORRELATION, TREATMENT, AND PROGNOSIS

Knowledge of clinical data, such as creatinine trends, medication compliance, or calcineurin inhibitor drug levels, recent antirejection treatment, serum or urine BK polyomavirus data, and so forth, is often very helpful, if not essential, for diagnosis in certain settings. For instance, in patients with recent noncompliance with medication, rejection is common, whereas BK polyomavirus nephropathy would be quite unlikely.

In general, treatment for acute T-cell–mediated rejection usually involves pulse steroid administration, although treatment protocols for acute rejection differ by center. Most patients experience a good response, with normalization of creatinine, and even resolution of inflammation on follow-up biopsy specimens. Refractory rejection may be treated with other agents, along with optimization of baseline immunosuppression.

ACUTE REJECTION: ANTIBODY-MEDIATED (HUMORAL REJECTION)

OVERVIEW

Although HLA-crossmatching has dramatically reduced the incidence of hyperacute rejection, some recipients develop antibodies to their kidney allograft over time after transplantation. Like T-cell–mediated rejection, antibody-mediated (humoral) rejection is common early after transplantation, but occurs at late time points as well, especially after periods of noncompliance with immunosuppression. In the past 15 years, diagnostic criteria for AbMR have been developed and refined in kidney transplantation,[6–8] and are now evolving for other solid organ allografts (heart, pancreas, lung, and so forth).[12] Nevertheless, many aspects of pathophysiology, diagnosis, and treatment of AbMR remain enigmatic.

The latest 2013 Banff criteria for diagnosis of AbMR include both pathologic and clinical laboratory elements (see **Box 1**): (1) evidence of recent/current antibody-to–vascular endothelium interaction, especially C4d deposition; (2) morphologic evidence of tissue injury; and (3) presence of donor-specific antibodies. The presence of 2 of 3 features is considered "suspicious" for AbMR.[12]

MICROSCOPIC DESCRIPTION

The most commonly recognized morphologic features of acute AbMR include peritubular capillaritis and glomerular capillaritis (glomerulitis). There is a rich network of peritubular capillaries between cortical tubules, yet they are usually inconspicuous in sections of normal kidney. The finding of dilated peritubular capillaries containing inflammatory cells should raise concern for acute AbMR. Recent updates to the Banff classification scheme suggest a threshold of 3 to 4 or more cells per cross section in more than 10% of peritubular capillaries, in non-atrophic cortex.[7,8,13] Capillaritis should not be scored in areas of atrophy, adjacent to infarcts, or in vessels surrounding lymphoid aggregates (these could be lymphatics); further, caution is needed in interpreting capillaritis in the medulla, as vasa recta infiltrates may be associated with acute tubular injury/necrosis (ATN).[7,13] Inflammatory cells congregating in glomerular capillaries (glomerulitis) also should be noted. The type of inflammatory cells may vary, including of neutrophils and mononuclear cells; capillaritis is often quite rich in monocytes.[14,15] An "ATN-like" histology with minimal inflammation also has been described in acute AbMR.[6–8] Fibrin thrombi in glomeruli, and arterial fibrinoid necrosis are sometimes sequelae of AbMR, with the latter indicating severe injury (see also acute T-cell–mediated rejection earlier in this article, and **Fig. 1E** and **Fig. 4F**). Recently, Lefaucheur and colleagues[16] characterized a group of patients with donor-specific antibodies, endothelialitis, and poor response to conventional treatment for T-cell–mediated rejection, which led them to propose the so-called "antibody-mediated vascular rejection."[16–18]

C4d STUDIES

For a number of years, immune markers of antibody-mediated damage in tissue were elusive; immunostaining for panels of immunoglobulins and complement generally proved unrevealing. However, in the 1990s, antibodies were developed specifically to the "d" peptide fragment of complement 4 (C4, C4d antibodies).[6,10] This C4d split product is unique in that it binds covalently to the cell (endothelial) surfaces at the site of antibody-mediated (also known as classical) complement pathway activation, where it accumulates, and can thus be detected in peritubular capillaries by immunostaining. Similarly, antibodies to C3d are used complementarily in some centers.

Techniques for C4d immunostaining include indirect immunofluorescence on frozen sections (IF), or indirect immunohistochemical staining on formalin-fixed paraffin-embedded tissue after antigen retrieval (IHC); a few centers use formalin-fixed, paraffin-embedded tissue with immunofluorescence detection. The different techniques have advantages and disadvantages, but are generally all reliable if appropriately validated and carefully controlled (**Fig. 2**). The IF method on frozen sections is generally considered most sensitive, but it requires separately submitted frozen tissue, and a fluorescence microscope.[19–22] Further, tissue context is less apparent with darkfield fluorescence,

such that deposits in peritubular capillaries may be difficult to distinguish from granular deposits along tubular basement membranes (see **Fig. 2**), especially in zones of atrophy, or cases with polyomavirus infection.[23] With the IF method, normal glomeruli show mild-to-moderate predominantly mesangial C4d staining, which may serve as a handy internal control (see **Fig. 2**). C4d glomerular staining in other specific patterns provides potential clues to immune complex–mediated glomerular disease that deserve further workup (see **Fig. 2**).

In evaluating C4d studies by either the IF or IHC method, circumferential staining of peritubular capillaries should be evaluated, including intensity and extent of staining. Historically, moderate to strong staining in more than 50% of peritubular capillaries was considered clinically significant using the IF method, but thresholds were recently lowered (10% or more for IF, 1% or more for IHC, **Table 3**).[7,12,22] Guidelines also recommend a minimum of 5 high-power microscopic fields of cortex and/or medulla without scarring or infarction[7]; as in other aspects of rejection, areas of atrophy are not assessed. C4d deposition in other endothelial compartments (eg, glomerular capillaries, arterial intimal) should be noted, but are of uncertain significance. The 2013 Banff criteria have incorporated the entity of C4d-negative AbMR (see **Box 1**).[12]

DIFFERENTIAL DIAGNOSIS

The histologic finding of peritubular capillaritis also may be seen as a response to acute tubular injury or necrosis, and can thus be difficult to dissect at short time points posttransplantation. In ATN, neither C4d nor DSA studies should be positive. Conversely, the "ATN-like" form of AbMR may present without capillaritis, with only subtle histologic findings of ATN, but with positive C4d and DSA studies.

The immunomicroscopic finding of C4d-positive peritubular capillaries is very commonly seen in patients who have received ABO blood group incompatible allografts; this was initially considered a form of "accommodation," as it was not associated with compromised allograft function.[7,24] However, long-term study will be needed to determine whether there is an impact on late graft survival.[7,24] The terminology "C4d deposition without morphologic evidence of active rejection" has been suggested for this situation; ATN, capillaritis, and peritubular or glomerular capillary multilayering (by EM analysis) preclude use of this category (see **Box 1**).[7,8]

DIAGNOSIS

Current criteria require the presence of all 3 of the following elements for a firm diagnosis of

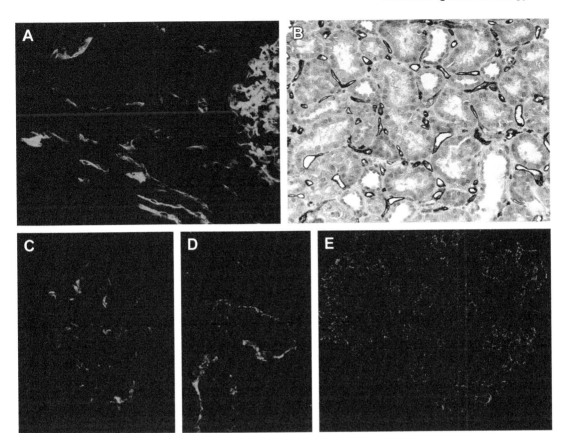

Fig. 2. C4d immunostaining. (*A*) Immunofluorescence staining for C4d is positive in peritubular capillaries, some with branching profiles. The intervening tubules have larger circumferences and are inapparent, as they are C4d negative. A portion of a glomerulus is at the far right, also with C4d staining of glomerular capillaries (C4d immunofluorescence on frozen tissue, original magnification ×400). (*B*) Immunohistochemical staining for C4d is positive (brown) in peritubular capillaries. The location of staining and tissue architecture is readily identified with the hematoxylin counterstain (C4d immunohistochemistry on formalin-fixed, paraffin-embedded tissue [FFPE], original magnification ×200). (*C*) Immunofluorescence staining for C4d shows weak-moderate mesangial staining of a normal glomerulus, a useful internal control. Glomerular staining in other patterns could indicate glomerular disease, as in *E*. This pattern of reactivity is not seen in FFPE C4d staining (C4d immunofluorescence on frozen tissue, original magnification ×400). (*D*) Immunofluorescence staining for C4d shows granular reactivity along tubular basement membranes, but peritubular capillaries are inapparent (negative). This pattern is not associated with rejection, and is sometimes seen in BK viral nephropathy.[23] Tubular basement membrane staining must be carefully distinguished from capillary staining (C4d immunofluorescence on frozen tissue, original magnification ×400). (*E*) C4d stains this glomerulus in a granular capillary loop pattern. The C4d reactivity was the first indication of early (recurrent) membranous lupus nephritis in this allograft (C4d immunofluorescence on frozen tissue, original magnification ×400).

Table 3
C4d scoring in peritubular capillaries

Score	% Biopsy Area Positive	Interpretation: Immunofluorescence	Interpretation: Immunohistochemistry
C4d0 negative	0	Negative	Negative
C4d1 minimal	1–9	Negative	Positive*
C4d2 focal	10–50	Positive*	Positive
C4d3 diffuse	>50	Positive	Positive

* Newly revised to positive.[12]
 Adapted from Solez K, Colvin RB, Racusen LC, et al. Banff 07 classification of renal allograft pathology: updates and future directions. Am J Transplant 2008;8:754.

AbMR: (1) evidence of antibody interaction with vascular endothelium, especially C4d deposition; (2) morphologic evidence of acute tissue injury (capillaritis, fibrin thrombi, ATN, and so forth); and (3) donor-specific antibodies.[6–8] If 2 of the 3 features are present, a diagnosis of "suspicious" for AbMR is indicated currently. Isolated reports have documented AbMR associated with deleterious non-HLA antibodies; however, such DSAs are not amenable to clinical testing in most centers, resulting in the unsatisfying profile: C4d-positive, capillaritis-positive, DSAs are not demonstrable.[25–27]

It is important to keep in mind that AbMR often coexists with T-cell–mediated rejection, in which case, both diagnoses are warranted.

CLINICAL CORRELATION, TREATMENT, AND PROGNOSIS

In practice, the finding of capillaritis or C4d staining in an allograft biopsy generally leads to a recommendation for serum DSA testing. In fact, even in patients with only weakly positive C4d staining, DSA studies may be valuable. Close communication with the transplant nephrology team and clinicopathologic correlation is necessary to appropriately manage patients with suspected AbMR. AbMR requires treatment different from acute T-cell–mediated rejection.[6,10] In AbMR, treatment is directed at B cells or plasma cells; steroids are usually ineffective. Protocols typically involve plasmapheresis, intravenous immunoglobulin, rituximab, and so on.[6,10] If AbMR is diagnosed early in its evolution, these therapies may be effective. Unfortunately, many instances of established AbMR are refractory to therapy.

POLYOMAVIRUS NEPHROPATHY

OVERVIEW

The pathogenic polyomavirus family includes simian virus 40 (SV40, BK, JC, and the recently described Merkel cell polyomavirus). Ninety percent of the adult population is seropositive for BK polyomavirus, and the virus generally remains latent in the urothelium.[28,29] The combination of reduced immune surveillance (or overimmunosuppression) and a foreign kidney makes the renal allograft especially susceptible to BK reactivation. Increasingly, patients undergo surveillance for BK in serum or urine by polymerase chain reaction, an alternative method is urine cytology to screen for infected urothelial cells ("decoy" cells).[28,29] The finding of increasing viral titers then leads to reduction in immunosuppression, with consideration for renal biopsy in refractory or unusual cases.

MICROSCOPIC DESCRIPTION

Polyomavirus nephropathy is characterized by interstitial inflammation, tubulitis, and tubular epithelial injury with viral cytopathic inclusions (**Fig. 3**). Polyomaviral inclusions are intranuclear with a glassy to granular texture, and basophilic to pale staining, sometimes surrounded by a clear halo (see **Fig. 3**).[10,28] Pale glassy casts may contain viral debris in severe cases. As infection may spread from the urothelium and medulla, inflammation and viral cytopathic changes may be more intense in the medulla, as compared with the cortex. Polyomavirus can be nicely demonstrated in tissue sections by immunohistochemistry, which has largely supplanted EM imaging of infected nuclei.

DIFFERENTIAL DIAGNOSIS

It is critically important to distinguish polyoma (or other) viral nephropathy from acute T-cell–mediated rejection, as treatment is essentially "opposite" in these scenarios. A high index of suspicion, along with a careful search for viral inclusions, and judicious application of immunostaining, is helpful in the inflamed renal biopsy specimen. The possibility of concomitant polyomavirus (or other viral) infection and rejection complicates matters further. A confident diagnosis of infection and rejection can be made when the biopsy shows evidence of virus, together with endothelialitis (type II T-cell–mediated rejection), or shows features of AbMR. However, the overlapping histology makes the diagnosis of type I (tubulointerstitial) rejection in the setting of viral infection difficult, if not impossible, to establish. Further complexities arise in patients with positive viral studies in whom immunosuppression was reduced before biopsy. Recent case series suggest that cellular-rejection–like inflammation lingers after polyomavirus has been cleared from the kidney and blood[30,31]; data from other centers are needed. Close collaboration with the clinical team and correlation with trends in viral load, serum creatinine, in addition to immunohistochemical studies, are necessary to plan treatment for these patients.

Immunostains for cytomegalovirus and adenovirus also may be used when suspicion for viral infection is high. Fungal, mycobacterial, and bacterial infections may involve the renal allograft, and can be further investigated by standard histochemical stains.

DIAGNOSIS

Tubulointerstitial inflammation, together with viral cytopathic nuclear change, and especially

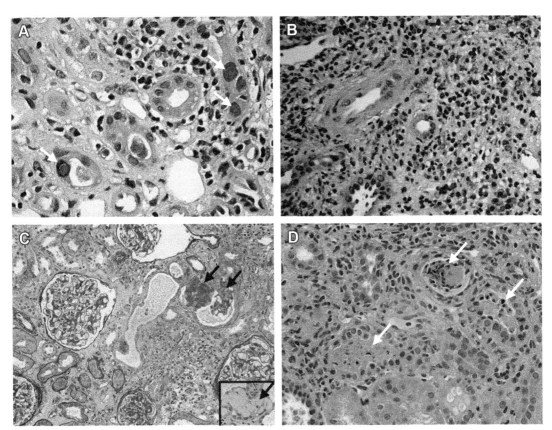

Fig. 3. Other inflammatory patterns in renal allograft biopsies. (*A*) BK viral nephropathy. Several tubular cells exhibit prominent viral cytopathic nuclear inclusions (*white arrows*). Viral inclusions may be subtle or inapparent, but immunohistochemical staining for polyomavirus can provide diagnostic confirmation (not shown). Inflammation accompanying BK viral nephropathy may mimic acute cellular rejection (H&E stain, original magnification ×400). (*B*) Acute interstitial nephritis. Infiltrates of rejection may include eosinophils, but the large numbers of eosinophils seen in this field also suggest the possibility of interstitial nephritis. Interstitial inflammation and tubulitis are common to both rejection and acute interstitial nephritis (H&E stain, original magnification ×200). (*C*) Tamm-Horsfall protein casts. Prominent PAS-positive Tamm-Horsfall protein casts are seen in ectatic tubules, center right (*black arrows*). These same casts are pale on H&E stain (*inset*). These changes may follow rejection-associated tubular injury, but may also be evidence of obstruction or reflux; clinical correlation is usually needed. An area of tubular atrophy is seen at bottom left, and interstitial inflammation on bottom right (PAS or H&E [*inset*] stain, original magnification ×200). (*D*) White blood cell casts and debris in several tubules (*white arrows*) often correlate with reflux or pyelonephritis. The background of tubulitis might otherwise mimic rejection (H&E stain, original magnification ×200).

immunohistochemical demonstration of virus in epithelial cell nuclei are needed to establish the diagnosis of polyoma viral nephropathy. Various classification systems for scoring combinations of acute infection and chronic allograft damage in polyomavirus nephropathy have been proposed.[28,32]

PROGNOSIS

In the current era of increased surveillance, many patients may clear polyomavirus infection with reduction of immunosuppression, even before coming to biopsy. Various antiviral pharmacologic agents (cidofovir, leflunomide, quinolones, intravenous immunoglobulin) have been used for established infections, with mixed results.[28] Once fibrosis is established in polyomavirus nephropathy, allograft prognosis is poor.[28,32]

DRUG TOXICITIES

OVERVIEW: CALCINEURIN INHIBITORS

A calcineurin inhibitor (cyclosporine, tacrolimus [FK506]) is a key component of immunosuppression for many patients who receive renal transplantation. Ironically, however, these agents themselves cause renal toxicity; thus, drug levels are carefully monitored. Assessment of renal allograft biopsy specimens should include attention to histopathologic findings associated with drug toxicity (**Fig. 4**). Unfortunately, none of these are specific, and their utility has been questioned.[33–36]

MICROSCOPIC DESCRIPTION: CALCINEURIN INHIBITORS

Classically (acute) calcineurin inhibitor toxicity is associated with so-called "isometric vacuolization" of tubular epithelial cytoplasm (see **Fig. 4**).[10] This is often quite focal, and stands out on trichrome stain, although it can be seen on any of the typical histochemical stains. Medial arteriolar hyalinosis is associated with (chronic) calcineurin inhibitor toxicity, attributed to injury of arteriolar myocytes. The first manifestation of this injury may be vacuolization of myocytes, which are later replaced by brightly PAS-positive (magenta) acellular hyaline material in nodules or in a beadlike pattern (see **Fig. 4**; **Fig. 5E–5F**).[10,35] Although beaded medial arteriolar hyalinosis was long considered to be relatively specific for drug toxicity, recent studies have associated this finding with many other mechanisms of vascular injury, including alloimmune (see later in this article).[33] So-called "striped" tubular atrophy and fibrosis denote a pattern of alternating atrophic and nonatrophic parenchyma, as might arise with focal

narrowing of small arteries/arterioles, and is classically associated with chronic calcineurin inhibitor toxicity.[10] Again, this pattern has poor specificity (see chronic allograft injury, later in this article), and it may be difficult to recognize in a core biopsy. Juxtaglomerular apparatus hypertrophy and calcification are also loosely associated with calcineurin inhibitor toxicity (see **Fig. 4**).[10,37]

Rarely, calcineurin inhibitors are associated with thrombotic microangiopathic (TMA) changes in glomeruli and/or vessels.[10] In TMA, glomeruli appear "bloodless," with swollen endothelial cells occluding capillary loops. Red blood cell fragments may be seen in glomeruli, or trapped under the endothelium of small arteries. Focal segmental glomerulosclerosis (FSGS) is another rare association of calcineurin inhibitor toxicity.

DIFFERENTIAL DIAGNOSIS: CALCINEURIN INHIBITORS

Features of calcineurin inhibitor toxicity, along with the differential diagnosis of the various histologic findings, are enumerated in the Key Features Box. Tubular epithelial cell vacuolization may result from other causes of tubular injury, including intravenous contrast agents, or osmotic agents, although those tend to be associated with more diffuse tubular epithelial changes as compared with the focal isometric vacuolization of acute calcineurin inhibitor toxicity. Importantly, arteriolar hyaline is frequently seen in diabetes and

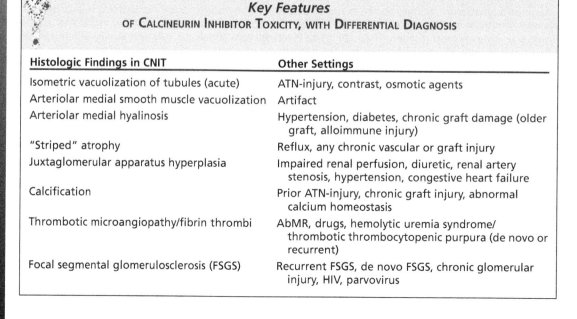

Key Features
OF CALCINEURIN INHIBITOR TOXICITY, WITH DIFFERENTIAL DIAGNOSIS

Histologic Findings in CNIT	Other Settings
Isometric vacuolization of tubules (acute)	ATN-injury, contrast, osmotic agents
Arteriolar medial smooth muscle vacuolization	Artifact
Arteriolar medial hyalinosis	Hypertension, diabetes, chronic graft damage (older graft, alloimmune injury)
"Striped" atrophy	Reflux, any chronic vascular or graft injury
Juxtaglomerular apparatus hyperplasia	Impaired renal perfusion, diuretic, renal artery stenosis, hypertension, congestive heart failure
Calcification	Prior ATN-injury, chronic graft injury, abnormal calcium homeostasis
Thrombotic microangiopathy/fibrin thrombi	AbMR, drugs, hemolytic uremia syndrome/ thrombotic thrombocytopenic purpura (de novo or recurrent)
Focal segmental glomerulosclerosis (FSGS)	Recurrent FSGS, de novo FSGS, chronic glomerular injury, HIV, parvovirus

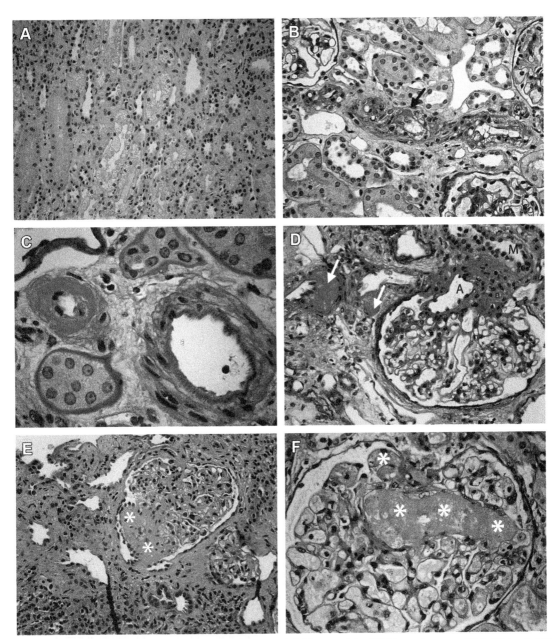

Fig. 4. Histologic findings that may indicate calcineurin-inhibitor toxicity (CNIT, most nonspecific). (*A*) Isometric vacuolization of tubular epithelial cells. Tubules in the center show cytoplasmic vacuolization. Isometric vacuolization associated with CNIT is typically focal. Vacuolization may be seen after other causes of acute tubular injury (H&E stain, original magnification ×200). (*B*) Arteriolar myocyte vacuolization and focal hyaline deposition. (*hyaline-black arrow*, PAS stain, original magnification ×400). (*C*) Arteriolar hyalinosis. The media of the small arteriole at left is replaced by PAS-positive hyaline. In contrast, the small artery at right has normal, intact myocytes (PAS stain, original magnification ×400). (*D*) Juxtaglomerular apparatus (JGA) hyperplasia and arteriolar hyalinosis. The distal tubule, including the macula densa, is labeled "M." The nearby arteriolar lumen is designated "A." The renin secreting juxtaglomerular granular cells of this hyperplastic JGA are located between the macula densa and arteriole. White arrows indicate large aggregates of arteriolar hyaline (PAS, original magnification ×200). (*E*) Focal segmental glomerulosclerosis (FSGS). There is a large segment of sclerosis (scarring), indicated by the 2 asterisks (H&E stain, original magnification ×200). (*F*) Glomerular fibrin thrombi. A large, PAS-pale fibrin thrombus is seen centrally within the glomerulus (*white asterisks*). Fibrin thrombi are brightly eosinophilic on H&E, and red on trichrome, with coarse fibrillary texture. Several neutrophils are seen in nearby capillary loops. In the allograft setting, fibrin thrombi are associated with a differential diagnosis of donor disseminated intravascular coagulation (DIC) or head trauma at short posttransplant time points, AbMR, calcineurin inhibitor toxicity, recurrent hemolytic uremia syndrome. However, the latter 2 entities often present with "bloodless" glomeruli and fragmentation of red blood cells (PAS stain, original magnification ×400).

380

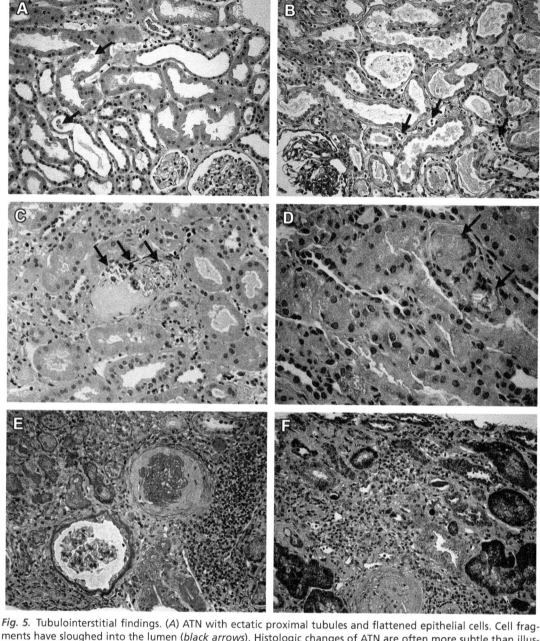

Fig. 5. Tubulointerstitial findings. (*A*) ATN with ectatic proximal tubules and flattened epithelial cells. Cell fragments have sloughed into the lumen (*black arrows*). Histologic changes of ATN are often more subtle than illustrated here (H&E, original magnification ×200). (*B*) Another example of ATN with ectatic tubules, flattened reactive epithelial cells with loss of brush border, and abundant granular debris in tubular lumens. Dilated peritubular capillaries contain nucleated cells (*black arrows*). The peritubular capillary cells associated with acute tubular injury may include nucleated red blood cells and immature myeloid cells, particularly in the medulla and deep cortex. In this case, the peritubular inflammation was thought to be a reaction to the tubular injury, rather than evidence of AbMR (PAS stain, original magnification ×200). (*C*) Tubulointerstitial calcification. The coarse light and dark purple amorphous material is consistent with calcium phosphate (*black arrows*). Calcifications are common in allograft biopsies, typically as remnants of prior tubular injury, with many nonspecific causes. They are unlikely to be of clinical significance unless present in large amounts (H&E, original magnification ×400). (*D*) Calcium oxalate crystals are translucent (*black arrows*), birefringent in polarized light (not shown), and inapparent on PAS, trichrome, and silver stains. Examination between polarizing filters may reveal many more of these crystals than is evident with conventional microscopy (H&E, original magnification ×400). (*E*) Tubular atrophy and interstitial fibrosis. Tubules in the left side of the field are atrophic, with thick wavy basement membranes. To the right, there is a dense lymphocytic infiltrate. There is abundant hyaline in the small arterioles heading toward the central globally sclerotic glomerulus (PAS, original magnification ×200). (*F*) Tubular atrophy and interstitial fibrosis. A trichrome stain highlights the interstitial fibrosis. There is a chronic inflammatory infiltrate, and a globally sclerotic glomerulus at bottom center (trichrome, original magnification ×200).

hypertension, although the hyaline deposits are more likely to be intimal in those settings.[34,36,38,39] Recent studies have found arteriolar hyaline in a high percentage of 5-year and 10-year surveillance biopsies; although involvement was seen in a greater percentage of calcineurin inhibitor–treated patients, it was also prevalent in groups without calcineurin inhibitor exposure.[34,36,38,39]

Besides the association with calcineurin inhibitors, TMA-like changes occur in AbMR, and very rarely in situations including recurrent hemolytic uremia syndrome, thrombotic thrombocytopenic purpura, malignant hypertension, scleroderma, radiation damage, viral infection, as in native kidneys.[10]

DIAGNOSIS: CALCINEURIN INHIBITORS

Histopathologic features associated with drug toxicity, such as isometric vacuolization, myocyte vacuolization, medial hyalinosis, striped fibrosis, and TMA, should be descriptively reported. Even with careful clinical correlation, it is difficult to determine whether histopathologic changes can be definitively attributed to calcineurin inhibitor toxicity.

SIROLIMUS

Sirolimus (rapamycin) is a newer immunosuppressive agent that affects the same molecular pathway as calcineurin inhibitors, with greater antiproliferative properties. In brief, histologic manifestation of sirolimus toxicity includes rare reports of FSGS and tubular vacuolization.[40,41] The combination of tacrolimus and sirolimus has been associated with delayed graft function and cast nephropathy.[42]

PROGNOSIS: DRUG TOXICITIES

Acute drug toxicity, such as tubular vacuolization or cast nephropathy in the case of sirolimus, is often reversible. However, interstitial fibrosis, tubular atrophy, and other chronic drug-related changes are often seen in progressive graft dysfunction.

ACUTE TUBULAR NECROSIS AND RELATED INJURY

OVERVIEW: ATN

In the process of transplantation, the donor organ experiences ischemia-reperfusion injury. This is generally mild in living donor transplantation procedures, but can be prolonged and severe in deceased donor organs, particularly those from extended criteria donors. This sort of preservation injury affects tubules most dramatically, and clinically manifests as delayed graft function, or poor graft function with higher than expected posttransplantation creatinine. Thus, an early biopsy is performed to distinguish preservation injury from early rejection (T-cell mediated, antibody mediated, or both). Other causes of ATN, such as hypotension/hypoperfusion, toxin exposure, and heavy proteinuria, are rarely seen in allograft kidneys, as in native kidneys.

MICROSCOPIC DESCRIPTION: ATN

When severe, ATN is dramatic, with epithelial cells sloughing, accumulation of luminal necrotic debris, flattening of tubular epithelial cells, and presence of tubular mitotic figures (see **Fig. 5**). In some cases, however, acute tubular injury can be quite subtle, with tubular dilation (ectasia), loss of proximal tubular brush border (normally a pale magenta layer apically on PAS), and granular casts. Although ATN is usually pauci-inflammatory and readily distinguished from rejection, there may be mild interstitial inflammation, or even peritubular capillaritis in the cortex, in response to tubular injury.[7,43]

DIFFERENTIAL DIAGNOSIS: ATN

Of note, renal biopsies that are not fixed promptly may show evidence of tubular injury. At early time points posttransplant, acute rejection, especially AbMR, may overlap with ATN in 2 different settings. First, ATN may be accompanied by mild interstitial inflammation and/or mild to prominent peritubular capillaritis. Conversely, AbMR may rarely present as the pauci-inflammatory "ATN-like" category. Both of these scenarios reinforce the need for correlation of histopathology, C4d results, clinical setting, and laboratory studies (DSA testing).

DIAGNOSIS: ATN

Attention to proximal tubular morphology is needed to establish a diagnosis of ATN, including features of tubular ectasia, loss of brush border, flattening of epithelial cells, mitotic figures, and so on. Clinical correlation can provide helpful clues in terms of risk of ATN, such as length of cold ischemic time and type of donor kidney.

TUBULOINTERSTITIAL CALCIFICATION

Coarse purple tubulointerstitial calcifications are often found in kidney allografts, particularly following recovery from delayed graft function or ATN (see **Fig. 5**), sometimes accompanied by areas of interstitial fibrosis and/or tubular atrophy. Translucent, birefringent oxalate crystals may form in tubules shortly after transplantation, especially in the setting of ATN. Typically, this is an incidental finding, but oxalate nephropathy has been recognized as an important, potentially reversible cause of kidney allograft injury (see **Fig. 5**). Thus, if oxalate crystals are numerous and accompanied by acute tubular injury, particularly more than 3 months posttransplantation, the risk factors for and implications of possible oxalate nephropathy should be discussed with the clinical team.[44–46]

PROGNOSIS: TUBULAR INJURY

Acute tubular injury is typically reversible, with good recovery of graft function. However, if prolonged, ATN may result in interstitial fibrosis and consequent reduced transplant functional lifespan.

CHRONIC REJECTION AND CHRONIC ALLOGRAFT INJURY

OVERVIEW

Chronic kidney transplant injury results in progressive irreversible renal dysfunction, including proteinuria, and the structural changes inevitably include global glomerulosclerosis, interstitial fibrosis, and tubular atrophy. Causes of chronic allograft injury include prior/repeated acute rejection episodes, chronic rejection, drug toxicity, arteriosclerosis-ischemia, postinfection, reflux, and hypertension.

MICROSCOPIC DESCRIPTION

Atrophic tubules have reduced tubular diameters and epithelial cell size, and thick wavy basement membranes (see **Fig. 5**). Tubular atrophy is often accompanied by interstitial fibrosis, with separation of tubules by collagen and other basement membrane matrix, which can be nicely demonstrated on trichrome stain (see **Fig. 5**). Histopathologic features that are thought to be somewhat specific for chronic alloimmune-mediated injury (chronic rejection) include allograft glomerulopathy and allograft vasculopathy.

Allograft glomerulopathy likely stems from antibody or T-cell–mediated glomerular endothelial injury, resulting in new basement membrane formation, variously described as glomerular basement membrane "double-contours," "tram-tracks," or "duplication" (**Fig. 6**).[10] Glomeruli may also appear mildly hypercellular and have increased mesangial matrix. C4d may outline glomerular capillaries of allograft glomerulopathy, but it should be otherwise essentially negative for immune complex deposition, in contrast to recurrent or de novo membranoproliferative glomerulonephritis (MPGN). Electron microscopy shows subendothelial new basement membrane formation often in fine layers (see **Fig. 6**) in allograft glomerulopathy. Peritubular capillary multilayering, as demonstrated by EM, is also a hallmark of antibody mediated and/or chronic rejection.[8,47,48]

Another feature of chronic T-cell rejection or AbMR is allograft vasculopathy (transplant arteriopathy), characterized by concentric layers of intimal fibrosis, pale matrix, and myofibroblastic cells, sometimes with admixed foam cells in larger arteries (see **Fig. 6**).[10] Lymphocytes also may be seen within the deeper neointimal layers of allograft vasculopathy; however, concomitant endothelialitis in this setting prompts a diagnosis of chronic active vascular rejection (Banff type 2).

DIFFERENTIAL DIAGNOSIS

The classic histologic changes of chronic allograft injury are remarkably similar regardless of etiology, and it may not be possible to determine the underlying cause once such changes are established. As described previously, inflammatory infiltrates in zones of atrophy and fibrosis are currently considered nonspecific, and should not factor in to assessment of acute T-cell–mediated rejection.

Allograft glomerulopathy should be distinguished from glomerular ischemia; on H&E stain, ischemic glomeruli appear small with expanded mesangial zones and thick capillary loops. However, PAS or Jones stains highlight the classic features of chronically underperfused glomeruli: periglomerular fibrosis, wrinkled glomerular basement membranes without double contours.

The differential diagnosis of allograft glomerulopathy also includes immune-complex–mediated MPGN, or the rare chronic thrombotic microangiopathy. As described previously, immunofluorescence studies for the standard panel of immunoglobulins and complement deposition will help address MPGN. Because the C4d and EM findings of allograft glomerulopathy are quite similar to those of chronic thrombotic microangiopathy, clinical and historical correlation may be needed.

Chronic vascular changes include arteriosclerosis, as well as allograft vasculopathy. Vasculopathy tends to be more cellular, with pale or myxoid matrix, and concentric, more symmetric intimal layers. Arteriosclerosis is less cellular, more eccentric, and has an elastotic component (see **Fig. 6, Table 4**). If implantation or early posttransplant biopsies show paucicellular elastotic changes, then the arteriosclerosis can be attributed to the donor organ. Alternatively, arteriosclerosis may evolve during the life of the graft due to

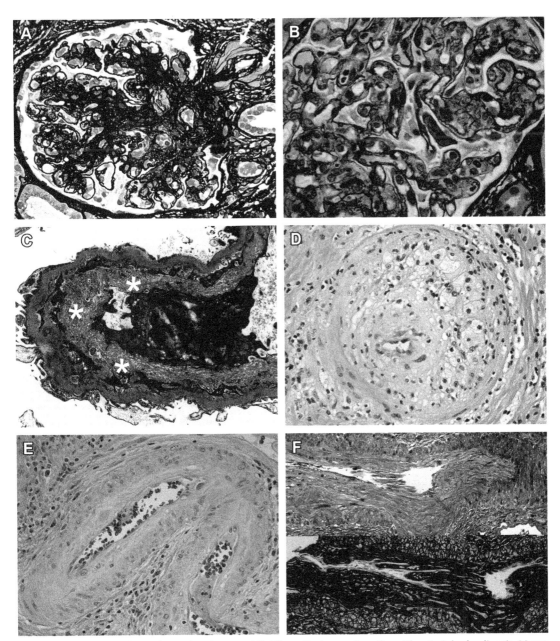

Fig. 6. Chronic glomerular and vascular changes. (*A*) Allograft glomerulopathy with arteriolar hyalinosis. Mesan-gial zones are expanded by argyrophilic sclerosis, and mildly increased cellularity. Many capillary loops have double contours ("tram tracks"). Full-panel immunofluorescence studies would help to rule out an immune com-plex–mediated glomerulonephritis. Arteriolar hyaline is denoted by *white arrows* (Jones silver stain, original magnification ×400). (*B*) Allograft glomerulopathy. Glomerular basement membranes show complicated double contours, a few with cellular interposition between layers. There is increased mesangial cellularity and glomer-ulitis. This recipient had AbMR due to major-histocompatibility-complex class I–related Chain A (MICA) anti-bodies[26] (Jones silver stain, original magnification ×630). (*C*) Allograft glomerulopathy, EM. This capillary wall is thickened by laminated new subendothelial layers of basal lamina (*asterisks*), separated from the original base-ment membrane by thin ("interposed") layers of cell cytoplasm. The nonfenestrated, enlarged endothelial cell nearly fills the capillary lumen (EM, original magnification ×10,500). (*D*) Allograft vasculopathy (allograft arterio-pathy). This artery is severely narrowed by foam cells (*right*). There is fibromyxoid substance and loose cellularity in the intima, with admixed lymphocytes deep in the wall, but no endothelialitis (H&E stain, original magnifica-tion ×200). (*E*) Allograft vasculopathy. The small artery is tortuous with concentric myofibroblastic intimal prolif-eration with myxoid quality (H&E stain, original magnification ×200). (*F*) Arteriosclerosis. In this artery, the fibrous intimal changes are much less cellular, and more collagenized as compared with those in *D* and *E*. Typi-cally, the intimal fibrosis of arteriosclerosis is eccentric within the vessel, and contains elastic fibers, best demon-strated on Van Gieson stain (VVG, EVG), but may also be seen on typical renal silver stains, as illustrated here by prominent black layers on Jones stain (trichrome [*top*], Jones silver [*bottom*]; original magnifications ×200).

Table 4
Histologic characteristics of allograft vasculopathy and arteriosclerosis

Feature	Arteriosclerosis	Allograft Vasculopathy
Cellularity	None/minimal	More cellular
Matrix	Dense	May be myxoid
Trichrome stain	Dense blue	Admixed cells or paler blue
Elastosis	Present	Absent/less
Pattern	Eccentric	Concentric

nonimmune-related insults, as in native kidneys. In many situations, the etiology of the chronic vascular changes is impossible to determine with certainty.

DIAGNOSIS

The histologic features of chronic allograft injury are generally straightforward to recognize: glomerulosclerosis, interstitial fibrosis, and tubular atrophy (see **Fig. 5**). Determining the etiology of chronic structural changes is more challenging, if not impossible. The number of total and sclerotic glomeruli (percent global sclerosis), along with the estimated percent interstitial fibrosis and tubular atrophy are elements that should be included in the renal allograft pathology report.[4]

PROGNOSIS

Fibrotic and atrophic changes in the renal allograft tubulointerstitium, vessels, and glomeruli are irreversible. Interstitial fibrosis and tubular atrophy correlate with poor graft survival in multiple large studies.

POSTTRANSPLANT LYMPHOPROLIFERATIVE DISORDER

Posttransplant lymphoproliferative disorder (PTLD) refers to a spectrum of lymphoproliferative lesions that occur in patients who have received transplantation, consequent to reduced immune surveillance. The incidence of PTLD varies with transplant type, and is relatively low after kidney transplantation (about 1%).[49] PTLD is commonly associated with Epstein-Barr virus (EBV), and may occur in the allograft organ, or elsewhere in the body.[49–51] In its least aggressive forms, PTLD manifests early as plasmacytic hyperplasia or as an infectious-mononucleosis like proliferation that may respond to reduced immunosuppression. At the other end of the spectrum,

monomorphic PTLD is a lymphoma requiring aggressive chemotherapy (**Box 3**).[50,51] Transplant biopsies with an unusually dense, plasma cell–rich, or cytologically atypical lymphoid proliferation deserve consideration of PTLD. Special studies for EBV, to assess clonality, and to identify lymphoma, along with hematopathology consultation, are essential in arriving at the correct diagnosis in this setting.

OTHER ALLOGRAFT BIOPSY FINDINGS

Pathologic changes relatively unique to the renal allograft have been discussed and illustrated in this section. However, it is important to keep in mind that any sort of renal disorder may affect the transplanted kidney; for example, tumors, hypertensive nephropathy, diabetes, pyelonephritis, reflux, and acute interstitial nephritis. Recurrent and de novo glomerulonephritis must be distinguished from allograft glomerulopathy. Some forms of glomerulonephritis commonly recur over time, but often have low impact on allograft survival (membranous glomerulonephritis, immunoglobulin [Ig]A nephropathy).[52,53] Other glomerulonephritides frequently recur, and portend poor graft outcome (dense deposit disease, C3 glomerulopathy, so-called "primary" FSGS in children).[52,53] The reader is referred to the accompanying articles for further details on these entities. De novo glomerulonephritis also occurs in the allograft, most commonly IgA nephropathy, membranous nephropathy, and FSGS.[52] FSGS is not infrequently seen during progressive chronic allograft damage, as nephron loss subjects the

Box 3
Classification of posttransplant lymphoproliferative disorder (PTLD)

Early PTLD

  Plasmacytic hyperplasia

  Infectious mononucleosislike

Polymorphic PTLD

Monomorphic PTLD

  Subclassify further as per lymphoma

Classical Hodgkin lymphoma–like PTLD

Data from Tsao L, Hsi ED. The clinicopathologic spectrum of posttransplantation lymphoproliferative disorders. Arch Pathol Lab Med 2007;131:1209–18 and Swerdlow SH, Webber SA, Chadburn A, et al. Posttransplant lymphoproliferative disorders. In: Swerdlow SH, Campo E, Harris NL, et al, editors. WHO classification of tumours of haematopoietic and lymphoid tissues. Lyon (France): IARC Press; 2008. p. 345–50.

remaining glomeruli to hyperfiltration injury and subsequent sclerosis (so-called "adaptive" etiology).[54] Recurrent or de novo crescentic glomerulonephritis is extremely rare, but very important to recognize.

SUMMARY

Renal allograft biopsy provides critical information in the management of patients with renal transplantation. However, pathologic interpretation must be performed in the context of the patient history, clinical as well as other laboratory studies, and in close collaboration with the clinical team. The histologic correlates of acute T-cell–mediated rejection are interstitial inflammation, tubulitis, and endothelialitis, and mimics of acute rejection have been discussed. In the past 2 decades, the diagnostic features of AbMR have been characterized and are under refinement. Drug toxicity, recurrent disease, chronic injury, and other entities affecting both native and transplanted kidneys must also be evaluated.

ACKNOWLEDGMENTS

The authors acknowledge Drs Ellen Flatley and Maylee Hsu for critical reading and helpful suggestions. Dr Douglas Norman contributed to the HLA vocabulary table.

REFERENCES

1. Delos Santos R, Langewisch E, Norman DJ. Immunological assessment of the transplant patient. In: Matthew Weir, Edgar Lerma, editors. Kidney transplantation: a practical guide to medical management. Newyork: Springer Science+Business Media, LLC; 2014. p. 23–34.
2. Walker PD, Cavallo T, Bonsib SM, et al. Practice guidelines for the renal biopsy. Mod Pathol 2004; 17:1555–63.
3. Walker PD. The renal biopsy. Arch Pathol Lab Med 2009;133:181–8.
4. Chang A, Gibson IW, Cohen AH, et al. A position paper on standardizing the nonneoplastic kidney biopsy report. Clin J Am Soc Nephrol 2012;7: 1365–8.
5. Racusen LC, Solez K, Colvin RB, et al. The Banff 97 working classification of renal allograft pathology. Kidney Int 1999;55:713–22.
6. Racusen LC, Colvin RB, Solez K, et al. Antibody-mediated rejection criteria—an addition to the Banff '97 classification of renal allograft rejection. Am J Transplant 2003;3:708–14.
7. Solez K, Colvin RB, Racusen LC, et al. Banff 07 classification of renal allograft pathology: updates and future directions. Am J Transplant 2008;8: 753–60.
8. Sis B, Mengel M, Haas M, et al. Banff '09 meeting report: antibody mediated graft deterioration and implementation of Banff working groups. Am J Transplant 2010;10:464–71.
9. Colvin RB, Cohen AH, Saiontz C, et al. Evaluation of pathologic criteria for acute renal allograft rejection: reproducibility, sensitivity and clinical correlation. J Am Soc Nephrol 1997;8:1930–41.
10. Colvin RB. Renal transplant pathology. In: Jennette JC, Olson JL, Schwartz MM, et al, editors. Heptinstall's pathology of the kidney. 5th edition. Philadelphia: Lippencott-Raven; 1998. p. 1409–540.
11. Nickeleit V. The pathology of kidney transplantation. In: Ruiz P, editor. Transplantation pathology. Cambridge (United Kingdom): Cambridge University Press; 2009. p. 45–110.
12. Haas M, Sis B, Racusen LC, et al. Banff 2013 meeting report: inclusion of C4d-negative antibody-mediated rejection and antibody-associated arterial lesions. Am J Transplant 2014;14:272–83.
13. Gibson IW, Gwinner W, Bröcker V, et al. Peritubular capillaritis in renal allografts: prevalence, scoring system, reproducibility and clinicopathological correlates. Am J Transplant 2008;8:819–25.
14. Magil AB, Tinckam K. Monocytes and peritubular capillary C4d deposition in acute renal allograft rejection. Kidney Int 2003;63:1888–93.
15. Tinckam KJ, Djurdjev O, Magil AB. Glomerular monocytes predict worse outcomes after acute renal allograft rejection independent of C4d status. Kidney Int 2005;68:1866–74.
16. Lefaucheur C, Loupy A, Vernerey D, et al. Antibody-mediated vascular rejection of kidney allografts: a population-based study. Lancet 2013; 381:313–9.
17. Nankivell BJ. Antibody-mediated vascular rejection: relation to causation. Lancet 2013;381: 275–7.
18. Loupy A, Lefaucheur C, Glotz D, et al. Diagnostic criteria for kidney transplant rejection: a call to action—Authors' reply. Lancet 2013;381:1458–9.
19. Nadasdy GM, Bott C, Cowden D, et al. Comparative study for the detection of peritubular capillary C4d deposition in human renal allografts using different methodologies. Hum Pathol 2005;36: 1178–85.
20. Troxell ML, Weintraub LA, Higgins JP, et al. Comparison of C4d immunostaining methods in renal allograft biopsies. Clin J Am Soc Nephrol 2006;1: 583–91.
21. Seemayer CA, Gaspert A, Nickeleit V, et al. C4d staining of renal allograft biopsies: a comparative analysis of different staining techniques. Nephrol Dial Transplant 2007;22:568–76.

22. Batal I, Girnita A, Zeevi A, et al. Clinical significance of the distribution of C4d deposits in different anatomic compartments of the allograft kidney. Mod Pathol 2008;2:1490–8.

23. Bracamonte E, Leca N, Smith KD, et al. Tubular basement membrane immune deposits in association with BK polyomavirus nephropathy. Am J Transplant 2007;7:1552–60.

24. Haas M. The significance of C4d staining with minimal histologic abnormalities. Curr Opin Organ Transplant 2010;15:21–7.

25. Dragun D, Müller DN, Bräsen JH. Angiotensin II type 1-receptor activating antibodies in renal-allograft rejection. N Engl J Med 2005;352:558–69.

26. Zou Y, Stastny P, Süsal C, et al. Antibodies against MICA antigens and kidney-transplant rejection. N Engl J Med 2007;357:1293–300.

27. Sigdel TK, Li L, Tran TQ. Non-HLA antibodies to immunogenic epitopes predict the evolution of chronic renal allograft injury. J Am Soc Nephrol 2012;23:750–63.

28. Ramos E, Drachenberg CB, Wali R, et al. The decade of polyomavirus BK-associated nephropathy: state of affairs. Transplantation 2009;87:621–30.

29. Hirsch HH, Randhawa P. BK polyomavirus in solid organ transplantation. Am J Transplant 2013; 13(Suppl 4):179–88.

30. Menter T, Mayr M, Schaub S, et al. Pathology of resolving polyomavirus-associated nephropathy. Am J Transplant 2013;13:1474–83.

31. Randhawa P. Incorporation of pathology and laboratory findings into management algorithms for polyomavirus nephropathy. Am J Transplant 2013;13: 1379–81.

32. Masutani K, Shapiro R, Basu A, et al. The Banff 2009 working proposal for polyomavirus nephropathy: a critical evaluation of its utility as a determinant of clinical outcome. Am J Transplant 2012; 12:907–19.

33. Issa N, Kukla A, Ibrahim HN. Calcineurin inhibitor nephrotoxicity: a review and perspective of the evidence. Am J Nephrol 2013;37:602–12.

34. Mengel M, Mihatsch M, Halloran PF. Histological characteristics of calcineurin inhibitor toxicity—there is no such thing as specificity! Am J Transplant 2011;11:2549–50.

35. Horike K, Takeda A, Yamaguchi Y, et al. Is arteriolar vacuolization a predictor of calcineurin inhibitor nephrotoxicity? Clin Transplant 2011;25(Suppl 23): 23–7.

36. Snanoudj R, Royal V, Elie C, et al. Specificity of histological markers of long-term CNI nephrotoxicity in kidney-transplant recipients under low-dose cyclosporine therapy. Am J Transplant 2011;11:2635–46.

37. Young BA, Burdmann EA, Johnson RJ, et al. Cellular proliferation and macrophage influx precede interstitial fibrosis in cyclosporine nephrotoxicity. Kidney Int 1995;48:439–48.

38. Nankivell BJ, Borrows RJ, Fung C, et al. The natural history of chronic allograft nephropathy. N Engl J Med 2003;349:2326–33.

39. Stegall MD, Park WD, Larson TS, et al. The histology of solitary renal allografts at 1 and 5 years after transplantation. Am J Transplant 2011;11: 698–707.

40. Laftavi MR, Weber-Shrikant E, Kohli R, et al. Sirolimus-induced isometric tubular vacuolization: a new sirolimus histopathologic manifestation. Transplant Proc 2010;42:2547–50.

41. Letavernier E, Bruneval P, Mandet C, et al. High sirolimus levels may induce focal segmental glomerulosclerosis de novo. Clin J Am Soc Nephrol 2007; 2:326–33.

42. Smith KD, Wrenshall LE, Nicosia RF, et al. Delayed graft function and cast nephropathy associated with tacrolimus plus rapamycin use. J Am Soc Nephrol 2003;14:1037–45.

43. Racusen L, Kashgarian M. Ischemic and toxic acute tubular injury and other ischemic renal injury. In: Jennette JC, Olson JL, Schwartz MM, et al, editors. Heptinstall's pathology of the kidney. 5th edition. Philadelphia: Lippencott-Raven; 1998. p. 1140–98.

44. Truong LD, Yakupoglu U, Feig D, et al. Calcium oxalate deposition in renal allografts: morphologic spectrum and clinical implications. Am J Transplant 2004;4:1338–44.

45. Bagnasco SM, Mohammed BS, Mani H, et al. Oxalate deposits in biopsies from native and transplanted kidneys, and impact on graft function. Nephrol Dial Transplant 2009;24:1319–25.

46. Troxell ML, Houghton DC, Hawkey M, et al. Enteric oxalate nephropathy in the renal allograft: an underrecognized complication of bariatric surgery. Am J Transplant 2013;13:501–9.

47. Ivanyi B, Kemeny E, Rago P, et al. Peritubular capillary basement membrane changes in chronic renal allograft rejection: comparison of light microscopic and ultrastructural observations. Virchows Arch 2011;459:321–30.

48. Roufosse CA, Shore I, Moss J, et al. Peritubular capillary basement membrane multilayering on electron microscopy: a useful marker of early chronic antibody-mediated damage. Transplantation 2012;94:269–74.

49. Opelz G, Döhler B. Lymphomas after solid organ transplantation: a collaborative transplant study report. Am J Transplant 2004;4:222–30.

50. Tsao L, Hsi ED. The clinicopathologic spectrum of posttransplantation lymphoproliferative disorders. Arch Pathol Lab Med 2007;131:1209–18.

51. Swerdlow SH, Webber SA, Chadburn A, et al. Post-transplant lymphoproliferative disorders. In: Swerdlow SH, Campo E, Harris NL, et al, editors.

WHO classification of tumours of haematopoietic and lymphoid tissues. Lyon (France): IARC Press; 2008. p. 345–50.

52. Ivanyi B. A primer on recurrent and de novo glomerulonephritis in renal allografts. Nat Clin Pract Nephrol 2008;4:446–57.

53. Choy BY, Chan TM, Lai KN. Recurrent glomerulonephritis after kidney transplantation. Am J Transplant 2006;6:2535–42.

54. D'Agati VD, Kaskel FJ, Falk RJ. Focal segmental glomerulosclerosis. N Engl J Med 2011;365: 2398–411.

Renal Infections

Jean Hou, MD[a], Leal C. Herlitz, MD[b],*

KEYWORDS

- Acute pyelonephritis • Chronic pyelonephritis • Xanthogranulomatous pyelonephritis
- Malacoplakia • Viral interstitial nephritis • Polyomavirus nephropathy • Fungal pyelonephritis

ABSTRACT

This review discusses the various gross and histologic findings seen in renal infections due to bacteria, viruses, fungi, and mycobacteria. It is crucially important to separate infectious processes in the kidney from other inflammatory or neoplastic processes, as this will have a major impact on therapy. We describe the diagnostic features of renal infections with a specific focus on the differential diagnosis and other processes that may mimic infection. The topics discussed include acute bacterial pyelonephritis, chronic bacterial pyelonephritis, xanthogranulomatous pyelonephritis, malacoplakia, viral infections in the kidney, fungal pyelonephritis and mycobacterial infection of the kidney.

OVERVIEW

Renal infections can be seen in a wide variety of settings, and identifying the cause of infection so that proper treatment can be pursued is critical. Also important is the recognition that inflammation in the kidney is not necessarily indicative of infection, and other processes, such as glomerulonephritis, transplant rejection, and vasculitis, can mimic infection. It is necessary for the pathologist to carefully examine renal specimens for histologic features of infection, and correlate with other pertinent clinical and laboratory data to arrive at an accurate diagnosis. This review addresses the main types and patterns of renal infections, their histologic appearances, the pitfalls of diagnosis and how to resolve them.

ACUTE BACTERIAL PYELONEPHRITIS

Direct infection of the renal parenchyma by bacterial organisms is the defining feature of acute bacterial pyelonephritis. In practice, acute bacterial pyelonephritis is most commonly encountered by the pathologist in specimens removed in the setting of urinary tract obstruction, which results in ascending infection from the lower urinary tract into the renal parenchyma. The most common organism in ascending forms of pyelonephritis is *Escherichia coli* but other common bacteria that cause lower urinary tract infections are also seen.[1] Less common than the obstructive form of pyelonephritis is direct infection of the renal parenchyma through the hematogenous spread of bacteria. The most common organisms in these cases tend to be staphylococci and streptococci. Some pathologists consider this to be such a sufficiently distinct entity from the ascending form of pyelonephritis described previously that they use diagnostic terms, such as "diffuse suppurative nephritis" or "multiple cortical abscesses" to describe these hematogenously spread cases.[2] Regardless of the route of infection, the key feature of acute bacterial pyelonephritis is the direct infection of the renal parenchyma by bacteria.

GROSS FEATURES

In acute bacterial pyelonephritis related to obstruction, the kidney is generally enlarged and displays whitish abscesses of varying size. Collecting ducts filled with pus may be visible as

Funding Sources and Conflict of Interest: None.
[a] Department of Pathology and Cell Biology, Columbia University Medical Center, New York Presbyterian Hospital, VC14-224, New York, NY 10032, USA; [b] Division of Renal Pathology, Department of Pathology and Cell Biology, Columbia University Medical Center, New York Presbyterian Hospital, VC14-224, New York, NY 10032, USA
* Corresponding author.
E-mail address: LB684@columbia.edu

surgpath.theclinics.com

thin yellow streaks running through the medulla. In a minority of cases, severe infection can result in papillary necrosis. The renal pelvis and calices may be dilated as a result of the obstruction, and in severe cases the renal pelvis may be filled with pus (termed pyonephrosis). In cases of hematogenous spread, both kidneys are typically involved. They are enlarged with numerous whitish abscesses visible on the subcapsular surface. On sectioning, the parenchymal surface will be diffusely involved by microabscesses of varying size. Calyceal dilatation is generally not seen in hematogenous spread, as urinary obstruction is not typical of these cases.

MICROSCOPIC FEATURES

Regardless of the route of infection, acute bacterial pyelonephritis is characterized by prominent neutrophilic inflammation of the renal tubules, which causes destruction of tubular basement membranes, resulting in inflammation spilling into the renal interstitium (**Fig. 1**A). Within days, the inflammatory infiltrate will become mixed, containing significant numbers of lymphocytes, plasma cells, histiocytes, and occasional eosinophils. Parenchymal involvement is often patchy, with areas of intense inflammation juxtaposed with relatively normal-appearing areas. Glomeruli and vessels are typically relatively preserved and may appear to "float" in a sea of neutrophils. In cases of ascending infection, sections of the renal pelvis will show severe inflammation of the mucosa. In hematogenously spread infection, the renal pelvis may be relatively uninvolved and numerous microabscesses can be seen diffusely throughout the renal parenchyma, particularly in the cortex (see **Fig. 1**B).

DIFFERENTIAL DIAGNOSIS

The differential diagnosis of acute tubulointerstitial inflammation includes noninfectious processes that can have a similar appearance to acute pyelonephritis. In severe cases of glomerulonephritis, there is often a significant element of associated tubulointerstitial inflammation by a mixed inflammatory infiltrate. In acute bacterial pyelonephritis, occasional glomeruli may be overtaken by the surrounding inflammatory infiltrate, but in the setting of more diffuse glomerular involvement, a thorough evaluation to exclude a primary glomerulonephritis should be undertaken. Likewise, various vasculitic processes, including antineutrophilic cytoplasmic antibody–mediated forms of disease, can be associated with prominent tubulointerstitial inflammation. Any evidence of artery

wall inflammation in the setting of tubulointerstitial inflammation should raise the possibility of vasculitis. Of note, fungal organisms can occasionally cause a necrotizing vasculitis when directly invading a vessel wall (addressed further in the section on fungal pyelonephritis), but arteritis is highly unusual in bacterial infection. Also in the differential diagnosis of acute tubulointerstitial nephritis is a drug-induced hypersensitivity reaction. Hypersensitivity reactions are classically eosinophil-rich but also can have prominent numbers of neutrophils. The presence of prominently dilated tubules filled with neutrophils (see **Fig. 1**A) or microabscesses (see **Fig. 1**B) strongly favors the diagnosis of pyelonephritis over noninfectious forms of disease. Clinical correlation with urine cultures, medication history, and appropriate serologic workup is often important in differentiating these entities.

Pitfalls
IN THE DIAGNOSIS OF ACUTE BACTERIAL PYELONEPHRITIS

! Not all neutrophil-rich inflammation in the kidney is infectious in origin.

! Severe acute glomerulonephritis can be accompanied by prominent tubulointerstitial inflammation containing neutrophils.

! Acute vasculitis can be associated with acute tubulointerstitial inflammation. Any evidence of arteritis favors the diagnosis of vasculitis over bacterial pyelonephritis.

! Fungal infections may have neutrophil-rich inflammation and may be overlooked unless appropriate stains are performed.

! Drug-induced or other hypersensitivity reactions can have significant numbers of neutrophils in the tubulointerstitial infiltrate, although eosinophils classically predominate in these cases.

CHRONIC PYELONEPHRITIS

Chronic pyelonephritis was liberally diagnosed in the past when significant lymphocytic inflammation of the renal interstitium was noted. It was presumed that this inflammation reflected prior bacterial infection that had caused destruction of the parenchyma. It is important to realize that scarring in the kidney from noninfectious conditions is also often accompanied by prominent, nonspecific chronic inflammation, and the presence of

Fig. 1. Acute bacterial pyelonephritis. (*A*) A dilated renal tubule filled with neutrophils that have caused rupture of the tubular basement membrane and can be seen spilling into the surrounding interstitium (original magnification ×400). (*B*) A cortical microabscess from a patient who developed acute pyelonephritis in the setting of staphylococcal bacteremia (HE, original magnification ×100).

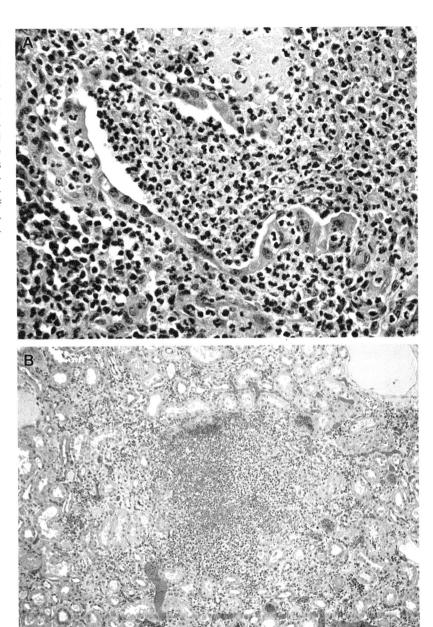

chronic inflammation in areas of tubulointerstitial scarring is not adequate to fully support the diagnosis of chronic pyelonephritis.[3] A clinical history of frequent or chronic urinary infections, a history of vesicoureteral reflux, or a history of past or present urinary obstruction is very helpful in making a more definitive diagnosis.

GROSS FEATURES

Gross examination of the kidney removed for chronic pyelonephritis can be crucial to definitively establishing the diagnosis. Often, broad "U-shaped" scars are seen on the capsular surface, and cut sections will reveal prominent cortical and medullary thinning in these scarred areas. Examination of the renal pelvis in the bivalved specimen should show dilated, blunted, or otherwise deformed calices. The ureteropelvic junction and attached portions of ureter should be grossly examined for evidence of narrowing or masses that could cause obstruction.

MICROSCOPIC FEATURES

The microscopic findings of chronic pyelonephritis are quite nonspecific and include mononuclear inflammation involving the tubulointerstitial compartment of both the cortex and medulla (**Fig. 2**A). Glomeruli are often surrounded by inflammation and may exhibit scarring as a result, but they should be less affected than the tubulointerstitial compartment. Severe tubular atrophy can result in "thyroidization," which is characterized by prominent hyaline casts in tubules with markedly thinned tubular epithelium (see **Fig. 2**B). Tubular thyroidization is not specific for chronic pyelonephritis and can be seen in the setting of severe tubular atrophy due to any number of causes. Sampling of the renal pelvis should reveal prominent lymphocytic inflammation of the submucosa, often with germinal center formation (see **Fig. 2**C).

XANTHOGRANULOMATOUS PYELONEPHRITIS

Xanthogranulomatous pyelonephritis (XGP) is a rare subtype of chronic tubulointerstitial nephritis characterized by suppurative granulomatous inflammation and progressive destruction of the renal parenchyma.[4] Although the disease primarily occurs in middle age[5] and with a female predominance, pediatric cases also have been reported.[6,7] The precise etiology of XGP is unknown; however, case series have demonstrated an association with positive urine cultures, most frequently E coli, Proteus mirabilis, and Klebsiella spp.[5,8] XGP is often associated with chronic urinary tract obstruction resulting from obstructive renal calculi (frequently staghorn type), as well as ureteropelvic junction obstruction, vesicoureteral reflux, and external compression from adjacent renal masses.[5,8,9] XGP is often misdiagnosed preoperatively because clinical and imaging features are often nonspecific and can mimic other pathologic conditions, such as pyelonephritis, interstitial nephritis, or renal cell carcinoma (RCC). Frequently, ultrasound imaging reveals a unilaterally enlarged kidney with renal calculi, multiple fluid-filled, hypoechoic intraparenchymal

collections, hydronephrosis, and dilated calices.[10] Computerized tomography (CT) can reveal perinephric fat accumulation and stranding, corresponding to inflammation and extrarenal disease.[11]

GROSS FEATURES OF XGP

XGP is almost always unilateral. On gross examination, the kidney is typically enlarged, with or without evidence of obstruction and resultant hydronephrosis. The kidney may display capsular and perirenal tissue thickening as a result of intrarenal and extrarenal inflammation. Although multiple renal calculi may be present, a single staghorn calculus completely filling the renal pelvis is often observed. Three forms of renal involvement have been described: focal, segmental, and diffuse.[12] In focal disease, the granulomatous inflammatory process may be localized to a discrete mass or form small discrete nodules. In diffuse disease, the collecting system is dilated, with medullary papillary necrosis and pus accumulation. The normal renal parenchyma surrounding the calices is eventually replaced by soft tissue with a yellow-orange color imparted by collections of xanthomatous histiocytes. Multiple fluid-filled cysts and abscesses of varying sizes are often present. In severe cases, the inflammatory process extends through the renal capsule and into adjacent soft tissue and structures. Three stages of XGP have been proposed, according to the extent of involvement of adjacent tissue: in stage I, nephric stage, the inflammatory process is confined to the renal parenchyma; in stage II, nephric and perinephric stage, the disease process extends beyond the parenchyma into Gerota fascia; and in stage III, nephric and perinephric stage, there is further extension into adjacent structures and/or the retroperitoneal tissues.[13]

MICROSCOPIC FEATURES OF XGP

Microscopic examination reveals a mixed inflammatory infiltrate composed of variable numbers of lymphocytes, neutrophils, plasma cells, and histiocytes. Cholesterol clefts are often seen within the fibrotic interstitium. The key pathologic feature in XGP is the appearance of "xanthomatous histiocytes," which are characterized by abundant foamy and lipid-laden cytoplasm (**Fig. 3**A). Periodic acid-Schiff (PAS) staining shows granular positivity of the histiocyte cytoplasm. Lesional areas will often display areas of central necrosis, surrounded by a granulomatous response with collections of palisading foamy histiocytes. In

Fig. 2. Chronic pyelonephritis. (*A*) A portion of kidney removed from an 8-month-old child with ureteropelvic junction obstruction causing chronic pyelonephritis. Diffuse lymphocytic inflammation of the cortex is seen. The fetal glomeruli appear to "float" in the sea of chronic inflammation (original magnification ×100). (*B*) Severe "thyroidization" of tubules in a case of chronic pyelonephritis. Although thyroidization is classically seen in chronic pyelonephritis, it is a nonspecific lesion that can be seen in any case of severe tubular atrophy (original magnification ×100). (*C*) Severe chronic inflammation of the mucosa of the renal pelvis in a case of chronic pyelonephritis. The urothelium is inflamed by lymphocytes, mucosal capillaries are dilated, and lymphoid follicle formation is present (HE, original magnification ×200).

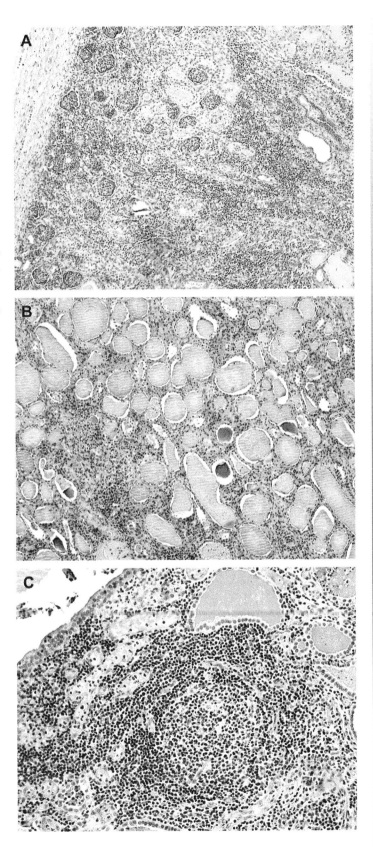

cases associated with chronic bacterial infection and/or staghorn calculi, the urothelium of the renal pelvis can display squamous metaplasia. Acute inflammation and microabscesses are often present. Immunohistochemical staining reveals diffuse cytoplasmic positivity for macrophage marker CD68 (see **Fig. 3B**) and negative staining for epithelial markers, which is important in distinguishing XGP from RCC. Staining of the xanthomatous histiocytes will show positive cytoplasmic staining for α-1 antitrypsin and lysozyme.[14]

DIFFERENTIAL DIAGNOSIS OF XGP

The differential diagnosis for XGP includes other causes of granulomatous inflammation in the kidney. XGP manifesting as a localized mass is often preoperatively misdiagnosed as RCC because of nonspecific imaging features. Recent case reports continue to describe this diagnostic challenge.[15,16] Grossly, the presence of renal obstruction with staghorn calculi and dilated calices with adjacent yellow-orange parenchymal replacement are suggestive of an inflammatory rather than a malignant lesion. Immunohistochemical staining is helpful in distinguishing between focal XGP and RCC. In XGP, the xanthomatous histiocytes display diffuse cytoplasmic expression of the macrophage marker CD68. RCC, clear-cell type, is characterized by plump cells with abundant clear to eosinophilic cytoplasm containing intracellular glycogen that also stains positively by PAS, mimicking the appearance of the xanthomatous histiocytes in XGP. However, the malignant cells in RCC arise from the proximal convoluted tubules and express epithelial cell markers, such as CD10, which are not expressed in cells of XGP.

A common diagnostic challenge is distinguishing XGP from renal malacoplakia (MCP), another rare granulomatous inflammatory disorder. Generally, XGP is unilateral, whereas MCP tends to display bilateral renal involvement. Unilateral involvement of perirenal and extrarenal soft tissue and adjacent structures by the inflammatory process is also more suggestive of XGP, which, in later stages, can be complicated by retroperitoneal spread and fistula formation. Grossly, XGP and MCP share overlapping features, with renal parenchymal replacement by yellow-orange soft tissue composed of granulomatous collections of foamy histiocytes. Microscopically, however, MCP is characterized by the presence of intracytoplasmic inclusions called Michaelis-Gutmann (MG) bodies, which are described in the next section.

MALACOPLAKIA

MCP is another rare cause of granulomatous inflammation that is typically seen in the lower urinary tract, but also can be seen in the genital tract, gastrointestinal system, lungs, and skin. The kidney is the primary site of involvement in 15% of patients with MCP.[17] Although the exact etiology of MCP is unknown, it is commonly associated with underlying immunosuppression or immunodeficiency. This is primarily seen following organ transplantation,[18] but also occurs in the setting of autoimmune disease, hematologic malignancy,[19] and HIV infection.[20] MCP is thought to result from the impaired phagocytic activity of macrophages, leading to incomplete bacterial elimination.[21] This results in the accumulation of partially digested bacterial fragments and antigens within the phagolysosomes of macrophages, which eventually form the characteristic intracytoplasmic MG bodies observable by light microscopy.[22] MCP is also associated with chronic gram-negative bacterial infections, most commonly *E coli*.[23] Renal MCP tends to occur in middle-aged women with chronic urinary tract infections and obstruction, whereas childhood MCP is exceedingly rare.

GROSS FEATURES OF MCP

MCP tends to manifest as bilateral disease. Gross examination reveals enlarged kidneys, often with dilated calices and other changes of obstructive uropathy. The capsule may be thickened and adherent to the underlying cortex, and renal

---

Causes of Granulomatous Kidney Disease

1. Drug hypersensitivity reaction
2. Infection
   a. Bacterial and mycobacterial
   b. Fungal infections
   c. Viral
3. Sarcoidosis
4. Granulomatosis with polyangiitis[a]
5. Tubulointerstitial nephritis with uveitis (TINU)
6. Idiopathic

[a] Formerly known as Wegener granulomatosis.

Fig. 3. Xanthogranuloma-tous pyelonephritis. (*A*) Light microscopy reveals granulomatous intersti-tial inflammation with collections of foamy xan-thomatous histiocytes (he-matoxylin-eosin [H&E], original magnification ×400). (*B*) Immunohisto-chemical staining with the macrophage marker CD68 shows diffuse cyto-plasmic staining of the xanthomatous cells, differ-entiating XGP from other lesions such as renal cell carcinoma (original magnification ×400).

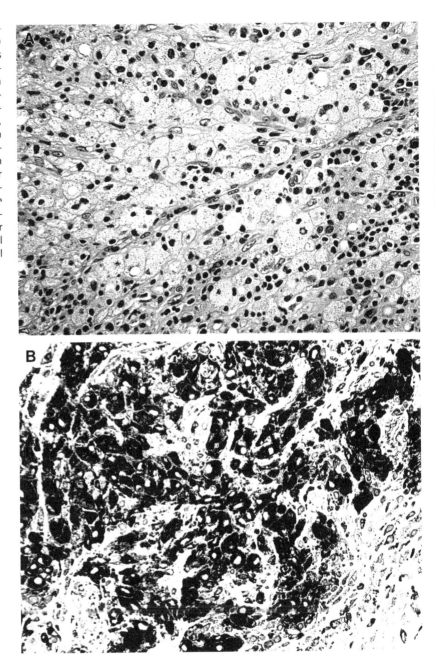

calculi are often identified. When observed in ex-trarenal sites, such as the bladder, lesions of MCP appear as a soft, yellow papules, plaques, or ulcerations in the urothelial lining.[21] Similarly, in renal MCP, the lining of the renal calices may be replaced by soft, yellowish tissue resulting from histiocytic infiltration. Within the cortex, the gross findings of MCP overlap considerably with those of XGP. Progressive granulomatous inflammation results in parenchymal damage, and the normal renal cortex is replaced by soft, yellow-orange tissue with areas of necrosis and hemorrhage. Although the disease process can be localized to a single discrete lesion, renal involvement in MCP is typically diffuse and bilat-eral, with multiple, occasionally confluent nodules that are often mistaken for tumor (pseudotumoral lesions).[24] In more severe disease, there is

	Key Features	

DIFFERENTIATING XANTHOGRANULOMATOUS PYELONEPHRITIS FROM MALACOPLAKIA

Features	Xanthogranulomatous Pyelonephritis	Malacoplakia
Laterality	Usually unilateral	Usually bilateral
Histiocytic cells	Xanthomatous	von Hansemann cells
Michaelis-Gutmann bodies	Not present	Numerous
Pathogenesis	Unknown	Defective macrophage phagocytosis

extensive replacement of the renal parenchyma by multiple, large abscesses with resultant cortical effacement and atrophy.

MICROSCOPIC FEATURES OF MCP

Microscopic evaluation reveals a mixed inflammatory infiltrate composed of lymphocytes, plasma cells, neutrophils, and histiocytes. Occasional multinucleated giant cells also can be seen. Similar to XGP, the histologic pattern of MCP is that of granulomatous inflammation characterized by dense collections of histiocytic cells with abundant granular cytoplasm that may be pale or eosinophilic. These cells also are known as von Hansemann cells.[25] The cytoplasm of these cells displays abundant phagolysosomes that stain positively by PAS (**Fig. 4**A). The characteristic feature of the von Hansemann cells are intracytoplasmic inclusions known as MG bodies (see **Fig. 4**B).[26] These bodies, which measure between 2 and 10 μM in diameter, appear basophilic, with concentric lamination and calcification, and therefore stain positively with calcium stains, such as von Kossa (see **Fig. 4**C). Due to ineffective phagocytosis, it is thought that incompletely degraded bacterial debris accumulates within the phagolysosomes and undergoes progressive calcification, resulting in the characteristic targetoid appearance of MG bodies. The tubulointerstitial compartment displays a variable degree of tubular atrophy and interstitial fibrosis.

DIFFERENTIAL DIAGNOSIS OF MCP

As with XGP, the differential diagnosis for MCP also includes other causes of granulomatous inflammation in the kidney. In terms of other infectious etiologies, mycobacterial and fungal involvement can be excluded with stains for these organisms. Key features that distinguish MCP from XGP include the laterality of involvement:

XGP is typically unilateral, whereas MCP tends to involve both kidneys. The extent of involvement of adjacent tissues also may be helpful in distinction. Extrarenal spread into adjacent structures, which can result in fistula formation, is a recognized complication of advanced XGP (stage III). MCP may involve other organ systems (such as the lungs or gastrointestinal tract); however, this is not the result of direct spread to adjacent structures. Histologically, both XGP and MCP are characterized by granulomatous inflammation with collections of foamy histiocytes and macrophages. However, defective phagocytic activity of macrophages in MCP result in the formation of MG bodies, which are not observed in XGP, and are therefore considered by some to be pathognomonic for this disease.[27]

VIRAL INFECTIONS IN THE KIDNEY

POLYOMAVIRUS NEPHROPATHY

JC virus (JCV) and BK virus (BKV) are members of the family Polyomaviridae, genus Orthopolyomavirus. Both are nonenveloped, double-stranded DNA viruses. The viruses were named according to the initials of the patients from whom they were first isolated: JC from the brain of a patient with progressive multifocal leukoencephalopathy (PML),[28] and BK from the urine of a patient who received a renal transplant.[29] Both viruses are widely prevalent in the general population. Seroconversion occurs in childhood or adolescence and may be associated with mild illness, although no acute disease has been associated with seroconversion. Shedding of JCV and BKV in the urine occurs in both healthy and immunocompromised hosts. However the incidence is higher for JCV, approximately 70%,[30] as opposed to BKV, which is approximately 5% to 10%.[31] Although infection in the healthy host is typically asymptomatic, viral reactivation can occur in the setting of

Fig. 4. Malacoplakia. (*A*) Light micro-scopy reveals granulomatous inflam-mation by histiocytes with cytoplasm (von Hansemann cells) containing numerous PAS-positive phagolyso-somes (PAS stain, original magnifica-tion ×200). (*B*) Higher magnification reveals the presence of targetoid, PAS-positive cytoplasmic inclusions (*arrows*), Michaelis-Gutmann bodies (PAS stain, original magnification ×400). (*C*) The calcified Michaelis-Gutmann bodies are highlighted with the von Kossa stain (original magnification ×600).

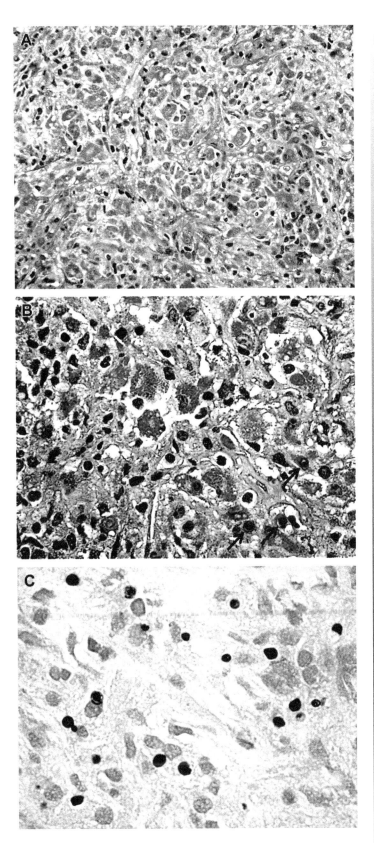

immunosuppression and cause opportunistic infections. The best-characterized associations are those of JCV reactivation occurring during HIV infection, resulting in the demyelinating disease PML, and BKV reactivation occurring during posttransplant immune suppression, resulting in BKV-associated nephropathy (BKVN) or polyomavirus-associated nephropathy (PVN). Although BKV infection in the kidney is well recognized, the impact of JCV reactivation on the renal allograft is not as well characterized.

When PVN complicates renal transplantation, it is typically an early event and occurs within the first year, often between 10 and 12 months.[32] Viral replication begins early after transplantation, followed by viruria, viremia, and PVN. In one prospective study, cytologic examination of the urine demonstrated the presence of "decoy cells," or infected tubular epithelial cells with viral inclusions, in approximately one-third of patients who receive renal transplantation and all of those patients diagnosed with PVN. Although these findings were 100% sensitive, they provided a relatively low positive predictive value for the diagnosis of PVN[33] because virus could be originating anywhere along the urinary tract. Polymerase chain reaction (PCR) analysis of the peripheral blood for viral DNA and quantification of viral load has emerged as a more useful marker for monitoring viral replication in patients who receive transplantation. Viral DNA has been reported in between 10% and 30% of renal transplant recipients in the first posttransplant year.[34,35] In one prospective study, viremia was detected in all patients with PVN, quantification of which demonstrated higher levels in patients with active PVN that decreased with resolution of nephropathy.[36] Although increased viral load, particularly in the setting of graft dysfunction, should heighten the index of suspicion for PVN, the gold standard remains a histologic diagnosis at renal biopsy.

GROSS FEATURES

Gross examination of kidneys in early polyomavirus-associated nephropathy is not well documented, and descriptions are limited to a few observations made after transplant nephrectomy. Failed grafts often exhibit nonspecific features that overlap with those seen in other nonviral causes of graft failure. Allografts may appear shrunken and fibrotic, with cortical scarring. On sectioning, the cortex can appear atrophic, with blurring of the cortico-medullary junction.[37]

MICROSCOPIC FEATURES

The key histologic findings in PVN are nuclear enlargement of tubular epithelial cells with prominent nucleoli and the identification of circumscribed basophilic intranuclear inclusions that often take on a "smudgy" or "ground-glass" appearance (**Fig. 5A**). Although these findings can be seen in the cortex and medulla, they tend to be more prominent in the tubules and collecting ducts of the deep cortex and medulla, with relative sparing of the superficial cortex. Tubular epithelial cells may show other signs of acute injury, including swelling, lysis with intraluminal cellular debris, and sloughing from the underlying basement membrane. The widely used immunohistochemical marker for polyomavirus infection, Simian Virus 40 (SV40) large T antigen (see **Fig. 5B**), cross-reacts not only with JCV and BKV, but also with SV40. The large T antigen is an early gene transcribed during viral infection that plays a role in viral genome replication[38] and oncogenic transformation.[39] Although virus-specific antibodies for immunohistochemical staining have been developed, to date, none are commercially available. Definitive viral identification in fixed tissue can be achieved by in situ DNA hybridization using specific DNA probes.[40,41]

Interstitial inflammation may be absent in the early stages of infection, but when present, is typically a mixed inflammatory infiltrate composed of lymphocytes, neutrophils, plasma cells, and eosinophils. Lymphocytes may focally cluster together to form aggregates. Although the proportions of each inflammatory cell type vary from case to case, there have been reports that plasma-cell-rich infiltrates are suggestive of polyomavirus infection.[42] The inflammatory infiltrate may cross basement membranes to produce foci of tubulitis. It has been observed that more severe tubulitis occurs in tubules lacking viral cytopathic changes.[43]

In chronic infection, viral inclusions, positive immunostaining for viral antigens, and viral cytopathic effects may no longer be visible. The background may show variable degrees of interstitial fibrosis and signs of tubular atrophy, including thickening of the basement membrane and simplification of the tubular epithelial cells. Three stages of PVN have been suggested. All stages can display visible intranuclear inclusion bodies and/or positive immunohistochemical or in situ hybridization signals. Stage A describes the early morphologic changes indicative of viral reactivation in the cortex and/or medulla: visible intranuclear inclusion bodies with minimal

Fig. 5. Polyoma virus nephropathy. (*A*) Light microscopy reveals tubular epithelial cells with characteristic circumscribed, "ground-glass" polyoma viral inclusions (HE, original magnification ×400). (*B*) Immunohistochemical staining for SV40 large T antigen (a marker for polyomavirus infection) highlights intranuclear inclusions (original magnification ×400).

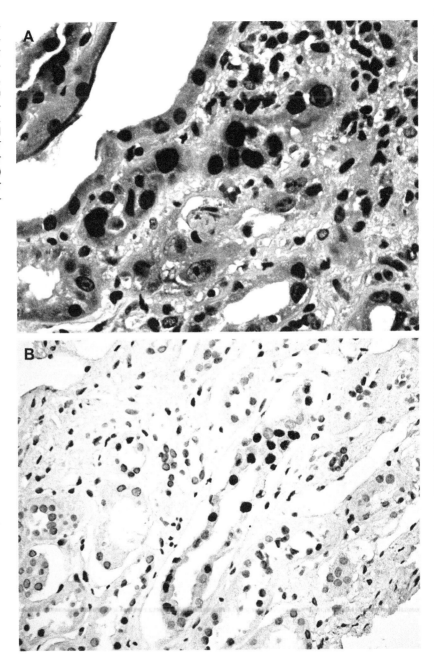

tubular injury and minimal or no interstitial inflammation, tubular atrophy, or interstitial fibrosis. Stage B describes florid changes of marked viral activation: marked tubular degenerative changes with variable degrees of interstitial inflammation, tubular atrophy, and interstitial fibrosis. Stage C describes the advanced sclerosing changes of viral activation: at least mild to moderate tubular atrophy and interstitial fibrosis and varying degrees of both tubular degenerative changes and interstitial inflammation.[44]

DIFFERENTIAL DIAGNOSIS

In terms of viral infection, the differential diagnosis for PVN includes nephropathy resulting from either

JCV or BKV, but also viruses such as cytomegalovirus (CMV) and adenovirus. Although JCV infection in renal transplant recipients has been reported,[45] the association with viruria and viremia has been met with some controversy.[46,47] A recent review suggests that JCV PVN may be a unique entity that should be differentiated from BKV PVN.[48] Immunohistochemical staining with specific viral markers can differentiate other viruses from the human polyomaviruses.

One common pitfall in the diagnosis of PVN arises from the overlapping histologic changes seen in acute cellular rejection, which is also characterized by interstitial inflammation and foci of tubulitis. The presence of abundant interstitial plasma cells is more suggestive of a diagnosis of PVN. In contrast, diffuse peritubular capillary C4d staining, vasculitis, glomerulitis, or interstitial hemorrhage would support a diagnosis of rejection.[43] Immunohistochemical staining for SV40, or another marker of PVN is key to differentiating infection from rejection. Notably, because BKV infects the tubular epithelial cells, cytopathic changes and interstitial inflammation can be very focal or localized to the renal medulla. Evaluation of a single core results in a missed diagnosis of PVN in up to one-third of cases,[49] underscoring the need for adequate sampling that includes renal medulla.

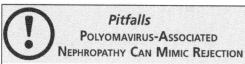

Pitfalls

POLYOMAVIRUS-ASSOCIATED NEPHROPATHY CAN MIMIC REJECTION

! PVN and rejection can occur in the same allograft biopsy.

! The presence of plasma-cell–rich interstitial inflammatory infiltrate is suggestive of infection.

! Tubular injury and tubulitis can be seen in both polyomavirus-associated nephropathy and rejection.

! Positive immunohistochemical staining for SV40 large T antigen demonstrates active polyomavirus infection.

! Adequate sampling for diagnosing PVN should include a portion of renal medulla.

ADENOVIRUS INFECTION OF THE KIDNEY

Members of the family Adenoviridae (AdV) are nonenveloped double-stranded DNA viruses. The family name is derived from the fact that the virus

was isolated from adenoid tissue.[50] Transmission primarily occurs via respiratory inhalation of aerosolized droplets, although fecal-oral transmission also is possible. AdV infection is most common in children, those living in close quarters, and in immunocompromised individuals. Viral infection typically causes respiratory illness, although different serotypes can manifest as a variety of illnesses, including pharynconjunctival fever, gastroenteritis, hepatitis, cystitis, and cutaneous rash. AdV is also a recognized cause of opportunistic infection in bone marrow and solid organ transplant recipients. In these cases, infection can occur de novo, or via reactivation of latent infection. Organs may be specifically targeted by viral infection, or be affected by disseminated infection.

MICROSCOPIC FEATURES

The spectrum of pathologic features in AdV nephritis varies widely. The characteristic findings are glassy, amphophilic to hyperchromatic intranuclear inclusions within tubular epithelial cells (**Fig. 6**). Immunohistochemical staining can demonstrate the presence of viral epitopes within these inclusions. Tubular epithelial cells can display signs of acute injury, including swelling, lysis, and detachment from underlying basement membranes. A varying degree of interstitial inflammation may be observed, with a mixture of lymphocytes, neutrophils, eosinophils, plasma cells, and macrophages. Lymphocytic tubulitis is also frequently seen, with disruption of tubular basement membranes. In many cases, AdV infection manifests as a pattern of severe necrotizing granulomatous inflammation, centered on infected tubules.[51,52] Interstitial hemorrhage may be identified. Rare reports of AdV nephritis presenting as a renal mass[53,54] demonstrate that this entity can also be misdiagnosed as a malignant lesion.

DIFFERENTIAL DIAGNOSIS

In terms of viral etiologies, the differential diagnosis for AdV nephritis includes other disease resulting from viruses, including CMV and polyomavirus. Immunohistochemical staining with specific antibodies can distinguish between the different viral pathogens. The pattern of inflammation may provide an additional clue to etiology. Although granulomatous inflammation also has been described in PVN, it is more commonly reported with AdV infection.[55] Similarly, the necrotizing features reported in several cases of AdV nephritis also may support a diagnosis of AdV nephritis over PVN.[56] Chronic changes, including

Fig. 6. Adenovirus. (*A*) Severe interstitial inflammation with necrotizing features, lymphocytic tubulitis, and an intact tubule (*upper left*) displaying characteristic intranuclear viral inclusions (JMS stain, original magnification ×400). (*B*) Higher magnification of intranuclear viral inclusions and surrounding acute inflammation with necrosis (H&E, original magnification ×600).

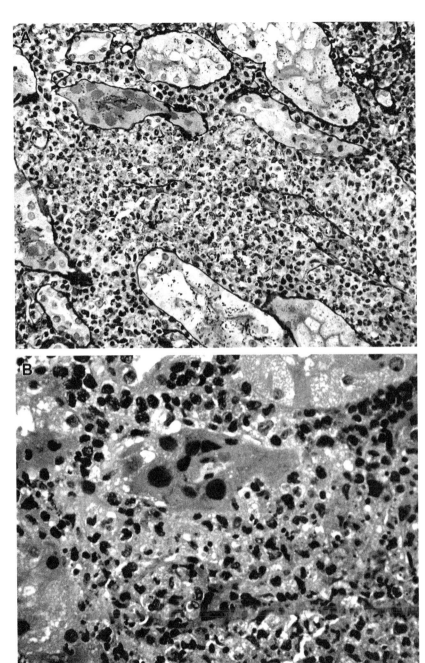

interstitial fibrosis and atrophy, are more commonly associated with PVN, as the course of the disease tends to be more indolent. The lack of these chronic changes in many of the cases of reported AdV nephritis may provide an additional clue in diagnosis.[57]

CYTOMEGALOVIRUS

CMV is a member of the family Herpesviridae, subfamily Betaherpesvirinae. CMV is an encapsulated, double-stranded DNA virus. Initial infection can occur in different stages in life. Congenital infection is associated with hepatosplenomegaly, hepatitis, and conjugated hyperbilirubinemia, thrombocytopenia, and pneumonitis, as well as numerous central nervous system abnormalities. Seroprevalence in the general population ranges from 50% to 80% in adults in the United States, with higher prevalence in developing countries. Initial infection typically occurs in childhood and adolescence, and is usually asymptomatic in immunocompetent individuals. In some, initial infection is associated with a mononucleosislike syndrome. The most common mode of transmission is via absorption through the mucous membranes, and can spread via saliva, urine, sexual contact, transfusion with human-derived blood products, and organ transplantation. CMV and BKV are the most common viral pathogens causing allograft dysfunction after renal transplantation.

MICROSCOPIC FEATURES

The most common histopathologic manifestation of CMV infection in the kidney is tubulointerstitial nephritis. Assessment of the inflammatory cells reveals a plasma-cell–rich infiltrate with variable numbers of lymphocytes and other mononuclear leukocytes. Prominent, eosinophilic intranuclear viral inclusions can be seen within tubular epithelial and endothelial cells. Granular, eosinophilic cytoplasmic viral inclusions also can be identified. Viral cytopathic effects in infected cells include nuclear enlargement, cytoplasmic swelling, epithelial cell

necrosis, and detachment from the underlying basement membrane. The pattern of interstitial inflammation also demonstrates a zonal preference for areas displaying cytopathic effects. CMV-induced cytopathy has been reported in the glomerular compartment as well, with viral cytopathic effects identified in the glomerular endothelial cells (**Fig. 7**) and podocytes.[58–60] Although the validity of CMV-induced glomerulopathy has been controversial, 2 reports identify characteristic intracytoplasmic inclusions within the glomeruli,[58] with immunohistochemical confirmation provided in one report.[61] Other atypical renal manifestations of CMV infection include thrombotic microangiopathy,[62] and 1 case of concomitant viral cytopathic effects and invasive fungal infection in an anastomosed graft artery, leading to graft failure.[58]

DIFFERENTIAL DIAGNOSIS

The differential diagnosis includes infection from other opportunistic viral pathogens, such as BKV and AdV, which can be identified by immunohistochemical staining with virus-specific antibodies. Unlike AdV and BKV, however, granular CMV viral inclusions often can be identified in the cytoplasm of infected cells. Although the presence of cytopathic effects within the glomerulus has been controversial, these findings also may be suggestive of CMV infection.

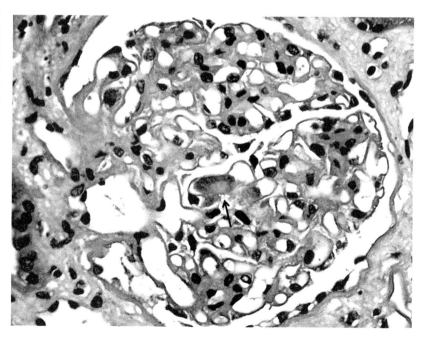

Fig. 7. Cytomegalovirus infection involving a glomerulus. A nuclear CMV inclusion in an endothelial cell (*arrow*) (H&E, original magnification ×400).

		Key Features	
		HISTOPATHOLOGIC FEATURES OF VIRAL INFECTION	
Features	Polyomavirus	Adenovirus	Cytomegalovirus
Viral inclusions	Nuclear	Nuclear	Nuclear and cytoplasmic
Interstitial inflammation	Plasma-cell–rich	Can be granulomatous	Plasma-cell–rich
Glomerular involvement	Not typical	Not typical	Has been described in some cases
Necrotizing features	Rare	More commonly seen	Rare

FUNGAL AND MYCOBACTERIAL INFECTIONS OF THE KIDNEY

The finding of granulomatous interstitial nephritis (GIN) must always raise the possibility of renal infection by mycobacterial or fungal organisms. GIN has been reported to occur in 0.5% to 0.9% of native renal biopsies[63–65] and 0.6% of transplant renal biopsies.[66] Drug-induced GIN and granulomatous inflammation related to sarcoidosis are the most common causes of GIN,[63,64] but mycobacterial and fungal infections are well described, predominantly in case reports and small series, as causes of GIN.[66–70]

MYCOBACTERIAL INFECTION OF THE KIDNEY

Renal tuberculosis can be caused by members of the Mycobacterium tuberculosis complex, most commonly M tuberculosis but occasionally by Mycobacterium bovis. Renal tuberculosis can be seen as a complication in patients who have received intravesical instillation of the vaccine strain Bacille Calmette-Guerin (BCG) for the treatment of bladder cancer.[63] Rare cases of renal infection by environmental mycobacteria (such as Mycobacterium avium-intracellulare) have been described in patients who have received transplantation or in patients with AIDS.[71] It is notable that the genitourinary tract is a common site of involvement in extrapulmonary tuberculosis,[72,73] and renal tuberculosis is easily overlooked because of the nonspecific presenting symptoms[74] and absence of positive urine cultures when using routine culture media.[75] Mycobacterial infection of the kidney is also an established complication of renal transplantation.[71]

GROSS FINDINGS

Two main gross patterns of renal tuberculosis can be seen. Renal involvement by diffuse military tuberculosis is often seen in patients with disseminated systemic infection.[76] In these cases, small white nodules, approximately 1 mm in diameter, are seen diffusely throughout the renal cortex. Alternatively, the kidney can develop a cavitary form of tuberculosis in which the renal medulla is the most prominently affected and renal papillae are replaced by caseous material that eventually fills and obliterates calyces. The caseous material can form large tumorlike masses. The cortex becomes atrophic with extensive parenchymal destruction.[3] Xanthogranulomatous pyelonephritis and renal medullary tuberculosis have prominent overlap of their gross features.

MICROSCOPIC FINDINGS

The light microscopic findings resemble those seen in other parts of the body involved by tuberculosis, including the presence of granulomatous inflammation, with or without caseous necrosis (Fig. 8). Organisms can be sparse and may be difficult to demonstrate, despite the prominent granulomatous reaction. The degree of granuloma formation and the presence of caseous necrosis will vary depending on the immunocompetence of the host. Highly immunocompromised individuals may not mount a well-developed granulomatous response to infection by mycobacteria, and in these cases organisms are typically plentiful and easily demonstrated with acid-fast stains, such as the Ziehl-Neelsen stain. The presence of granulomatous interstitial nephritis should always prompt special staining for acid-fast bacilli and fungal organisms. If necrotizing granulomata are present, but staining for acid-fast bacilli and fungal organisms is negative, PCR-based techniques can be used to increase sensitivity and more specifically identify mycobacteria.[77]

FUNGAL INFECTIONS OF THE KIDNEY

Fungal pyelonephritis is rare and is predominantly found in immunocompromised patients, most frequently transplant patients. A consortium of

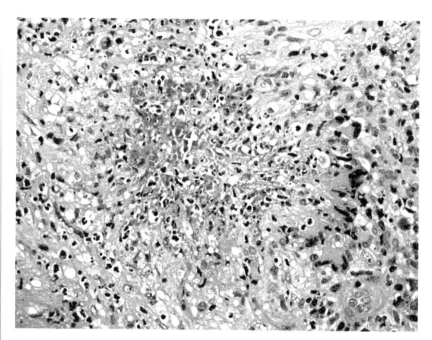

Fig. 8. A tuberculous granuloma within the renal parenchyma. Multinucleated giant cells are seen at the periphery (HE, original magnification ×400). There is central caseous necrosis. In this case, only rare acid-fast bacilli were detectable at the periphery of the granuloma with the Ziehl-Neelsen stain.

23 US transplant centers reports the 1-year cumulative incidence of invasive fungal infections ranges from 11.6% in small bowel transplant recipients to 1.3% for kidney transplant recipients. The most common invasive fungal infections were candidiasis (53%), aspergillosis (19%), and cryptococcosis (8%).[78] There are also reports of fungal infections involving the kidneys of immunocompetent individuals by organisms such as histoplasmosis.[68,69] In nontransplant patients, mycobacterial renal infection is typically due to hematogenous spread of the organism in the setting of systemic infection. However, it also can be seen as an ascending infection, especially when there are foreign bodies in the lower urinary tract.

Renal biopsies performed for medical renal and transplant indications are routinely stained with PAS, which stains many types of fungi (**Fig. 9**). Greater sensitivity is obtained with fungal stains, such as Gomori methenamine silver (GMS), which should be applied in any case where granulomatous inflammation is present. The morphologic characteristics of fungi are typical of what is seen elsewhere in the body.

RENAL CANDIDIASIS

Renal infection by *Candida* can occur either as an ascending infection from the lower urinary tract,[79] or in the setting of disseminated candidiasis. In the setting of renal transplantation, there is evidence that much of the invasive candidiasis is the result of contamination during the process of recovery of organs from the donor.[80] As in cases of bacterial pyelonephritis due to ascending infection, candidal infections that arise in this manner show disproportionately severe involvement of the renal pelvis and medulla, and when untreated, can lead to abscess development and/or "fungus ball" formation, which can obstruct the urinary tract. When *Candida* infects the kidney through hematogenous spread, numerous microabscesses develop throughout the renal parenchyma and may resemble acute bacterial pyelonephritis both grossly and microscopically. In the setting of hematogenous spread, glomerular capillaries may contain clumps of candidal organisms. In these cases, prominent glomerular inflammation can be seen within the glomeruli that show large numbers of fungal organisms, mimicking acute glomerulonephritis. The tubulointerstitium often reveals a granulomatous interstitial nephritis similar to what can be seen in mycobacterial infection; however, the granulomas associated with *Candida* infection are typically noncaseating. *Candida* can cause mycotic aneurisms and fungal arteritis, most commonly seen in the setting of transplantation.[80] Candidal organisms are easily visualized with PAS or GMS stains and are typically composed of budding yeast with pseudohyphae.

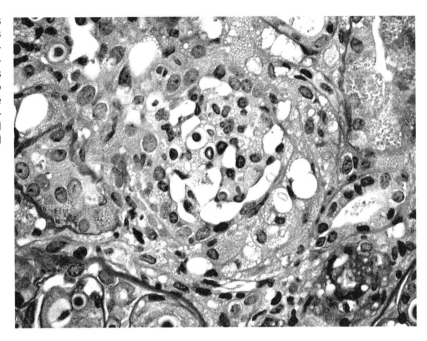

Fig. 9. Granulomatous interstitial nephritis showing PAS-positive organisms within the granuloma. This biopsy was taken in a patient who was later found to be HIV-positive and had disseminated cryptococcal infection (PAS, original magnification ×400).

ASPERGILLOSIS IN THE KIDNEY

Renal involvement by *Aspergillus* is most commonly seen in the setting of disseminated aspergillosis spread hematogenously. As in candidal infection, the gross and histologic pattern is that of multiple microabscesses bilaterally throughout the kidneys, often associated with a granulomatous interstitial reaction. Special stains for fungi, such as Gomori silver, reveal septate hyphae with acute angle branching, characteristic of *Aspergillus* species. *Aspergillus* infection localized to the urinary tract is rare, but can be seen in immunocompromised patients, such as those with diabetes and those who abuse intravenous drugs.[81] Localized infections may evolve into

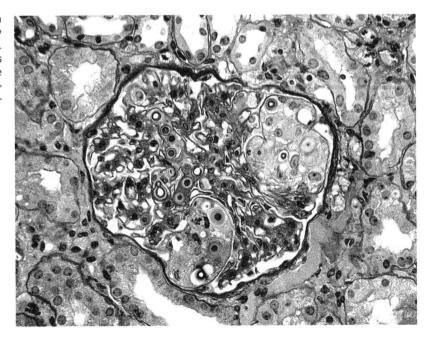

Fig. 10. Glomerulus with numerous intracapillary cryptococcal organisms. The PAS stain highlights the prominent capsule surrounding most *Cryptococci* (original magnification ×400).

fungus balls within the renal pelvis or ureters, which can lead to urinary obstruction.[82] In the renal transplantation setting, *Aspergillus* infection may be acquired as a subclinical infection that is donor-transmitted or can be iatrogenically introduced during handling and preservation of the organ. Infection can involve the renal parenchyma, but also has been noted to cause mycotic aneurysms and necrotizing arteritis at sites of infections in transplant patients.[83,84]

RENAL INFECTION BY *CRYPTOCOCCUS*

Cryptococcal infection of the kidney is almost exclusively found in patients with significant immunocompromise, including transplant recipients and patients with HIV. Infection is typically disseminated and spread hematogenously. Granulomatous interstitial nephritis is the characteristic pattern of injury (see **Fig. 9**) and organisms are readily demonstrated with the PAS stain. In some cases, large numbers of cryptococcal organisms may be seen within glomerular capillaries (**Fig. 10**).

REFERENCES

1. Czaja CA, Scholes D, Hooton TM, et al. Population-based epidemiologic analysis of acute pyelonephritis. Clin Infect Dis 2007;45:273–80.
2. Weiss M, Liapis H, Tomaszewski J, et al. Heptinstall's pathology of the kidney. 6th edition. Philadelphia: Lippincott Williams & Wilkins; 2007. p. 991–1081.
3. D'Agati VD, Jennette JC, Silva FG, et al. Non-neoplastic kidney diseases. Atlas of nontumor pathology, first series. Washington, DC: American Registry of Pathology in collaboration with the Armed Forces Institute of Pathology; 2005. p. 547–71.
4. Li L, Parwani AV. Xanthogranulomatous pyelonephritis. Arch Pathol Lab Med 2011;135:671–4.
5. Kuo CC, Wu CF, Huang CC, et al. Xanthogranulomatous pyelonephritis: critical analysis of 30 patients. Int Urol Nephrol 2011;43:15–22.
6. Goyal A, Gadodia A, Sharma R. Xanthogranulomatous pyelonephritis: an uncommon pediatric renal mass. Pediatr Radiol 2010;40:1962–3.
7. Ozkayin N, Inan M, Aladag N, et al. Complicated xanthogranulomatous pyelonephritis in a child. Pediatr Int 2010;52:e20–2.
8. Kim SW, Yoon BI, Ha US, et al. Xanthogranulomatous pyelonephritis: clinical experience with 21 cases. J Infect Chemother 2013;19:1221–4.
9. Levy M, Baumal R, Eddy AA. Xanthogranulomatous pyelonephritis in children. Etiology, pathogenesis, clinical and radiologic features, and management. Clin Pediatr (Phila) 1994;33:360–6.
10. Craig WD, Wagner BJ, Travis MD. Pyelonephritis: radiologic-pathologic review. Radiographics 2008; 28:255–77 [quiz: 327–8].
11. Claes H, Vereecken R, Oyen R, et al. Xanthogranulomatous pyelonephritis with emphasis on computerized tomography scan. Retrospective study of 20 cases and literature review. Urology 1987;29: 389–93.
12. Schlagenhaufer F. Uber epigentumliche Staphylmykosen der Nieven und der pararenalen Bindegewebes. Frankf Z Pathol 1916;19:139–48.
13. Elder JS, Marshall FF. Focal xanthogranulomatous pyelonephritis in adulthood. Johns Hopkins Med J 1980;146:141–7.
14. Parsons MA, Harris SC, Longstaff AJ, et al. Xanthogranulomatous pyelonephritis: a pathological, clinical and aetiological analysis of 87 cases. Diagn Histopathol 1983;6:203–19.
15. Chandrankunnel J, Cunha BA, Petelin A, et al. Fever of unknown origin (FUO) and a renal mass: renal cell carcinoma, renal tuberculosis, renal malakoplakia, or xanthogranulomatous pyelonephritis? Heart Lung 2012;41:606–9.
16. Hyuga T, Nakamura S, Ishino T, et al. A case of renal malacoplakia that was difficult to distinguish from cystic renal cell carcinoma. Nihon Hinyokika Gakkai Zasshi 2011;102:591–4 [in Japanese].
17. Singh PB, Gupta RC, Dwivedi US, et al. Renal parenchymal malakoplakia. Br J Urol 1989;63: 99–100.
18. Leao CA, Duarte MI, Gamba C, et al. Malakoplakia after renal transplantation in the current era of immunosuppressive therapy: case report and literature review. Transpl Infect Dis 2012;14:E137–41.
19. El Jamal SM, Malak SF, Cox RM, et al. Extragenitourinary malakoplakia in a patient with myeloma clinically mimicking extramedullary myelomatous disease. Hum Pathol 2011;42:602–4.
20. Savant SR, Amladi ST, Kangle SD, et al. Cutaneous malakoplakia in an HIV-positive patient. Int J STD AIDS 2007;18:435–6.
21. Stanton MJ, Maxted W. Malacoplakia: a study of the literature and current concepts of pathogenesis, diagnosis and treatment. J Urol 1981;125: 139–46.
22. Sagaert X, Tousseyn T, De Hertogh G, et al. Macrophage-related diseases of the gut: a pathologist's perspective. Virchows Arch 2012;460:555–67.
23. Dobyan DC, Truong LD, Eknoyan G. Renal malacoplakia reappraised. Am J Kidney Dis 1993;22: 243–52.
24. Puerto IM, Mojarrieta JC, Martinez IB, et al. Renal malakoplakia as a pseudotumoral lesion in a renal transplant patient: a case report. Int J Urol 2007; 14:655–7.
25. von Hasemann D. Ueber malacoplakia der harnblase. Virchows Arch A Pathol Anat 1903;173:302–8.

26. Michaelis L, Gutmann C. Ueber einsclusse in bla-sentumoren. Klein Med 1902;47:208–15.

27. An T, Ferenczy A, Wilens SL, et al. Observations on the formation of Michaelis-Gutmann bodies. Hum Pathol 1974;5:753–8.

28. Padgett BL, Walker DL, ZuRhein GM, et al. Cultivation of papova-like virus from human brain with progressive multifocal leucoencephalopathy. Lancet 1971;1:1257–60.

29. Gardner SD, Field AM, Coleman DV, et al. New human papovavirus (B.K.) isolated from urine after renal transplantation. Lancet 1971;1:1253–7.

30. Berger JR, Miller CS, Mootoor Y, et al. JC virus detection in bodily fluids: clues to transmission. Clin Infect Dis 2006;43:e9–12.

31. Hirsch HH, Knowles W, Dickenmann M, et al. Prospective study of polyomavirus type BK replication and nephropathy in renal-transplant recipients. N Engl J Med 2002;347:488–96.

32. Ahuja M, Cohen EP, Dayer AM, et al. Polyoma virus infection after renal transplantation. Use of immunostaining as a guide to diagnosis. Transplantation 2001;71:896–9.

33. Dall A, Hariharan S. BK virus nephritis after renal transplantation. Clin J Am Soc Nephrol 2008; 3(Suppl 2):S68–75.

34. Hussain S, Bresnahan BA, Cohen EP, et al. Rapid kidney allograft failure in patients with polyoma virus nephritis with prior treatment with antilymphocyte agents. Clin Transplant 2002;16:43–7.

35. Brennan DC, Agha I, Bohl DL, et al. Incidence of BK with tacrolimus versus cyclosporine and impact of preemptive immunosuppression reduction. Am J Transplant 2005;5:582–94.

36. Randhawa P, Ho A, Shapiro R, et al. Correlates of quantitative measurement of BK polyomavirus (BKV) DNA with clinical course of BKV infection in renal transplant patients. J Clin Microbiol 2004;42: 1176–80.

37. Nickeleit V, Hirsch HH, Binet IF, et al. Polyomavirus infection of renal allograft recipients: from latent infection to manifest disease. J Am Soc Nephrol 1999;10:1080–9.

38. Frisque RJ, Rifkin DB, Topp WC. Requirement for the large T and small T proteins of SV40 in the maintenance of the transformed state. Cold Spring Harb Symp Quant Biol 1980;44(Pt 1):325–31.

39. Ali SH, DeCaprio JA. Cellular transformation by SV40 large T antigen: interaction with host proteins. Semin Cancer Biol 2001;11:15–23.

40. Aksamit AJ, Mourrain P, Sever JL, et al. Progressive multifocal leukoencephalopathy: investigation of three cases using in situ hybridization with JC virus biotinylated DNA probe. Ann Neurol 1985;18: 490–6.

41. Arthur RR, Beckmann AM, Li CC, et al. Direct detection of the human papovavirus BK in urine of bone marrow transplant recipients: comparison of DNA hybridization with ELISA. J Med Virol 1985;16:29–36.

42. Kemeny E, Hirsch HH, Eller J, et al. Plasma cell infiltrates in polyomavirus nephropathy. Transpl Int 2010;23:397–406.

43. Meehan SM, Kadambi PV, Manaligod JR, et al. Polyoma virus infection of renal allografts: relationships of the distribution of viral infection, tubulointerstitial inflammation, and fibrosis suggesting viral interstitial nephritis in untreated disease. Hum Pathol 2005;36:1256–64.

44. Gaber LW, Egidi MF, Stratta RJ, et al. Clinical utility of histological features of polyomavirus allograft nephropathy. Transplantation 2006;82:196–204.

45. Hogan TF, Borden EC, McBain JA, et al. Human polyomavirus infections with JC virus and BK virus in renal transplant patients. Ann Intern Med 1980; 92:373–8.

46. Husseiny MI, Anastasi B, Singer J, et al. A comparative study of Merkel cell, BK and JC polyomavirus infections in renal transplant recipients and healthy subjects. J Clin Virol 2010;49:137–40.

47. Yin WY, Lu MC, Lee MC, et al. A correlation between polyomavirus JC virus quantification and genotypes in renal transplantation. Am J Surg 2010;200:53–8.

48. Delbue S, Ferraresso M, Ghio L, et al. A review on JC virus infection in kidney transplant recipients. Clin Dev Immunol 2013;2013:926391.

49. Drachenberg RC, Drachenberg CB, Papadimitriou JC, et al. Morphological spectrum of polyoma virus disease in renal allografts: diagnostic accuracy of urine cytology. Am J Transplant 2001;1:373–81.

50. Rowe WP, Huebner RJ, Gilmore LK, et al. Isolation of a cytopathogenic agent from human adenoids undergoing spontaneous degeneration in tissue culture. Proc Soc Exp Biol Med 1953;84:570–3.

51. Storsley L, Gibson IW. Adenovirus interstitial nephritis and rejection in an allograft. J Am Soc Nephrol 2011;22:1423–7.

52. Parasuraman R, Zhang PL, Samarapungavan D, et al. Severe necrotizing adenovirus tubulointerstitial nephritis in a kidney transplant recipient. Case Rep Transplant 2013;2013:969186.

53. Teague MW, Glick AD, Fogo AB. Adenovirus infection of the kidney: mass formation in a patient with Hodgkin's disease. Am J Kidney Dis 1991;18: 499–502.

54. Lim AK, Parsons S, Ierino F. Adenovirus tubulointerstitial nephritis presenting as a renal allograft space occupying lesion. Am J Transplant 2005; 5:2062–6.

55. Colvin RB, Nickeleit V. Renal transplant pathology. In: Jennette JC, Olson JL, Schwartz MM, et al, editors. Hepinstall's pathology of the

kidney. 6th edition. Lippincott, Williams, and Wilkins; 2007. p. 1441–9.

56. Koankiewicz LM, Pullman J, Raffeld M, et al. Adenovirus nephritis and obstructive uropathy in a renal transplant recipient: case report and literature review. Nephrol Dial Transplant 2010;3:388–92.

57. Kolankiewicz LM, Weinberg DA, Rothstein M, et al. Effects of erythropoietin stimulating agent (ESA) automated adjustment protocols on hemoglobin levels and mortality in end stage renal disease patients. Med Health R I 2012;95:172–5.

58. Rane S, Nada R, Minz M, et al. Spectrum of cytomegalovirus-induced renal pathology in renal allograft recipients. Transplant Proc 2012;44:713–6.

59. Richardson WP, Colvin RB, Cheeseman SH, et al. Glomerulopathy associated with cytomegalovirus viremia in renal allografts. N Engl J Med 1981; 305:57–63.

60. Birk PE, Chavers BM. Does cytomegalovirus cause glomerular injury in renal allograft recipients? J Am Soc Nephrol 1997;8:1801–8.

61. Payton D, Thorner P, Eddy A, et al. Demonstration by light microscopy of cytomegalovirus on a renal biopsy of a renal allograft recipient: confirmation by immunohistochemistry and in situ hybridization. Nephron 1987;47:205–8.

62. Jeejeebhoy FM, Zaltzman JS. Thrombotic microangiopathy in association with cytomegalovirus infection in a renal transplant patient: a new treatment strategy. Transplantation 1998;65:1645–8.

63. Bijol V, Mendez GP, Nose V, et al. Granulomatous interstitial nephritis: a clinicopathologic study of 46 cases from a single institution. Int J Surg Pathol 2006;14:57–63.

64. Joss N, Morris S, Young B, et al. Granulomatous interstitial nephritis. Clin J Am Soc Nephrol 2007; 2:222–30.

65. Mignon F, Mery JP, Mougenot B, et al. Granulomatous interstitial nephritis. Adv Nephrol Necker Hosp 1984;13:219–45.

66. Meehan SM, Josephson MA, Haas M. Granulomatous tubulointerstitial nephritis in the renal allograft. Am J Kidney Dis 2000;36:E27.

67. Bagnasco SM, Subramanian AK, Desai NM. Fungal infection presenting as giant cell tubulointerstitial nephritis in kidney allograft. Transpl Infect Dis 2012;14:288–91.

68. Chung S, Park CW, Chung HW, et al. Acute renal failure presenting as a granulomatous interstitial nephritis due to cryptococcal infection. Kidney Int 2009;76:453–8.

69. Nasr SH, Koscica J, Markowitz GS, et al. Granulomatous interstitial nephritis. Am J Kidney Dis 2003; 41:714–9.

70. Ogura M, Kagami S, Nakao M, et al. Fungal granulomatous interstitial nephritis presenting as acute kidney injury diagnosed by renal histology including PCR assay. Clin Kidney J 2012;5:459–62.

71. Qunibi WY, al-Sibai MB, Taher S, et al. Mycobacterial infection after renal transplantation–report of 14 cases and review of the literature. Q J Med 1990; 77:1039–60.

72. Alvarez S, McCabe WR. Extrapulmonary tuberculosis revisited: a review of experience at Boston City and other hospitals. Medicine 1984;63:25–55.

73. Horsburgh CR Jr. Mycobacterium avium complex infection in the acquired immunodeficiency syndrome. N Engl J Med 1991;324:1332–8.

74. Lattimer JK. Renal tuberculosis. N Engl J Med 1965;273:208–11.

75. Eastwood JB, Corbishley CM, Grange JM. Tuberculosis and the kidney. J Am Soc Nephrol 2001; 12:1307–14.

76. Simon HB, Weinstein AJ, Pasternak MS, et al. Genitourinary tuberculosis. Clinical features in a general hospital population. Am J Med 1977;63: 410–20.

77. Ikonomopoulos JA, Gorgoulis VG, Zacharatos PV, et al. Multiplex polymerase chain reaction for the detection of mycobacterial DNA in cases of tuberculosis and sarcoidosis. Mod Pathol 1999;12: 854–62.

78. Pappas PG, Alexander BD, Andes DR, et al. Invasive fungal infections among organ transplant recipients: results of the Transplant-Associated Infection Surveillance Network (TRANSNET). Clin Infect Dis 2010;50:1101–11.

79. Sadegi BJ, Patel BK, Wilbur AC, et al. Primary renal candidiasis: importance of imaging and clinical history in diagnosis and management. J Ultrasound Med 2009;28:507–14.

80. Albano L, Bretagne S, Mamzer-Bruneel MF, et al. Evidence that graft-site candidiasis after kidney transplantation is acquired during organ recovery: a multicenter study in France. Clin Infect Dis 2009;48:194–202.

81. Flechner SM, McAninch JW. Aspergillosis of the urinary tract: ascending route of infection and evolving patterns of disease. J Urol 1981;125: 598–601.

82. Kueter JC, MacDiarmid SA, Redman JF. Anuria due to bilateral ureteral obstruction by Aspergillus flavus in an adult male. Urology 2002;59:601.

83. Garrido J, Lerma JL, Heras M, et al. Pseudoaneurysm of the iliac artery secondary to Aspergillus infection in two recipients of kidney transplants from the same donor. Am J Kidney Dis 2003;41: 488–92.

84. Keating MR, Guerrero MA, Daly RC, et al. Transmission of invasive aspergillosis from a subclinically infected donor to three different organ transplant recipients. Chest 1996;109:1119–24.

Renal Amyloidosis

Nasreen Mohamed, MD, FRCPA[a], Samih H. Nasr, MD[b],*

KEYWORDS

- Amyloidosis • AL amyloidosis • AA amyloidosis • Amyloid types
- Laser microdissection and mass spectrometry • Renal biopsy

ABSTRACT

Amyloidosis is an uncommon group of diseases in which soluble proteins aggregate and deposit extracellularly in tissue as insoluble fibrils, leading to tissue destruction and progressive organ dysfunction. More than 25 proteins have been identified as amyloid precursor proteins. Amyloid fibrils have a characteristic appearance on ultrastructural examination and generate anomalous colors under polarized light. Amyloidosis can be systemic or localized. The kidney is a prime site for amyloid deposition. Immunofluorescence, immunoperoxidase, and more recently laser microdissection and mass spectrometry are important tools used in the typing of renal amyloidosis.

OVERVIEW

Amyloidosis constitutes a large group of uncommon diseases that share a common trait characterized by distinctive extracellular deposition of pathologic insoluble fibrillar proteins in which protein misfolding has an essential role in the pathogenesis.[1] The term was first adopted by Virchow in the nineteenth century to describe an abnormal extracellular material in autopsy cases, and later it was discovered to stain for Congo red and exhibit anomalous colors under polarized light. Its unique β-pleated sheet configuration confers on the amyloid the typical staining properties and stability under physiologic conditions.

Amyloid is characterized by deposition of homogenous and amorphous pale eosinophilic material, which ultimately leads to destruction of tissues and progressive disease. Besides its peculiar staining pattern, it is characterized by the presence of rigid, nonbranching, randomly oriented fibrils ranging in diameter from 7 to 14 nm on ultrastructural examination.[1]

In the United States and Europe, amyloidosis derived from immunoglobulin (Ig) light chain (AL) is the most prevalent form, followed by AA amyloidosis (AA). The incidence of AL is 6 to 10 cases per million population.[2] In a series of 1315 patients with amyloidosis seen at the Mayo Clinic (Rochester, Minnesota) between 1981 and 1992, 70% had AL, 19% localized amyloidosis, 4% familial amyloidosis, 4% senile amyloidosis, and 3% AA.[3] In developing countries, however, AA is more common than AL.[4]

Renal involvement is frequent in most types of systemic amyloidosis with AL, previously called primary amyloidosis, being the most common type involving the kidney. It has been reported that 50% to 80% of patients with AL have kidney involvement,[3] whereas in patients with AA, the kidney shows variable involvement. The overall renal biopsy incidence of amyloidosis ranges from 1.3% to 4%.[5–8]

AMYLOIDOSIS TYPES THAT AFFECT THE KIDNEY

There are more than 25 precursor proteins identified leading to amyloid deposition. The types of systemic amyloidosis that may be associated

Disclosure and Conflict of Interest: None.
[a] Department of Pathology and Laboratory Medicine, King Fahad Specialist Hospital-Dammam, Omar Bin Thabit Street, Dammam, Kingdom of Saudi Arabia; [b] Department of Laboratory Medicine and Pathology, Mayo Clinic, 200 First Street Southwest, Rochester, MN 55905, USA
* Corresponding author. Division of Anatomic Pathology, Mayo Clinic, 200 First Street Southwest, Hilton 10-20, Rochester, MN 55905.
E-mail address: nasr.samih@mayo.edu

Surgical Pathology 7 (2014) 409–425
http://dx.doi.org/10.1016/j.path.2014.04.006

surgpath.theclinics.com

with clinically significant kidney involvement are listed in **Table 1**. **Fig. 1** depicts the origin of renal amyloidosis in 474 cases diagnosed by renal biopsy at the Mayo Clinic Renal Biopsy Laboratory between 2007 and 2011. Ig-related amyloidosis (AIg) is by far the most common form affecting the kidney.[6–9] AIg is associated with B-cell lymphoproliferative disorders encompassing multiple myeloma–plasma cell dyscrasia, malignant lymphoma, and macroglobulinemia. AIg in most cases is derived from fragments of monoclonal light chains (AL) but rarely is derived from fragments of the Ig-heavy chain and light chain (AHL) or Ig heavy chain only (AH).[10–12]

AA is the second most common form of renal amyloidosis[6,8]; it is associated with chronic inflammatory diseases, such as chronic infection, rheumatoid arthritis, ankylosing spondylitis, inflammatory bowel disease, familial Mediterranean fever, bronchiectasis, and chronic osteomyelitis.[13–15] The kidney may also be affected by several forms of familial or hereditary amyloidosis, most of which have an autosomal dominant mode of inheritance and start in midlife with a slow rate of progression. These include amyloid derived from a mutant protein of transthyretin (TTR) (ATTR),[7,8] fibrinogen A-α chain (AFib),[6,16] gelsolin (AGel),[17] lysozyme (ALys),[18] apolipoprotein A-I (AApo AI),[19] apolipoprotein A-II (AApo AII),[20] and apolipoprotein A-IV (AApo AIV).[21] In 2008, a new member was added to the amyloid family, ALECT2—amyloid derived from leukocyte chemotactic factor 2 protein (LECT2).[22] ALECT2 is now the third most

common type of renal amyloidosis in the United States, accounting for 2.5% to 2.7% of cases.[6,8] It affects mainly the kidney and liver but can rarely involve other organs.[23–25]

CLINICAL PRESENTATION

The clinical presentation of patients with amyloidosis varies, reflecting the presence of different types of amyloidosis, with wavering predilection for organ involvement, making a diagnosis difficult.

Table 1
Systemic amyloidoses with clinically significance kidney involvement

Amyloid Precursor Protein	Name
Ig light chain	AL
Ig heavy chain	AH
Ig heavy and light chain	AHL
SAA	AA
Leukocyte chemotactic factor 2	ALECT2
Fibrinogen A-α chain	AFib
TTR	ATTR
Apolipoprotein A-I	AApo AI
Apolipoprotein A-II	AApo AII
Apolipoprotein A-IV	AApo AIV
Gelsolin	AGel
Lysozyme	ALys

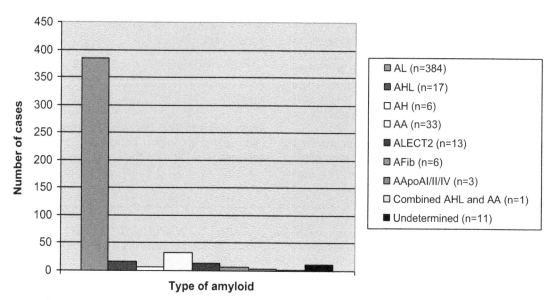

Fig. 1. The origin of renal amyloidosis in 474 cases diagnosed by renal biopsy at the Mayo Clinic Renal Biopsy Laboratory between 2007 and 2011.

The initial symptoms are vague with a subtle decrease in exercise capacity to fatigue and weight loss, but definite diagnosis is made when particular organ involvement appears. Other presenting features include dyspnea, lower extremity edema, syncope, ascites, and anasarca.[26] Amyloidosis can also affect the autonomic nervous system, leading to hemodynamic fragility and orthostatic hypotension. The development of nephrogenic diabetes insipidus secondary to peri-collecting duct tissue involvement by amyloid is another unusual manifestation.[27,28] The amyloid can be localized, confined to one site, and usually nonlethal, as in skin amyloidosis, or can be systemic, when it involves multiple visceral organs.[29] Generally, amyloidosis is more common in men than women, with a median age at presentation of 59.5 to 63 years.[6,30] Patients with AA usually present at a younger age, whereas AL and ALECT2 are more common in older patients.[6] ALECT2 mainly affects Hispanics of Mexican origin,[24,31] whereas AL and AA do not show clear ethnic bias.

Renal involvement is a frequent manifestation of amyloidosis, mainly AL, AA, and hereditary amyloidosis,[3,16,32] and it is a major source of morbidity in these patients. It is characterized by proteinuria ranging from subnephrotic range to massive with or without renal insufficiency. Proteinuria is present in 73% of cases, with 30% of patients exhibiting full nephrotic syndrome. Patients with AIg more commonly present with high levels of proteinuria than other types of amyloidosis, with approximately 68% of the cases presenting with full nephrotic syndrome.[6] When the amyloid involves primarily the interstitium, as typically seen in ALECT2,[31] or vasculature, as in vascular-limited AL,[33] the proteinuria can be negligible and reduced glomerular filtration rate (GFR) is the principal renal manifestation.

PATHOGENESIS

The initial step for fibrillogenesis and amyloid formation includes protein misfolding, which can occur as a result of proteolytic cleavage. The misfolded protein has a tendency for self-aggregation and subsequent fibrils generation.[1] During the amyloid formation, the intermediate protein takes on more β-sheet structures that enable aggregation and self-propagation. This is followed by a process where β-sheet regions from different molecules align themselves and interdigitate to form a dry interface. The end product is a protofibril, which is more resistant to degradation.[34]

Amyloid might form via different mechanisms, one of which is amino acid substitution. In AL, the substitution of a particular amino acid at a specific position in the light chain variable region occurs at a higher frequency in comparison with nonamyloidogenic Igs, leading to destabilization of light chains and increasing their likelihood of fibrillogenesis.[35,36] Similarly, in hereditary amyloidosis, the genetic mutation with amino acid substitution is the base for amyloid fibrils formation.[29] The unstable protein produced by substitution of amino acids may allow the protein to precipitate when stimulated by physical or chemical factors, such as local surface pH, electric field, and hydration forces on cellular surfaces.

Another mechanism is the excessive concentration of amyloidogenic protein due to unregulated production. When the protein precursor reaches a critical local concentration, it triggers fibrils formation, which is enhanced further by environmental factors and interaction with extracellular matrix,[1,37] as may occur in AA associated with chronic inflammation or familial Mediterranean fever. The excessive concentration of amyloidogenic protein may also be caused by decreased removal from the body. For example, amyloidosis derived from β2-microglobulin (Aβ2M) develops in patients with end-stage renal disease who are on long-term dialysis, because β_2-microglobulin is not efficiently cleared from the circulation during dialysis.[38] ALECT2 is derived from LECT2, which is a multifunctional factor involved in damage and repair, chemotaxis, inflammation, and immunomodulation.[39–41] The pathogenesis of ALECT2 is still unknown but may be due to increased synthesis of LECT2 by hepatocytes or involve an interference, possibly due to a genetic defect, in the LECT2 catabolic pathway or LECT2 transport, which may cause an increased local tissue concentration of LECT2, ultimately leading to amyloid fibril formation.[24,31,42] Moreover, amyloid protein may have an intrinsic propensity to assume a pathologic conformational change which becomes evident with aging (eg, TTR).[43]

Amyloid can be deposited in multiple organs, and this tendency might depend on several factors, such as high local protein concentration, low pH, presence of proteolytic processing, and the presence of fibrils seeds.[1] The amyloid deposits cause significant disruption of the tissue architecture, which might be the underlying mechanism of organ dysfunction.[1] Moreover, the amyloidogenic precursor proteins, folding intermediates, and protofilaments have toxicities independent of amyloid deposits. Amyloid can regress over time by endogenous degradation.[44]

The specific uptake of light chains by mesangial cells underlies the predominant kidney tropism and is a crucial step in amyloid formation in AL.

Factors that might promote or retard amyloid deposition in the kidney include the negative charge and the high glycosaminoglycan content of the glomerular basement membrane with the presence of certain proteases that could render a protein amyloidogenic.[45,46] Mesangial cells are modified smooth muscle cells expressing smooth muscle actin and muscle-specific actin.[47] Upon interaction with light chains, the light chains are avidly internalized and are delivered to the mature lysosomal compartment where amyloid fibrils are primarily formed.[47] During this process, the mesangial cell undergoes transformation into a macrophage phenotype with a prominent lysosomal system, making it capable of processing internalized amyloidogenic light chains and fibrils formation.[47] The amyloid deposition within the mesangium later stimulates metalloproteinase activity causing mesangial matrix destruction, inhibits transforming growth factor β impairing the repair of mesangial matrix,[48] and enhances apoptosis, ultimately leading to significant mesangial cell deletion and replacement by amyloid deposits.[49]

RENAL BIOPSY

LIGHT MICROSCOPY

Amyloid can involve any compartment within the kidney, but glomerular involvement predominates in the majority of cases.[30] Glomerular involvement is present in 97% of cases and vascular involvement is identified in 85% of the cases, whereas the interstitium is affected in 58% of cases.[6] Different types of amyloid have variable predilection to kidney compartments (**Fig. 2**).[24] For example, AFib shows massive glomerular obliteration by amyloid deposits (**Fig. 3**) with milder or absent vascular and interstitial involvement.[6,16] In contrast, AApo AI and AApo AIV show predominant involvement of medullary interstitium (**Fig. 4**).[6,21,28] ALECT2, on the other hand, is

characterized by extensive cortical interstitial amyloid deposits with variable, occasionally absent altogether, involvement of glomeruli and vessels; the medullary interstitial involvement is absent or trivial (**Fig. 5**).[6,24]

On hematoxylin-eosin (H&E)–stained sections, amyloid appears as amorphous pale eosinophilic material, which starts in the mesangium, eventually replacing the normal mesangial matrix and extending into the peripheral capillary walls (**Fig. 6**). The deposits are negative or weakly positive for periodic acid–Schiff (PAS) (**Fig. 7**) and are typically nonargyrophilic on silver stain (**Box 1**, see **Fig. 4**; **Fig. 8**). On trichrome stain, they may appear gray, which is a helpful clue to the diagnosis, or stain blue similar to collagen.[6] A minority of cases, particularly AH/AHL, show light microscopic features atypical for amyloid, such as PAS or silver positivity, mesangial hypercellularity, or more extensive glomerular basement membrane than mesangial involvement, mimicking fibrillary glomerulonephritis (FGN).[12] The early stage of AL shows small, segmental deposits within the mesangium, which can be easily missed if no immunofluorescence (IF) or electron microscopy (EM) is performed. In the more advanced stage, the mesangium exhibits uniform expansion with compression of the capillary spaces and occasional nodule formation resembling diabetic nephropathy or monoclonal Ig deposition disease. The nodular pattern is more frequent in AA.[15] When amyloid affects the glomerular basement membrane, it may form spicules—a characteristic feature of this disease, which can be readily identified on a good-quality silver stain (**Fig. 9**). Amyloid spicules are more common in AL than AA and the other forms of amyloidosis.[6,50] Rarely, cellular crescents can be seen in both AA and AL,[6,15,51,52] highlighting that capillary wall rupture can occur. Vasculature is another important site for amyloid deposition, frequently involving the arteriolar walls, followed by arteries, peritubular

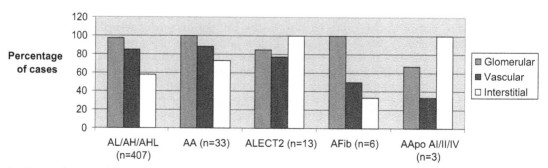

Fig. 2. Distribution of renal amyloid deposits according to type in 474 cases diagnosed by renal biopsy at the Mayo Clinic Renal Biopsy Laboratory between 2007 and 2011.

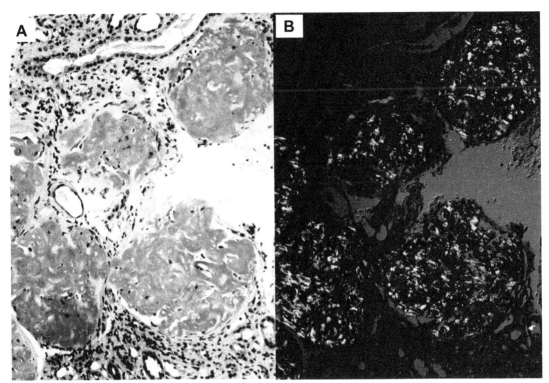

Fig. 3. Renal AFib. There is diffuse and global obliterative glomerular involvement by amyloid (Congo red stain) (*A*). (*B*) The congophilic deposits from the case (*A*) exhibit anomalous colors when viewed under polarized light (original magnification ×200).

capillaries, and veins.[6] In rare cases, particularly those of AL or ATTR types, the vessels are the only site in the kidney where amyloid is demonstrated, which can be distributed in a segmental or circular pattern.[30] Interstitial deposits are seen in approximately 50% of cases overall but are seen in every case of ALECT2 (see **Fig. 5**). As progressive amyloid deposition occurs, the percentage of obsolescent glomeruli and the degree of interstitial fibrosis and tubular atrophy increase.[30]

Fig. 4. A case of renal AApo A1 showing extensive deposition of silver-negative amyloid deposits in the medullary interstitium (×100).

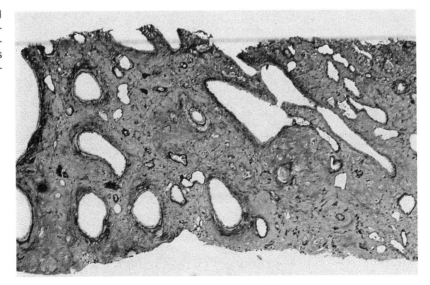

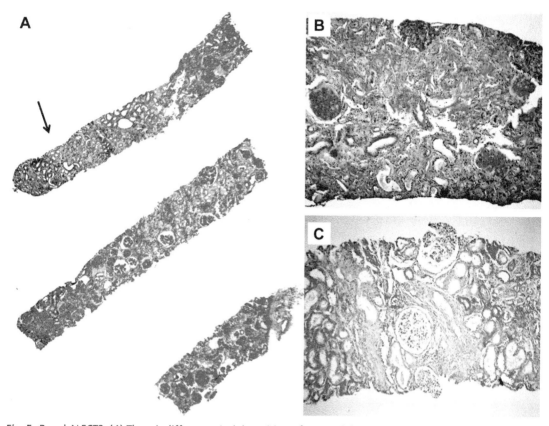

Fig. 5. Renal ALECT2. (*A*) There is diffuse cortical deposition of congophilic amyloid, both interstitial and glomerular, with sparing of medullary interstitium (*arrow*) (Congo red ×20). (*B*) This case shows extensive interstitial, glomerular and vascular amyloid deposits (Congo red ×100). (*C*) A different case exhibits extensive interstitial and focal arteriolar amyloid deposits; glomeruli and interlobular arteries are spared (Congo red ×100).

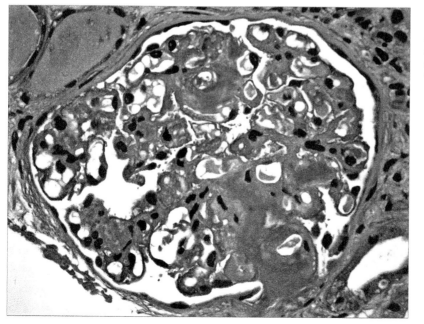

Fig. 6. There is variable mesangial expansion by amorphous, acellular, eosinophilic material, which segmentally extends to the glomerular capillary loops (H&E ×400).

Fig. 7. Mesangial areas are globally expanded by acellular, PAS-weak amyloid deposits (×400).

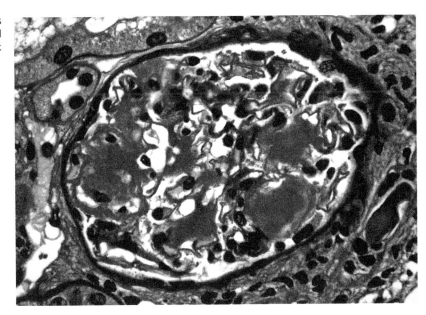

Interstitial inflammation is absent or trivial in pure renal amyloidosis, although interstitial foam cells and giant cells surrounding amyloid deposits may be seen.[6,30]

Amyloid has a characteristic Congo red–positive staining (salmon pink) (see **Fig. 5**) and fluorescence with thioflavin T or S. The Congo red–positive material must polarize and produce anomalous colors (yellow/orange/green) under polarized light to be considered diagnostic of amyloidosis (see **Fig. 3**).[53] This striking optical morphology, traditionally referred to as *apple green birefringence*, occurs as a result of ordered intercalation of Congo red dye and amyloid fibrils and is best obtained by using a strong light source and examination in the dark.[54] In cases of small amounts of amyloid, it might be difficult to demonstrate Congo red positivity. An alternative way of demonstrating small amount of deposits is to perform a Congo red stain and place the stained section under fluorescence light; amyloid then becomes bright red.[55] Rarely, in cases of hereditary amyloidosis, amyloid can be Congo red negative.[56] This may also occur if a section examined is less than 5 μm in thickness (**Box 2**). Overstaining might result, however, in false positivity.[44] Thioflavin T produces yellow-green fluorescence upon binding to amyloid. Although it is more sensitive in detecting small amount of amyloid,[49] it is less specific and is used less frequently than Congo red stain.[44]

Other renal pathologies that might coexist with amyloidosis include myeloma cast nephropathy, acute tubular necrosis, monoclonal Ig deposition disease, diabetic glomerulosclerosis, and thin basement membrane nephropathy.[6]

IMMUNOFLUORESCENCE

IF is essential for confirming the presence and for typing of renal amyloidosis. IF staining for kappa and lambda should be routinely performed on all native kidney biopsies. The finding of an intense staining for a single Ig light chain with negativity for Ig heavy chains is diagnostic of AL, with three-quarters of AL cases expressing lambda light chain (**Fig. 10**).[6] The diagnosis of AH is based

---

Box 1
Pathologic key features

Amyloid deposits are pale on H&E, PAS negative, nonargyrophilic, and congophilic.

Amyloid most commonly affects glomeruli and vessels; predominant cortical interstitial involvement is seen in ALECT2, and predominant medullary involvement is seen in AApo AI and Apo AIV.

The characteristic amyloid spicules are more common in AL than other types.

Amyloid typing is crucial for assessing prognosis and initiating proper therapy.

LMD/MS is required for typing renal amyloidosis in 16% of cases.

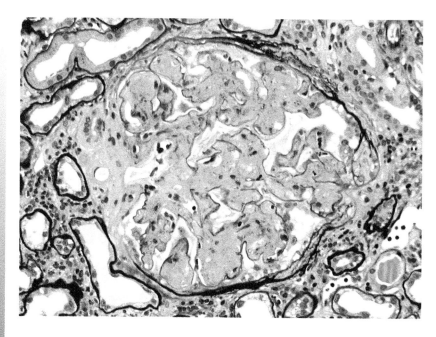

Fig. 8. Amyloid deposits are typically silver negative (ie, stain pink on silver stain). The glomerulus depicted exhibits extensive mesangial, glomerular capillary wall, and hilar nonargyrophilic amyloid deposits (×200).

on the presence of intense staining for a single Ig heavy chain with negativity for kappa and lambda light chains (**Fig. 11**), whereas the diagnosis of AHL is reserved for intense staining for a single Ig heavy chain and a single Ig light chain.[12] Amyloid deposits have a distinctive appearance on IF: they appear smudgy with fuzzy borders. In early renal AL, the mesangial or vascular deposits can be missed by light microscopy and EM but unequivocally identified by IF.

ELECTRON MICROSCOPY

Ultrastructurally, amyloid deposits, regardless of type, show a cottony appearance at low magnification (**Fig. 12A**). At high magnification, they appear

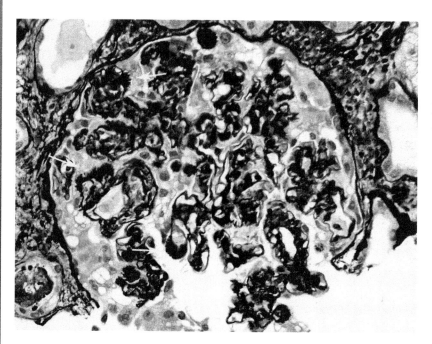

Fig. 9. Amyloid spicules are a characteristics feature of renal amyloidosis, which are seen more frequently in AIg (70% of cases) than other forms of amyloidosis. They are best seen on silver stain (*arrows*) and EM (silver stain ×400).

as randomly arranged, nonbranching fibrils, ranging in thickness between 7 and 14 nm (see **Fig. 12B**). The fibrils can be seen within the mesangium, glomerular basement membranes, interstitium, tubular basement membranes, and/or vessels. A notable deviation from the haphazard orientation of amyloid fibrils is the formation of amyloid spicules, which result from parallel alignment of amyloid fibrils in the subepithelial zone perpendicular to the glomerular basement membrane (see **Fig. 12C**). In few documented cases of amyloid regression, the glomerular basement membrane may exhibit few remaining fibrils or amorphous debris within lacunae left behind in the lamellated lamina densa. Podocytes overlying segments of glomerular basement membranes with amyloid deposits typically show foot process effacement and condensation of actin cytoskeleton.

DIFFERENTIAL DIAGNOSIS

The diagnosis of amyloidosis can be made with certainty in a majority of cases using a combined approach including light microscopy, IF, IP, and ultrastructural analysis. The differential diagnosis from other infiltrative glomerular processes is listed in **Table 2**. The renal disease most likely to be confused with amyloidosis is FGN. It may show mesangial expansion and loss of argyrophilia with thick capillary loops as in amyloidosis. Contrary to amyloidosis, the deposits in FGN are Congo red negative and most cases exhibit mesangial hypercellularity with/without duplication of the glomerular basement membranes. On IF, most cases of FGN show polyclonal deposits of IgG, kappa, and lambda. The FGN deposits ultrastructurally are composed of randomly oriented fibrils, similar to amyloid; however, they differ from amyloid fibrils in 3 aspects: (1) they are generally (but not always) thicker than amyloid fibrils, ranging from 9 to 26 nm in diameter; (2) they usually do not form spicules; and (3) they are only rarely seen outside the glomerulus (identified focally in tubular basement membranes in minority of cases).[57] A helpful internal point of reference for fibril thickness is the intracellular cytoskeletal filaments of adjacent podocytes, endothelial cells, and mesangial cells, which range in thickness from 5 nm (actin microfilament) to 10 nm (myosin and vimentin intermediate filaments). Amyloid

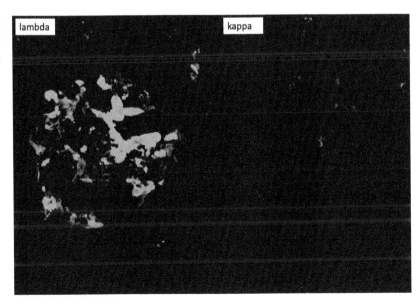

Fig. 10. This case of AL-lambda shows smudgy mesangial positivity for lambda with negative kappa (IF ×400).

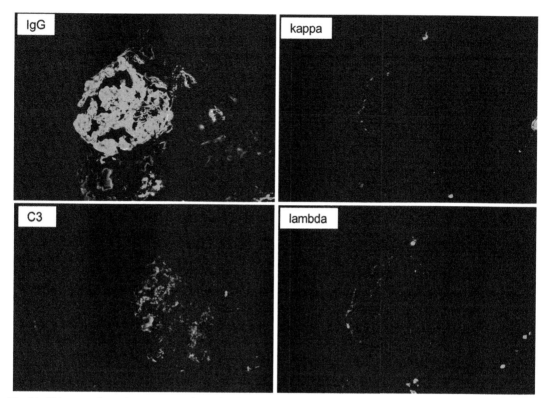

Fig. 11. This case of renal AH-gamma shows bright glomerular staining for IgG with weak staining for C3. Staining for kappa and lambda is negative (IF ×200).

fibrils should be comparable in size to cytoskeletal filaments (**Fig. 13**A) whereas FGN fibrils should be thicker (see **Fig. 13**B). Immunotactoid glomerulonephritis is easily distinguished from amyloidosis: the deposits are noncongophilic and are composed of thick hollow microtubules or cylindrical structures, arranged in parallel arrays and ranging in size between 10 and 90 nm.[58]

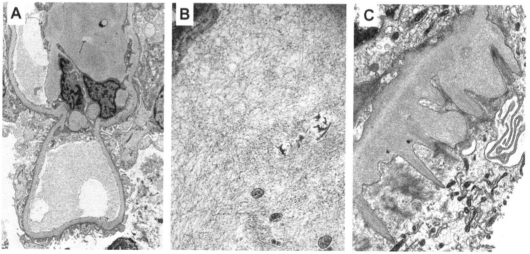

Fig. 12. Ultrastructural appearance of amyloid. (*A*) Low-magnification image showing mesangial expansion by cottony amyloid material. The peripheral capillaries are not involved (×6000). (*B*) On high magnification, amyloid deposits are composed of randomly oriented, nonbranching fibrils (×46,000). (*C*) Amyloid spicules develop as a result of parallel alignment of amyloid fibrils in the subepithelial space perpendicular to the glomerular basement membrane (×20,000).

Table 2
Histologic differential diagnosis of renal amyloidosis

Differential Diagnosis	Congo Red Stain	Light Microscopy	Immunofluorescence	Electron Microscopy
Light chain deposition disease	Negative	Mesangial matrix expansion, occasional nodule formation, PAS positive and argyrophilic, thick tubular basement membranes, crescents can be seen	Diffuse and dominant positive staining for 1 light chain (more kappa) involving mesangium, capillary loops (linear), vessels, and tubular basement membranes (linear)	Finely granular (punctate) electron dense deposits along the inner aspect of glomerular basement membranes and outer aspect of tubular basement membranes
FGN	Negative	Mesangial expansion and hypercellularity, PAS positive and nonargyrophilic, occasionally glomerular basement membrane duplication	Smudgy staining for IgG, C3, kappa, and lambda along glomerular capillary loops and mesangium	Randomly arranged fibrils with a size of 9–26 nm in diameter within mesangium, outer aspect of glomerular basement membranes and rarely in tubular basement membranes, spicules are exceptional
Immunotactoid glomerulonephritis	Negative	Variable mesangial expansion with thickened capillary loops, nonargyrophilic, might show mesangial proliferation with lobular accentuation or a membranous pattern	Smudgy to granular staining for IgG, C3, with light chain restriction (more kappa), staining mesangium and capillary loops	Hollow microtubular or cylindrical structure measuring 10–90 nm in diameter, arranged in parallel arrays, predominantly present within mesangium and subepithelial space
Diabetic glomerulosclerosis	Negative	Mesangial expansion with Kimmelstiel-Wilson nodules, intensely argyrophilic	Negative staining	Diabetic fibrillosis show fibrils of a size of 10–25 nm in diameter in the mesangium
Collagenofibrotic glomerulopathy	Negative	Increase in mesangial matrix, argyrophilic, occasional thickening of capillary loops	Negative staining	Curved, frayed, worm, comma-shaped fibrils, distinct periodicity from 43 to 65 nm
Fibronectin glomerulopathy	Negative	Mesangial expansion with no increase in cellularity, accentuation of lobular architecture, nonargyrophilic, and bright red on trichrome stain	Weak mesangial staining for IgG, IgM, and C3	Mesangial electron dense deposits, granular to fibrillary material, fibrils measures 14–16 nm in diameter

Other uncommon diseases that show fibrils on the ultrastructural level and may be confused with amyloidosis include fibronectin glomerulopathy and collagenofibrotic glomerulopathy, both of which share similar light microscopy findings with expanded mesangial matrix by nonargyrophilic deposits. On IF, fibronectin glomerulopathy shows bright staining for fibronectin and may exhibit weak glomerular staining for IgG, IgM, and C3. On EM, the deposits appear granular and/or fibrillar, with the fibrils measuring 14 to 16 in diameter. The presence of curved, worm-shaped, and comma-shaped fibrils with a periodicity of 43 to 65 nm is the hallmark of collagenofibrotic glomerulopathy, which can be confirmed by a positive immunohistochemical staining for type III collagen. Occasional cases of nodular diabetic glomerulosclerosis show mesangial expansion by nonargyrophilic matrix material, which on EM corresponds to randomly oriented precollagen fibrils measuring 10 to 25 nm in diameter.[49] This is referred to as *diabetic fibrillosis* and is distinguished from amyloidosis by its coexistence with typical diabetic mesangial sclerotic nodules, negativity for Congo red, restriction to the mesangium (without extending to the glomerular capillary walls), having shorter fibrils, and by showing linear staining of basement membranes for albumin and IgG with negativity for

light chains by IF. The interstitial amyloid fibrils in ALECT2 can readily be distinguished from collagen fibrils. The latter are much thicker (mean 65 nm) and show characteristic periodicity. Finally, in thrombotic microangiopathy, mesangial matrix collagen fibrils occasionally become accentuated in areas of mesangiolysis, which should not be interpreted as evidence of an infiltrative process.

AMYLOID TYPING (CLASSIFICATION)

Amyloid typing is not a trivial matter and misinterpretation may have profound consequences. It is crucial for assessing prognosis, genetic counseling, and initiating proper therapy.[59] The classification is based purely on the nature of the precursor plasma protein. The first step is direct IF, which is a convenient method for AL amyloid typing. IF is performed routinely on native kidney biopsies using fluorescein isothiocyanate (FITC)-labeled antibodies against IgG, IgM, IgA, kappa, and lambda light chains, which are directed against epitopes on the constant domains of these proteins.[29] In AL, there is a clear predominance and bright staining for 1 light chain in comparison to the other one (see **Fig. 10**). In AH, the deposits stain for a single subclass of Ig heavy chain without light chain (see **Fig. 11**), whereas a single heavy

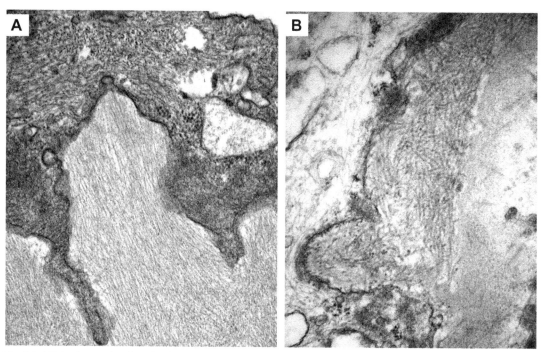

Fig. 13. (*A*) An internal point of reference for fibril thickness is the cellular filamentous cytoskeleton. This high-magnification image shows that the thickness of amyloid fibrils is comparable to the podocyte intracellular filaments (×49,000). (*B*) In contrast, the fibrils in FGN are thicker than the podocyte intracellular filaments (×46,000).

chain and a single light chain stain positive in cases of AHL.[29] In cases lacking frozen tissue, IF can be performed on pronase-digested, paraffin-embedded tissue, with excellent results.[60] The negativity of staining for Ig light chains or heavy chains suggest another type of amyloidosis, requiring further exploration using other modalities.

Immunohistochemistry using the IP technique can be performed for renal amyloid typing using commercially available antibodies against amyloid of the classes AL, AH, AA, AFib, ATTR, AApo AI, and Aβ2M.[29] Of these antibodies, serum amyloid A (SAA) IP on formalin-fixed, paraffin-embedded tissue is the most widely used and is considered the gold standard pathologic technique for diagnosing AA (**Fig. 14**). In general, IP is inferior to IF for diagnosing AL, AH, and AHL due to a higher background staining in the former.[12,29]

Despite the availability of IF and IP, they have multiple drawbacks, such as unavailability of antibodies to less common forms of amyloidosis as well as sensitivity and specificity of antibodies especially that they are designed against wild-type proteins. In cases of mutant protein or proteins with conformational changes, they might be less reactive.[29] In the vast majority of AL cases, the deposits are composed of the variable domain (VL) of the light chain, in particular VL VI,[61,62] but they also include a portion of the constant domain (CL) of the light chain.[63–65] In a minority of AL cases, due to light chain truncation, amyloid fibrils are composed of VL that is devoid of CL; therefore,

these proteins might not be reactive to commercial antibodies and hence a false negativity of IF.[54,66] For example, in renal AL, the amyloid deposits can be negative for both kappa and lambda in 7% to 35% of cases.[6,54,67] The authors' unpublished experience is that IF has a sensitivity of 82% and a specificity of 100% for diagnosing AL but has lower sensitivity and specificity for diagnosing AHL and AH. Thus, a negative or equivocal staining for light and/or heavy chain does not exclude AIg (see **Box 2**).[66,68] Amyloid typing by IF might also be difficult due to charge interaction of amyloid and the reagent antibody or contamination of the amyloid deposits by serum proteins, which result in a nonspecific false-positive staining.[68] This phenomenon is frequently observed in AA.[54,66,68,69] Up to 21% of renal AA cases show nonspecific IF staining for 1 or more Ig light chains and/or heavy chains.[6] False-positive staining for Ig light chains and/or heavy chains may also occur in renal ALECT2[24] but to a lesser extent than AA. Although rare, deposition of more than one type of amyloid protein can occur leading to difficulty in typing.[68,70–72]

PROTEOMICS

The direct method of amyloid demonstration is proteomics using LMD/MS, which has the capability for high throughput and identification of the entire proteome.[29] This new technique for amyloid typing has a high sensitivity and

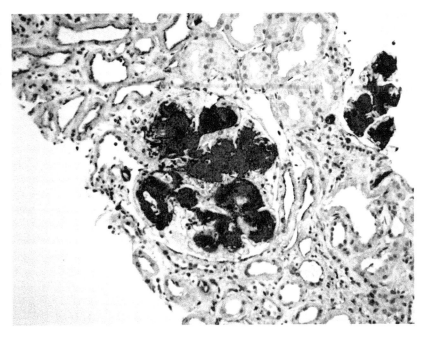

Fig. 14. Nodular glomerular amyloid deposits in this patient with AA secondary to rheumatoid arthritis show bright staining for SAA by immunohistochemistry (×400).

specificity and overcomes many of the problems presented by the other methods.[59,73] LMD/MS involves microdissecting the formalin-fixed, paraffin-embedded, Congo red–positive amyloid deposits under laser dissecting microscopy followed by tryptic digestion of the dissected material (**Fig. 15**A, B).[73] The digested peptides are then analyzed by liquid chromatography electrospray tandem mass spectrometry (see **Fig. 15**C).[73] Amyloid type identification is based on the presence of the peptide spectra that correspond to the specific type of amyloid. For example, in AL lambda, the deposits show large spectra of Ig lambda light chain with very small or absent spectra for kappa light chain.[59] In AH, there are large spectra of Ig heavy chain with very small or absent spectra for kappa and lambda light chains (see **Fig. 15**C).[74] In cases of ALECT2, there are large spectra for LECT2 protein.[59] The presence of serum amyloid P component (SAP) is essential for amyloid diagnosis on proteomic level.[59] In addition, large spectra of apolipoprotein E are typically seen in all forms of amyloidosis.[59]

The advantages of LMD/MS over the conventional methods of amyloid typing are as follows: (1) it is a single test that can identify the amyloid protein in question instead of testing for multiple proteins using IF or IP; (2) it is performed on formalin-fixed, paraffin-embedded tissue and there is no need for fresh frozen tissue or special tissue preservation; and, (3) certain types of amyloidosis, such as hereditary amyloidosis and ALECT2, are easier to diagnose by LMD/MS methodology than IF or IP. LMD/MS is not used routinely for the diagnosis and typing of renal amyloidosis because most cases affecting the kidney are AL that can be diagnosed with confidence by IF and because this technique is only available in few selected centers, such as the Mayo Clinic. In certain situations (listed in **Box 3**), however, LMD/MS is essential for amyloid typing and should be performed. Overall, LMD/MS is required for amyloid typing in 16% of cases of renal amyloidosis.[6]

TREATMENT AND OUTCOME

Patients with AIg are typically treated with chemotherapy. A regimen of melphalan-dexamethasone-bortezomib is used for patients with stage I and II cardiac involvement.[75,76] Patients with stage III cardiac involvement or advanced CKD are

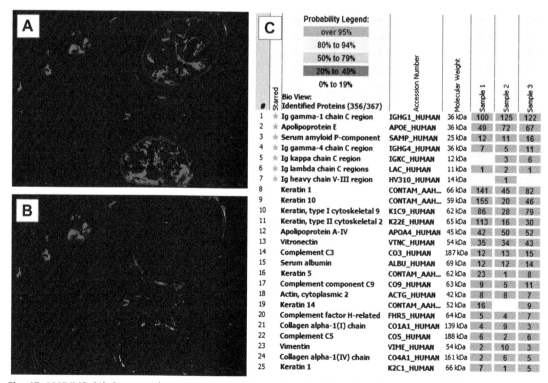

Probability Legend:
- over 95%
- 80% to 94%
- 50% to 79%
- 20% to 49%
- 0% to 19%

#	Starred	Bio View: Identified Proteins (356/367)	Accession Number	Molecular Weight	Sample 1	Sample 2	Sample 3
1	★	Ig gamma-1 chain C region	IGHG1_HUMAN	36 kDa	100	125	122
2	★	Apolipoprotein E	APOE_HUMAN	36 kDa	49	72	67
3	★	Serum amyloid P-component	SAMP_HUMAN	25 kDa	12	11	16
4	★	Ig gamma-4 chain C region	IGHG4_HUMAN	36 kDa	7	5	11
5	★	Ig kappa chain C region	IGKC_HUMAN	12 kDa		3	6
6	★	Ig lambda chain C regions	LAC_HUMAN	11 kDa	1	2	1
7	★	Ig heavy chain V-III region	HV310_HUMAN	14 kDa		1	
8		Keratin 1	CONTAM_AAH...	66 kDa	141	45	82
9		Keratin 10	CONTAM_AAH...	59 kDa	155	20	46
10		Keratin, type I cytoskeletal 9	K1C9_HUMAN	62 kDa	86	28	79
11		Keratin, type II cytoskeletal 2	K22E_HUMAN	65 kDa	113	16	30
12		Apolipoprotein A-IV	APOA4_HUMAN	45 kDa	42	50	52
13		Vitronectin	VTNC_HUMAN	54 kDa	35	34	43
14		Complement C3	CO3_HUMAN	187 kDa	12	13	15
15		Serum albumin	ALBU_HUMAN	69 kDa	12	12	14
16		Keratin 5	CONTAM_AAH...	62 kDa	23	1	8
17		Complement component C9	CO9_HUMAN	63 kDa	9	5	11
18		Actin, cytoplasmic 2	ACTG_HUMAN	42 kDa	8	8	7
19		Keratin 14	CONTAM_AAH...	52 kDa	16		9
20		Complement factor H-related	FHR5_HUMAN	64 kDa	5	4	7
21		Collagen alpha-1(I) chain	CO1A1_HUMAN	139 kDa	4	9	3
22		Complement C5	CO5_HUMAN	188 kDa	6	2	6
23		Vimentin	VIME_HUMAN	54 kDa	2	10	3
24		Collagen alpha-1(IV) chain	CO4A1_HUMAN	161 kDa	2	6	5
25		Keratin 1	K2C1_HUMAN	66 kDa	7	1	5

Fig. 15. LMD/MS. (*A*) Congo red–positive amyloid deposits marked for microdissection (×200). (*B*) Vacant space on slide after glomerular LMD (×200). (*C*) Scaffold readout showing the top 25 spectra in case of AH. There are large spectra for Ig gamma 1 constant region, SAP, and apolipoprotein E (>95% probability), with very small spectra for Ig kappa and lambda constant regions.

generally treated with cyclophosphamide-bortezomib-dexamethasone.[76,77] High-dose melphalan–autologous stem cell transplant is generally offered to patients with stage I or II cardiac involvement who have a GFR greater than or equal to 30 mL/min in the absence of advanced other organ failure.[76] The treatment of AA is directed toward the underlying condition, including antiinflammatory therapy, antibiotics, or surgery. Patients with hereditary amyloidosis, including those with AFib, ATTR, and AApo AI, in whom the liver is the source of precursor protein, are treated with liver transplantation. Thus far, there is no specific therapy for ALECT2.

The prognosis of amyloidosis varies but generally it is poor if the disease is untreated. Patients with AL have the worst prognosis, with a median overall survival of 1 to 2 years, and the prognosis depends on the extent of organ involvement.[2,78] Cardiac involvement is an independent negative predictor of patient survival in AL and AA.[79] The median survival for AL is 16 months when it occurs in combination with multiple myeloma.[79] AA, AH, AHL, AFib, and ALECT2 have longer overall survival compared with AL, largely due to a lower frequency of cardiac involvement.[12,16,24,31,79] For AA type, the median survival is reported between 2 and 10 years,[13,79,80] whereas the median survival for AFib is 15 years.[16]

REFERENCES

1. Merlini G, Bellotti V. Molecular mechanisms of amyloidosis. N Engl J Med 2003;349:583–96.
2. Kyle RA, Linos A, Beard CM, et al. Incidence and natural history of primary systemic amyloidosis in Olmsted County, Minnesota, 1950 through 1989. Blood 1992;79:1817–22.
3. Kyle RA, Gertz MA. Primary systemic amyloidosis: clinical and laboratory features in 474 cases. Semin Hematol 1995;32:45–59.
4. Tuglular S, Yalcinkaya F, Paydas S, et al. A retrospective analysis for aetiology and clinical findings of 287 secondary amyloidosis cases in Turkey. Nephrol Dial Transplant 2002;17:2003–5.
5. Rivera F, Lopez-Gomez JM, Perez-Garcia R. Frequency of renal pathology in Spain 1994-1999. Nephrol Dial Transplant 2002;17:1594–602.
6. Said SM, Sethi S, Valeri AM, et al. Renal amyloidosis: origin and clinicopathologic correlations of 474 recent cases. Clin J Am Soc Nephrol 2013;8: 1515–23.
7. von Hutten H, Mihatsch M, Lobeck H, et al. Prevalence and origin of amyloid in kidney biopsies. Am J Surg Pathol 2009;33:1198–205.
8. Larsen CP, Walker PD, Weiss DT, et al. Prevalence and morphology of leukocyte chemotactic factor 2-associated amyloid in renal biopsies. Kidney Int 2010;77:816–9.
9. Bergesio F, Ciciani AM, Santostefano M, et al. Renal involvement in systemic amyloidosis–an Italian retrospective study on epidemiological and clinical data at diagnosis. Nephrol Dial Transplant 2007;22:1608–18.
10. Eulitz M, Weiss DT, Solomon A. Immunoglobulin heavy-chain-associated amyloidosis. Proc Natl Acad Sci U S A 1990;87:6542–6.
11. Nasr SH, Colvin R, Markowitz GS. IgG1 lambda light and heavy chain renal amyloidosis. Kidney Int 2006;70:7.
12. Nasr SH, Said SM, Valeri AM, et al. The diagnosis and characteristics of renal heavy-chain and heavy/light-chain amyloidosis and their comparison with renal light-chain amyloidosis. Kidney Int 2013; 83:463–70.
13. Gertz MA, Kyle RA. Secondary systemic amyloidosis: response and survival in 64 patients. Medicine (Baltimore) 1991;70:246–56.
14. Strege RJ, Saeger W, Linke RP. Diagnosis and immunohistochemical classification of systemic amyloidoses. Report of 43 cases in an unselected autopsy series. Virchows Arch 1998;433:19–27.
15. Verine J, Mourad N, Desseaux K, et al. Clinical and histological characteristics of renal AA amyloidosis: a retrospective study of 68 cases with a special interest to amyloid-associated inflammatory response. Hum Pathol 2007;38:1798–809.
16. Gillmore JD, Lachmann HJ, Rowczenio D, et al. Diagnosis, pathogenesis, treatment, and prognosis of hereditary fibrinogen A alpha-chain amyloidosis. J Am Soc Nephrol 2009;20:444–51.
17. Maury CP. Homozygous familial amyloidosis, Finnish type: demonstration of glomerular gelsolin-derived amyloid and non-amyloid tubular gelsolin. Clin Nephrol 1993;40:53–6.

18. Pepys MB, Hawkins PN, Booth DR, et al. Human lysozyme gene mutations cause hereditary systemic amyloidosis. Nature 1993;362:553–7.

19. Soutar AK, Hawkins PN, Vigushin DM, et al. Apolipoprotein AI mutation Arg-60 causes autosomal dominant amyloidosis. Proc Natl Acad Sci U S A 1992;89:7389–93.

20. Benson MD, Liepnieks JJ, Yazaki M, et al. A new human hereditary amyloidosis: the result of a stop-codon mutation in the apolipoprotein AII gene. Genomics 2001;72:272–7.

21. Sethi S, Theis JD, Shiller SM, et al. Medullary amyloidosis associated with apolipoprotein A-IV deposition. Kidney Int 2012;81:201–6.

22. Benson MD, James S, Scott K, et al. Leukocyte chemotactic factor 2: A novel renal amyloid protein. Kidney Int 2008;74:218–22.

23. Dogan A, Theis JD, Vrana JA, et al. Clinical and pathological phenotype of leukocyte cell-derived chemo- taxin-2 (LECT2) amyloidosis (ALECT2). Amyloid 2010;17(Suppl 1):69–70 [abstract: OP-058].

24. Said SM, Sethi S, Valeri AM, et al. Characterization and outcomes of renal leukocyte chemotactic factor 2-associated amyloidosis. Kidney Int 2014 Jan 22. http://dx.doi.org/10.1038/ki.2013. 558. [Epub ahead of print].

25. Khalighi MA, Yue A, Hwang M, et al. Leukocyte chemotactic factor 2 (LECT2) amyloidosis presenting as pulmonary-renal syndrome: a case report and review of the literature. Clin Kidney J 2013;6:618–21.

26. Kapoor P, Thenappan T, Singh E, et al. Cardiac amyloidosis: a practical approach to diagnosis and management. Am J Med 2011;124:1006–15.

27. Carone FA, Epstein FH. Nephrogenic diabetes insipidus caused by amyloid disease. Evidence in man of the role of the collecting ducts in concentrating urine. Am J Med 1960;29:539–44.

28. Gregorini G, Izzi C, Obici L, et al. Renal apolipoprotein A-I amyloidosis: a rare and usually ignored cause of hereditary tubulointerstitial nephritis. J Am Soc Nephrol 2005;16:3680–6.

29. Leung N, Nasr SH, Sethi S. How I treat amyloidosis: the importance of accurate diagnosis and amyloid typing. Blood 2012;120:3206–13.

30. Hopfer H, Wiech T, Mihatsch MJ. Renal amyloidosis revisited: amyloid distribution, dynamics and biochemical type. Nephrol Dial Transplant 2011; 26:2877–84.

31. Murphy CL, Wang S, Kestler D, et al. Leukocyte chemotactic factor 2 (LECT2)-associated renal amyloidosis: a case series. Am J Kidney Dis 2010;56:1100–7.

32. Lachmann HJ, Goodman HJ, Gilbertson JA, et al. Natural history and outcome in systemic AA amyloidosis. N Engl J Med 2007;356:2361–71.

33. Eirin A, Irazabal MV, Gertz MA, et al. Clinical features of patients with immunoglobulin light chain amyloidosis (AL) with vascular-limited deposition in the kidney. Nephrol Dial Transplant 2012;27: 1097–101.

34. Sawaya MR, Sambashivan S, Nelson R, et al. Atomic structures of amyloid cross-beta spines reveal varied steric zippers. Nature 2007;447:453–7.

35. Bellotti V, Merlini G, Bucciarelli E, et al. Relevance of class, molecular weight and isoelectric point in predicting human light chain amyloidogenicity. Br J Haematol 1990;74:65–9.

36. Hurle MR, Helms LR, Li L, et al. A role for destabilizing amino acid replacements in light-chain amyloidosis. Proc Natl Acad Sci U S A 1994;91: 5446–50.

37. McLaurin J, Yang D, Yip CM, et al. Review: modulating factors in amyloid-beta fibril formation. J Struct Biol 2000;130:259–70.

38. Verdone G, Corazza A, Viglino P, et al. The solution structure of human beta2-microglobulin reveals the prodromes of its amyloid transition. Protein Sci 2002;11:487–99.

39. Yamagoe S, Yamakawa Y, Matsuo Y, et al. Purification and primary amino acid sequence of a novel neutrophil chemotactic factor LECT2. Immunol Lett 1996;52:9–13.

40. Lu XJ, Chen J, Yu CH, et al. LECT2 protects mice against bacterial sepsis by activating macrophages via the CD209a receptor. J Exp Med 2013;210:5–13.

41. Okumura A, Saito T, Otani I, et al. Suppressive role of leukocyte cell-derived chemotaxin 2 in mouse anti-type II collagen antibody-induced arthritis. Arthritis Rheum 2008;58:413–21.

42. Benson MD. LECT2 amyloidosis. Kidney Int 2010; 77:757–9.

43. Saraiva MJ. Transthyretin amyloidosis: a tale of weak interactions. FEBS Lett 2001;498:201–3.

44. Dember LM. Amyloidosis-associated kidney disease. J Am Soc Nephrol 2006;17:3458–71.

45. Scholefield Z, Yates EA, Wayne G, et al. Heparan sulfate regulates amyloid precursor protein processing by BACE1, the Alzheimer's beta-secretase. J Cell Biol 2003;163:97–107.

46. Zhu H, Yu J, Kindy MS. Inhibition of amyloidosis using low-molecular-weight heparins. Mol Med 2001; 7:517–22.

47. Teng J, Russell WJ, Gu X, et al. Different types of glomerulopathic light chains interact with mesangial cells using a common receptor but exhibit different intracellular trafficking patterns. Lab Invest 2004;84:440–51.

48. Teng J, Turbat-Herrera EA, Herrera GA. Role of translational research advancing the understanding of the pathogenesis of light chain-mediated glomerulopathies. Pathol Int 2007;57:398–412.

49. Herrera GA, Turbat-Herrera EA. Renal diseases with organized deposits: an algorithmic approach

to classification and clinicopathologic diagnosis. Arch Pathol Lab Med 2010;134:512–31.

50. Shiiki H, Shimokama T, Yoshikawa Y, et al. Renal amyloidosis. Correlations between morphology, chemical types of amyloid protein and clinical features. Virchows Arch A Pathol Anat Histopathol 1988;412:197–204.

51. Nagata M, Shimokama T, Harada A, et al. Glomerular crescents in renal amyloidosis: an epiphenomenon or distinct pathology? Pathol Int 2001;51:179–86.

52. Masutani K, Nagata M, Ikeda H, et al. Glomerular crescent formation in renal amyloidosis. A clinicopathological study and demonstration of upregulated cell-mediated immunity. Clin Nephrol 2008; 70:464–74.

53. Howie AJ, Brewer DB. Optical properties of amyloid stained by Congo red: history and mechanisms. Micron 2009;40:285–301.

54. Picken MM. Immunoglobulin light and heavy chain amyloidosis AL/AH: renal pathology and differential diagnosis. Contrib Nephrol 2007;153:135–55.

55. Puchtler H, Sweat F. Congo red as a stain for fluorescence microscopy of amyloid. J Histochem Cytochem 1965;13:693–4.

56. Koike H, Misu K, Sugiura M, et al. Pathology of early- vs late-onset TTR Met30 familial amyloid polyneuropathy. Neurology 2004;63:129–38.

57. Nasr SH, Valeri AM, Cornell LD, et al. Fibrillary glomerulonephritis: a report of 66 cases from a single institution. Clin J Am Soc Nephrol 2011;6:775–84.

58. Nasr SH, Fidler ME, Cornell LD, et al. Immunotactoid glomerulopathy: clinicopathologic and proteomic study. Nephrol Dial Transplant 2012;27:4137–46.

59. Sethi S, Vrana JA, Theis JD, et al. Laser microdissection and mass spectrometry-based proteomics aids the diagnosis and typing of renal amyloidosis. Kidney Int 2012;82:226–34.

60. Nasr SH, Galgano SJ, Markowitz GS, et al. Immunofluorescence on pronase-digested paraffin sections: a valuable salvage technique for renal biopsies. Kidney Int 2006;70:2148–51.

61. Solomon A, Frangione B, Franklin EC. Bence Jones proteins and light chains of immunoglobulins. Preferential association of the V lambda VI subgroup of human light chains with amyloidosis AL (lambda). J Clin Invest 1982;70:453–60.

62. Glenner GG. Amyloid deposits and amyloidosis. The beta-fibrilloses (first of two parts). N Engl J Med 1980;302:1283–92.

63. Olsen KE, Sletten K, Westermark P. Fragments of the constant region of immunoglobulin light chains are constituents of AL-amyloid proteins. Biochem Biophys Res Commun 1998;251:642–7.

64. Klimtchuk ES, Gursky O, Patel RS, et al. The critical role of the constant region in thermal stability and aggregation of amyloidogenic immunoglobulin light chain. Biochemistry 2010;49:9848–57.

65. Engvig JP, Olsen KE, Gislefoss RE, et al. Constant region of a kappa III immunoglobulin light chain as a major AL-amyloid protein. Scand J Immunol 1998;48:92–8.

66. Satoskar AA, Burdge K, Cowden DJ, et al. Typing of amyloidosis in renal biopsies: diagnostic pitfalls. Arch Pathol Lab Med 2007;131:917–22.

67. Novak L, Cook WJ, Herrera GA, et al. AL-amyloidosis is underdiagnosed in renal biopsies. Nephrol Dial Transplant 2004;19:3050–3.

68. Kebbel A, Rocken C. Immunohistochemical classification of amyloid in surgical pathology revisited. Am J Surg Pathol 2006;30:673–83.

69. D'Agati VD, Jennette JC, Silva FG. Atlas of Nontumor Pathology: Non-Neoplastic Kidney Diseases. Washington (DC): American Registry of Pathology-Armed Forces Institute of Pathology; 2005. p. 189–237.

70. Sakata N, Hoshii Y, Nakamura T, et al. Colocalization of apolipoprotein AI in various kinds of systemic amyloidosis. J Histochem Cytochem 2005;53:237–42.

71. Picken MM, Herrera GA. The burden of "sticky" amyloid: typing challenges. Arch Pathol Lab Med 2007;131:850–1.

72. Comenzo RL, Zhou P, Fleisher M, et al. Seeking confidence in the diagnosis of systemic AL (Ig light-chain) amyloidosis: patients can have both monoclonal gammopathies and hereditary amyloid proteins. Blood 2006;107:3489–91.

73. Vrana JA, Gamez JD, Madden BJ, et al. Classification of amyloidosis by laser microdissection and mass spectrometry-based proteomic analysis in clinical biopsy specimens. Blood 2009;114:4957–9.

74. Sethi S, Theis JD, Leung N, et al. Mass spectrometry-based proteomic diagnosis of renal immunoglobulin heavy chain amyloidosis. Clin J Am Soc Nephrol 2010;5:2180–7.

75. Reece DE, Sanchorawala V, Hegenbart U, et al. Weekly and twice-weekly bortezomib in patients with systemic AL amyloidosis: results of a phase 1 dose-escalation study. Blood 2009;114:1489–97.

76. Fermand JP, Bridoux F, Kyle RA, et al. How I treat monoclonal gammopathy of renal significance (MGRS). Blood 2013;122:3583–90.

77. Venner CP, Lane T, Foard D, et al. Cyclophosphamide, bortezomib, and dexamethasone therapy in AL amyloidosis is associated with high clonal response rates and prolonged progression-free survival. Blood 2012;119:4387–90.

78. Falk RH, Comenzo RL, Skinner M. The systemic amyloidoses. N Engl J Med 1997;337:898–909.

79. Bergesio F, Ciciani AM, Manganaro M, et al. Renal involvement in systemic amyloidosis: an Italian collaborative study on survival and renal outcome. Nephrol Dial Transplant 2008;23:941–51.

80. Joss N, McLaughlin K, Simpson K, et al. Presentation, survival and prognostic markers in AA amyloidosis. QJM 2000;93:535–42.

Classification Systems in Renal Pathology
Promises and Problems

M. Barry Stokes, MD

KEYWORDS

- Kidney disease • Renal biopsy • Pathologic classification

ABSTRACT

Kidney diseases are morphologically heterogeneous. Pathologic classifications of renal disease permit standardization of diagnosis and may identify clinical-pathologic subgroups with different outcomes and/or responses to treatment. To date, classifications have been proposed for lupus nephritis, allograft rejection, IgA nephropathy, focal segmental glomerulosclerosis, antineutrophil cytoplasmic antibody -related glomerulonephritis, and diabetic glomerulosclerosis. These classifications share several limitations related to lack of specificity, reproducibility, validation, and relevance to clinical practice. They offer a standardized approach to diagnosis, however, which should facilitate communication and clinical research.

OVERVIEW

Since the introduction of the kidney biopsy to nephrology practice in the 1950s, pathologic diagnosis has played a central role in defining the spectrum of medical kidney diseases and guiding patient management. It was quickly noted that kidney diseases are morphologically heterogeneous, with variable acute (inflammatory) and chronic (fibrosing and sclerosing) lesions that might contribute to the diverse clinical manifestations and variable outcomes in individual patients with the same disease. This observation led to the introduction of semiquantitative grading of pathologic findings and the development of morphologic classifications of renal disease, beginning with the original World Health Organization (WHO) classification of LN in 1974.[1] Morphologic classifications have since been proposed for renal allograft rejection,[2] IgA nephropathy,[3,4] FSGS,[5] diabetic nephropathy,[6] and pauci-immune glomerulonephritis.[7] This review considers the strengths and weaknesses of these pathologic classifications in relationship to clinical practice.

PATHOLOGIC CLASSIFICATION: GOALS AND GENERAL LIMITATIONS

Key Features
GENERAL PROBLEMS WITH RENAL PATHOLOGIC CLASSIFICATIONS

- Pathologic criteria based on expert opinion, not empiric evidence.

- Independence of clinical variables not demonstrated

- Nonspecificity of pathologic findings

- Variable reproducibility

- Imperfect validation studies

The primary goal of any pathologic classification is to identify subgroups of disease that have different natural histories and/or responses to therapy.

Funding Source: None.
Conflict of Interest: None.
Department of Pathology, Columbia University College of Physicians and Surgeons, 630 West 168th Street, VC14-224, New York, NY 10032, USA
E-mail address: Mbs2101@columbia.edu

Surgical Pathology 7 (2014) 427–441
http://dx.doi.org/10.1016/j.path.2014.04.007

surgpath.theclinics.com

Standardization of pathologic diagnosis is also important for communication and research. An ideal pathologic classification should be biologically plausible and clinically relevant, applicable to all subjects with the disease, reproducible and easy to use, and validated in independent studies. For kidney diseases, morphologic categories should predict clinical outcomes independently of other variables that are known to influence outcome, such as age, race, disease severity, and therapy. Finally, the classification system should be updated periodically, to incorporate new discoveries from clinical and experimental research.

All of the current pathologic classifications of kidney disease suffer from several limitations, including nonspecificity of pathologic findings, inconsistent reproducibility, lack of an external standard to verify pathologic diagnoses, and validation problems. The causes and pathogenesis of most renal diseases are poorly understood but are clearly multifactorial, involving a host of genetic predisposing factors and environmental triggers, which are not the same in all populations. The reproducibility of pathologic classifications is less than perfect,[8–11] reflecting the subjectivity of pathologic diagnosis, even for clearly defined pathologic variables. Sampling error is a problem in small biopsy specimens, and many disease processes have focal or patchy tissue involvement. In addition, segmental lesions (involving less than the entire glomerular tuft) may be missed due to the random orientation of the glomerulus in individual tissue sections. Moreover, exhaustive tissue sectioning is not feasible in routine diagnostic practice. Most pathologic classifications are heuristic, relying on expert opinion rather than empiric or experimental evidence. With the notable exception of the Oxford classification of IgA nephropathy,[3,4] the prognostic significance of pathologic variables has not been shown independent of clinical covariates. In addition, the Oxford classification is the only glomerular disease classification that scores tubulointerstitial lesions, which, together with vascular lesions, have been shown to have predictive value.[12–14] Lastly, morphologic classifications do not include information from genetic, transcriptomosal, and proteomic studies, which might better illuminate the underlying pathogenetic mechanisms.[15]

Glomerular diseases are uncommon and progress slowly and the development of end-stage renal disease (ESRD) is influenced by multiple variables, including demographic and socioeconomic factors (reflecting genetic risk factors and access to medical care), clinical disease severity, presence of comorbid conditions (eg, diabetes and hypertension), and choice of treatment. Therefore, studies with sufficient power to identify the prognostic significance of pathologic variants are difficult to accomplish. In addition, retrospective validation studies are subject to biases, including case selection criteria and choice of therapy, and which limits their generalizability. For individual patients with glomerular disease, morphologic variants have limited relevance to clinical management, with the exception of broad categories, such as proliferative LN.

With these caveats in mind, the individual pathologic classifications of renal disease are reviewed.

LUPUS NEPHRITIS

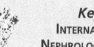

Key Features
INTERNATIONAL SOCIETY OF NEPHROLOGY/RENAL PATHOLOGY SOCIETY LUPUS NEPHRITIS CLASSIFICATION

- Definitions are not evidence based
- Improved reproducibility compared with earlier classifications
- Definition of segmental lesions requires further study
- Tubulointerstitial and vascular lesions are not incorporated
- Does not include nonimmune complex–mediated glomerular disease

The 2003 International Society of Nephrology (ISN)/Renal Pathology Society (RPS) classification of LN[16] is based on the original 1974 WHO classification,[1] which was previously updated in 1982[17] and 1995.[18] This classification is predicated on the presence of glomerular immune deposits by immunofluorescence microscopy and is categorized based on the light microscopic findings, with a minimum sample size of 10 glomeruli (Table 1). Mesangial LN is subdivided into class I (minimal mesangial) and class II (mesangial), depending on the absence or presence of histologically identifiable mesangial expansion. Class III (focal) and IV (diffuse) LN are distinguished based on the percentage of glomeruli demonstrating endocapillary and/or extracapillary proliferative lesions (<50% or ≥50%, respectively). Sclerotic glomeruli representing scarred LN are included in the count of proliferative lesions. Class III and class IV are categorized as purely active (A), mixed (A + C), or purely chronic (C). Class IV is further subclassified into segmental (S) or global categories (G), based

Table 1
ISN/RPS (2003) classification of lupus nephritis

Class I	Minimal mesangial LN
Class II	Mesangial proliferative LN
Class III	Focal LN (<50% of glomeruli) III (A): active lesions III (A/C): active and chronic lesions III (C): chronic lesions
Class IV	Diffuse LN (50% of glomeruli) Diffuse segmental (IV-S) or global (IV-G) LN IV (Λ): active lesions IV (A/C): active and chronic lesions IV (C): chronic lesions
Class V	Membranous LN
Class VI	Advanced sclerosing LN (90% globally sclerosed glomeruli without residual activity)

Adapted from Weening JJ, D'Agati VD, Schwartz MM, et al. The classification of glomerulonephritis in systemic lupus erythematosus revisited. Kidney Int 2004;65(2):525, Table 3; with permission from Macmillan Publishers Ltd.

on whether the lesions are predominantly segmental or global (ie, involving <50% or ≥50% of the glomerular tuft, respectively). The criteria for diagnosing membranous (class V) LN, alone or superimposed on class III or IV LN, are clearly defined. Class VI (advanced-stage LN) is defined as greater than or equal to 90% global glomerulosclerosis attributable to LN, provided that there is no residual activity.

Compared with the earlier WHO classifications, the ISN/RPS classification has shown improved interobserver reproducibility, due to more precise definition of each class of LN.[10,19,20] The percentage of class IV cases increased from 23% by the WHO 1982 classification to 46% by the ISN/RPS classification, with fewer diagnoses of class III and class V, due to the elimination of class Vd membranous LN and the inclusion of sclerotic glomeruli in calculating the total number of glomeruli affected. At least 1 study found poor interobserver agreement (intraclass correlation coefficient<0.2) for the ISN/RPS classification when a study set of 126 biopsies were reviewed independently by a group of 5 specialized renal pathologists without knowledge of the clinical status, but agreement was readily forthcoming when the pathologists met as a group.[20] The investigators speculated that the low initial reproducibility might have reflected inclusion of small samples with variable technical quality. The inclusion of modifiers reflecting activity (A) and chronicity (C) has been shown more predictive of outcomes in the ISN/RPS classification.[21]

The LN classes and pathologic characteristics were never formally tested for reproducibility or independent prognostic significance, although collective experience and subsequent validation studies[19,22] strongly suggest that these classes behave differently. Classes I and II are typically associated with asymptomatic disease or mild clinical features (eg, microscopic hematuria and subnephrotic proteinuria), class III and IV usually have more severe, nephritic features (acute renal insufficiency, hematuria and more proteinuria), whereas class V has the highest rate of nephrotic syndrome. The distinction between class III and class IV, however, based on 50% glomerular involvement, lacks a clearcut biologic basis. This distinction has the merit of simplicity but implies a continuum of disease severity from focal to diffuse glomerular involvement. Given the vagaries of sampling, however, it is difficult to conceive how a patient whose renal biopsy shows endocapillary hypercellularity in 5 of 10 glomeruli (class IV) has a more aggressive disease than one whose biopsy has proliferative lesions in 9 of 20 glomeruli (class III). In clinical practice, this distinction may not be meaningful, because the current treatment guidelines for treating class III and class IV disease are identical.[23–25]

A more important marker of biologic difference in severe LN might be the distinction of cases with predominantly necrotizing and crescentic lesions, which may be focal or diffuse and segmental or global (ie, involving >50% of the tuft). The Collaborative Study Group clinical trial reported worse outcomes for cases of severe LN with predominantly segmental lessons,[26] and 1 validation study using the ISN/RPS classification showed a trend to wore outcomes in cases of IV-S compared with IV-G.[19] Several other studies, however, found similar or worse outcomes in IV-G cases.[20–22,27–31] Thus, although cases of IV-G and IV-S may have different clinical presenting features their overall outcome is similar, which undercuts the rationale for making this distinction. The Collaborative Study, however, used a different definition of segmental (<90% tuft involvement) than the ISN/RPS classification (<50% tuft involvement), and, therefore, the ISN/RPS definitions may inadvertently minimize important pathologic and prognostic differences between subgroups of diffuse LN.[32] Thus, the definition of segmental lesions in the ISN-RPS classification may need to be reevaluated with this possibility in mind.

Another limitation of the ISN/RPS classification is that it is restricted to immune complex–mediated glomerulonephritis (the most common manifestation of glomerular disease in systemic lupus erythematosus [SLE]). Other pathologic entities, however, such as thrombotic microangiopathy,[13,33] nonimmune complex–mediated podocytopathy,[34,35] pauci-immune necrotizing and crescentic glomerulonephritis,[36] and collapsing glomerulopathy,[37,38] also cause kidney disease in some patients with SLE. In addition, grading of tubulointerstitial and vascular lesions, although strongly recommended, is not a part of the classification, even though these variables have a significant impact on outcome, irrespective of glomerular disease class.[12,14,33,39]

In summary, the ISN/RPS classification of LN remains one of the most successful and broadly accepted pathologic classifications, as evidenced by its inclusion in recent treatment guidelines issued by both the American College of Rheumatology[23] and the European League Against Rheumatism[24,25] for the management of SLE. Ongoing areas of study include the definition of segmental lesions, the role of activity and chronicity indices, and the use of immunofluorescence and electron microscopic findings to refine the diagnosis and broaden the spectrum of renal disease in patients with SLE.

RENAL ALLOGRAFT REJECTION

The first systematic classification of renal allograft pathology emerged from a 1991 meeting of a group of nephrologists, nephropathologists, and transplant surgeons in Banff, Alberta, Canada.[2] Since then, the Banff study group has met every 2 years and has issued multiple revisions and updates to the original classification, reflecting new pathogenetic insights. A separate classification, based on Banff, was developed by investigators in the National Institutes of Health–sponsored Cooperative Clinical Trials in Transplantation[40] and subsequently merged into the Banff 1997 revision. Details of the Banff classification schema are beyond the scope of this article and are reviewed by Troxell and colleagues elsewhere in this issue. Similar to the ISN/RPS classification of LN, the Banff classification has been broadly adopted worldwide and plays a major role in patient management and in the study of renal allograft disease.

The strengths of the Banff classification include that pathologic lesions of acute and chronic rejection have been verified in clinical studies[41,42] and experimental models,[43] confirming their biologic and clinical relevance. The biannual meetings facilitate consensus-based updates and help identify areas needing more study, thus ensuring that the classification continually reflects the best available knowledge.

The major limits of the Banff classification include lack of specificity and sensitivity of the pathologic criteria, the absence of a nonpathologic external standard for confirming the diagnosis of rejection, and variable reproducibility. Rejection is a patchy, focal process and thus subject to sampling error. Tubulitis and interstitial inflammation, the hallmarks of cell-mediated rejection, may also result from ischemia, infection, and drug allergies. Endarteritis, however, is relatively specific for rejection but may result from both T cell–mediated and antibody-mediated rejection,[44,45] which require different treatment. In the past, only severe endarteritis (v3) was considered a feature of antibody-mediated rejection whereas mild and moderate endarteritis (v1 and v2) were attributed to T cell–mediated rejection. There is growing evidence, however, that v1 and v2 endarteritis lesions may also result from antibody-mediated injury, as evidenced by their association with donor-specific antibodies (DSAs) to HLA antigens,[44] and gene expression of antibody-mediated rejection transcripts by microarray analysis.[46] The molecular phenotype identified by microarray analysis may correlate better with graft dysfunction than morphologic changes.[46] Studies have also shown that many cases of antibody-mediated rejection are C4d negative and may be misclassified using Banff criteria, leading to under-recognition and failure to treat appropriately.[44] In addition, de novo DSAs, although associated with worse long-term graft survival, are not always accompanied by antibody-mediated rejection[47] and not all cases of C4d positive rejection are accompanied by DSAs.[48] Similarly, tubulointerstitial scarring and chronic arterial disease may result from both alloimmune[49] and nonalloimmune mechanisms, including drug toxicity, infection, aging, and hypertension.

Intraobserver reproducibility (based on kappa statistics) for the Banff criteria is generally good or excellent but interobserver variability tends to be high,[9] which limits comparison of studies from different centers. The absence of an independent standard to diagnose rejection is another major drawback.[50] Urinary mRNA markers[51] and gene transcript microarrays[46] may provide more detailed insights into pathogenesis but the broad use of these techniques is limited by cost, availability, the need for inter-laboratory standardization, and the ongoing need for pathologic confirmation of the diagnosis of rejection. In conclusion, it is likely that the Banff classification will remain the gold standard for classifying renal allograft rejection in the foreseeable future.

FOCAL SEGMENTAL GLOMERULOSCLEROSIS

> ### Key Features
> #### COLUMBIA CLASSIFICATION OF FSGS
>
> - Derived from expert opinion, not evidence based
> - Applicable to primary and secondary forms of FSGS
> - Poor reproducibility for cellular variant
> - Primary collapsing and tip lesion variants have distinct outcomes
> - Tubulointerstitial and vascular lesions are not incorporated.

FSGS is not a single disease but a pattern of injury defined by segmental glomerular accumulation of extracellular matrix and/or hyaline. FSGS lesions are morphologically heterogeneous with respect to their location within the glomerular tuft and may also show features of endo- or extracapillary hypercellularity and capillary collapse. The Columbia classification of FSGS (**Table 2**) uses a stepwise, hierarchical approach to define 5 mutually exclusive morphologic variants of FSGS: collapsing, tip, cellular, perihilar, and not otherwise specified (NOS). This schema may be applied to both primary and secondary forms of FSGS. Several studies from around the world have shown that morphologic variants of primary FSGS have distinctive clinical presenting features and outcomes.[52–54]

All cases of FSGS seem to involve podocyte injury and/or loss (podocytopenia), which may result from diverse causes and pathogenetic mechanisms, including circulating permeability factors, genetic mutations, viruses, drugs, hyperfiltration, and progression of other kidney diseases.[55] The causes of most cases of FSGS identified by renal biopsy are, however, unknown (idiopathic or primary FSGS). A recent study identified elevated serum levels of soluble urokinase-type plasminogen activator (suPAR) in a majority of patients with primary FSGS; however, elevated suPAR levels have also been reported in cases of secondary FSGS.[56]

Table 2
Columbia classification variants of FSGS

Variant	Inclusion Criteria	Exclusion Criteria
FSGS (NOS)	At least 1 glomerulus with segmental increase in matrix obliterating the capillary lumina. There may be segmental glomerular capillary wall collapse *without* overlying podocyte hyperplasia.	Exclude perihilar, cellular, tip, and collapsing variants
Perihilar variant	At least 1 glomerulus with perihilar hyalinosis, with or without sclerosis >50% of glomeruli with segmental lesions must have perihilar sclerosis and/or hyalinosis.	Exclude cellular, tip, and collapsing variants
Cellular variant	At least 1 glomerulus with segmental endocapillary hypercellularity occluding lumina, with or without foam cells and karyorrhexis.	Exclude tip and collapsing variants
Tip variant	At least 1 segmental lesion involving the tip domain (outer 25% of tuft next to origin of proximal tubule). The tubular pole must be identified in the defining lesion. The lesion must have either an adhesion or confluence of podocytes with parietal or tubular cells at the tubular lumen or neck. The tip lesion may be cellular or sclerosing.	Exclude collapsing variant and any perihilar sclerosis
Collapsing variant	At least 1 glomerulus with segmental or global collapse *and* overlying podocyte hypertrophy and hyperplasia.	None

From D'Agati VD, Fogo AB, Bruijn JA, et al. Pathologic classification of focal segmental glomerulosclerosis: a working proposal. Am J Kidney Dis 2004;43(2):371, Table 3; with permission from Elsevier.

The major strength of the Columbia classification is that it provides clear definitions and a systematic, hierarchical approach that permits categorization of cases containing multiple different types of lesion, which is not uncommon in FSGS. In addition, it encompasses podocytopathies that have predominantly collapsing or cellular characteristics, in addition to those with purely sclerosing features. Several clinical studies have demonstrated significant clinical and prognostic differences among these variants of primary FSGS.[52–54] Collapsing variant predominantly affects individuals of African descent whereas tip variant is more commonly seen in older whites. Collapsing and tip variants have the heaviest initial proteinuria but collapsing variant has the highest initial serum creatinine and the worst prognosis, with lowest rates of remission and highest rate of ESRD. By comparison, tip variant tends to have the best outcomes, despite similarly high levels of proteinuria at initial presentation.

A major criticism of the Columbia classification is that FSGS is not a single disease but may result from diverse causes and pathogenetic pathways, which may be more important determinants of outcome than the morphologic variant. Collapsing FSGS may be primary or secondary to viruses (HIV[57] and parvovirus B19[58]), hemophagocytic syndrome,[59] pamidronate therapy,[60] interferon therapy,[61] and acute vasoocclusive disease.[62] In African Americans with HIV infection[63] and SLE,[38] collapsing variant has been associated with apolipoprotein (APO)-L1 risk alleles. Most cases of tip variant are primary but tip lesions may also occur in other glomerular diseases, such as diabetic nephropathy,[64] preeclampsia, and membranous glomerulonephritis,[65] perhaps reflecting podocyte injury at the tubular pole in the setting of efflux of a protein-enriched ultrafiltrate. Perihilar variant accompanied by glomerulomegaly is commonly encountered in secondary adaptive FSGS, such as related to obesity,[66] body building,[67] oligomeganephronia,[68] solitary kidney,[69] prematurity,[70] systemic hypertension,[71] and sickle cell anemia.[72] In these settings, perhilar FSGS may reflect glomerular hypertension due to reflex dilatation of the afferent arteriole leading to stress on the perihilar segment.[73] One study showed low levels of suPAR in the tip lesion variant, however, compared with perihilar and cellular variants, suggesting that tip lesion variant might be biologically different from other variants.[56] This long list emphasizes the diversity of potential causes among the pathologic variants of FSGS and supports the proposition that the term *variants* is misleading, because it implies that FSGS is a single disease that has different morphologic features.[74]

It has been suggested that collapsing glomerulopathy (ie, collapsing variant FSGS) and "pure" tip lesion (ie, without any other type of FSGS lesion, according to the original description by Howie and Brewster[75]) should not even be included within the general rubric of FSGS, given that both of these conditions often lack evidence of sclerosis and possess such distinctive clinical and pathologic characteristics.[74,76] Glomerular tip lesion might conceivably be a nonspecific response to heavy proteinuria and occur in diverse podocytopathies, including minimal change disease, thereby explaining the steroid responsiveness and preserved renal function in most cases and presumably reflecting a different pathogenesis from primary FSGS. Based on a review of autopsy slides from patients dying with probable minimal change disease prior to 1950, Haas and Yousefzadeh[77] identified tip lesions in 5 of 8 cases, but these were exceedingly focal (involving 0.7%–4% of glomeruli). Given that both collapsing lesions and tip lesions typically display segmental glomerular involvement, however, and are often accompanied by other FSGS lesions (74% of tip variant FSGS in 1 study[78]), it seems appropriate to include them within this classification. In cases of tip lesion, it is impractical to exclude all cases that display any nontip segmental lesions, given the possibility that the latter might reflect the vagaries of sampling, due to the random orientation of the glomerular globe and proximal tubule origin within the tissue block. Instead of excluding such cases, it might be better to compare pure tip lesion cases versus those with other (nontip) segmental lesions in future studies, given their apparent different outcomes.[78] Cellular variant is rare in most studies of adult FSGS (3%–4.6%),[52,53,79] and, therefore, its significance has been difficult to determine. Whether cellular variant should continue to be recognized as a distinct variant or might usefully be merged with NOS (after carefully excluding collapsing and tip lesion variant) also needs to be considered in future iterations of the Columbia classification.

Another weakness of this classification is that the pathologic categories were never formally tested for independent predictive value or reproducibility.[5] An independent study by Meehan and colleagues,[8] however, found overall good interobserver reproducibility (kappa 0.676) among a group of 6 renal pathologists, with lowest agreement for the cellular variant (kappa 0.53). In addition, the relationship of the different morphologic phenotypes to each another remains unproved.

NOS FSGS is likely heterogeneous, with some cases arising ab initio and others resulting from evolution of cellular, tip, and collapsing variants, where the defining characteristics are no longer present. Cellular features (endocapillary and/or extracapillary hypercellularity) may be seen in cases of NOS, collapsing, tip, and cellular variants, and it is likely that some cases of cellular variant and NOS variant include cases in which the defining features of the other variants are not sampled, even after exhaustive tissue sectioning.[52]

As discussed previously, several studies have shown different clinical outcomes among these variants in cases of primary FSGS, with best outcomes for tip lesion variant and worst outcomes for collapsing variant.[52–54] Chun and colleagues[80] reported that remission of proteinuria, either spontaneously or in response to therapy, was the sole factor that predicted outcome in primary FSGS, irrespective of morphologic variant (collapsing/cellular, tip lesion, or NOS). On the other hand, for participants in an FSGS clinical trial, all of whom had steroid-resistant FSGS, the rate of ESRD at 3 years' follow-up was 47% for collapsing variant, 20% for NOS variant, and 7% for tip variant ($P = .005$).[54] In multivariate analysis after controlling for baseline kidney function, degree of proteinuria, and age, however, only the percentage of tubular atrophy and interstitial fibrosis, not FSGS variant, significantly predicted ESRD ($P = .02$). This study is important because patients were randomly assigned to 1 of 2 treatment protocols, thus FSGS variant did not affect the treatment decision.

In summary, morphologic variants of FSGS are associated with distinctive clinical-pathologic profiles, with significantly different outcomes for the collapsing and tip variants of primary FSGS. These differences in outcome may reflect differences in the underlying (unknown) cause, pathogenesis, and severity of tubulointerstitial injury, rather than the morphologic variant of FSGS per se. The relationship of morphologic subtypes of FSGS to cause and pathogenesis remain to be demonstrated. Pathologic classification does not obviate excluding secondary causes in all patients with FSGS.

IgA NEPHROPATHY

The Oxford classification of IgA nephropathy represents a novel approach to glomerular disease classification. This schema, which might more accurately be termed a scoring system than a classification, was created by a working group of experts from the International IgA Nephropathy Network and the RPS, with the express purpose

Key Features
OXFORD CLASSIFICATION OF IgA NEPHROPATHY

- Pathologic features were independently predictive of outcome in initial test cohort.
- Most validations studies support some predictive value for the pathologic features.
- Tubulointerstitial injury is scored.
- Mild and severe disease were not included in the initial test cohort.
- Role of endocapillary hypercellularity, segmental sclerosis lesions, and crescents requires further study.

of providing an evidence-based pathologic classification of IgA nephropathy that predicts clinical outcomes.[3,4] The study began with a clinical data set of IgA nephropathy cases whose outcomes were known, then developed reproducible pathologic definitions and scoring methods that were linked to clinical outcomes (ESRD or $\geq$50% decline in estimated glomerular filtration rate [GFR]) independently of initial serum creatinine, mean arterial pressure, and level of proteinuria in the index population.

The clinical data set consisted of 265 IgA nephropathy cases from Asia, North America, and Europe, 30% of whom were children. Exclusion criteria included proteinuria less than 0.5 g/d, estimated GFR less than 30 mL/min, and follow-up of less than 12 months (thus excluding cases with very mild disease, advanced chronic disease, and rapidly progressive disease). A broad array of pathologic variables was first tested for reproducibility and lack of inter-relatedness before being applied to the clinical data set. Three pathologic variables were identified as independently predictive of outcome: mesangial hypercellularity (M), segmental glomerulosclerosis (S), and tubular atrophy/interstitial fibrosis involving greater than 25% of the cortical area (T). In addition, endocapillary proliferation (E) was associated with response to steroids and immunosuppressive therapy. These 4 pathologic features were included in the final MEST scoring system (**Table 3**).

The most compelling strength of the Oxford classification is that the pathologic variables were first tested for reproducibility, lack of interrelatedness, and prognostic value, independently of clinical characteristics. This classification has been tested in multiple independent cohorts (discussed in detail in 2 recent reviews[81,82]), including children[83,84] and

Table 3
Oxford classification of IgA nephropathy

Pathologic Feature	Score
Mesangial hypercellularity	M0: <50% glomeruli M1: >50% glomeruli
Segmental glomerulosclerosis	S0: absent S1: present
Endocapillary hypercellularity	E0: absent E1: present
Tubular atrophy/ interstitial fibrosis	T0: 25% T1: 26%–50% T2: >50%

patients who were excluded from the original test cohort (eg, those with rapidly progressive disease[85] or very mild disease[86]). Although none of these studies has shown complete concordance with the initial study, all but one[87] showed prognostic significance for at least 1 MEST lesion by multivariate analysis. These different results likely reflect differences in selection criteria for renal biopsy, therapies, and definition of outcomes in the various validation studies. Crescents, which were not found significant in the initial test cohort, have been demonstrated to be prognostically significant in cases with rapidly progressive disease.[85] There is some evidence that endocapillary hypercellularity and crescents may respond to immunosuppressive therapy,[85,88] but this requires confirmation in prospective studies. The results of a large study involving 1147 IgA nephropathy patients confirm the validity of the Oxford classification across a broad clinical spectrum of IgA nephropathy.[89] However, the predictive value of the MEST scores was reduced by immunosuppressive/corticosteroid therapy.[89]

A weakness of both the initial study and subsequent validation studies is that these were retrospective and may have confounding biases, particularly with respect to the use of corticosteroids and other immunosuppressive therapies. Crescents and endocapillary hypercellularity (E) are associated with use of corticosteroids and cytotoxic agents, thus introducing a treatment bias. As discussed previously, patients with mild disease or rapidly progressive disease were deliberately excluded from the initial cohort. The thickness of tissue sections was not specified, but even minor variations (eg, 3 μm vs 2 μm) may have a significant impact on the recognition of mesangial hypercellularity. The relevance of the Oxford classification to Henoch-Schönlein purpura

nephritis and other subgroups of IgA nephropathy remains unproved, including among patients with black African ancestry (who comprised only 3% of the Oxford cohort), secondary IgA nephropathy (eg, related to gastrointestinal disease, bacterial and HIV infection, and other causes), and coexistent renal disease (eg, diabetic glomerulosclerosis and hypertensive nephrosclerosis). Segmental sclerosis (S lesions) may result from scarring of proliferative lesions or coexistent podocytopathy, which may have different implications for treatment and effect on outcomes.[90] Finally, the Oxford classification does not address the role of genetic factors, which both predispose to the development of IgA nephropathy and may contribute to different outcomes in different populations.[91]

In summary, the Oxford IgA scoring system is the only truly evidence-based renal pathologic classification in existence and offers a template for future classification systems. Its role in guiding the clinical management of individual patients with IgA nephropathy remains, however, unclear.

DIABETIC NEPHROPATHY

Key Features
RPS CLASSIFICATION OF DIABETIC GLOMERULOSCLEROSIS

- Pathologic criteria are based on expert opinion, not empiric evidence.
- Reproducibility has not been tested independently.
- Diagnosis of class I requires electron microscopy.
- Only 2 validation studies have been performed, with variable findings.
- Tubulointerstitial injury is not scored.
- Clinical relevance is unclear.

Diabetes mellitus is the single leading cause of end-stage kidney disease in the United States and the incidence of diabetes-related ESRD has been rising. Previous research studies have sought to classify the pathologic features of diabetic glomerulosclerosis, but none of these classifications has been adopted in clinical practice. Therefore, in 2006, the Research Committee of the RPS set out to develop, with international consensus, "a uniform classification system containing specific categories that discriminate lesions with various prognostic severities that would be easy to use."[6] The proposed classification includes 4 classes of glomerular disease (**Table 4**) and can be applied to both type 1 and type 2 diabetes mellitus. This classification is based mainly on light microscopic assessment of glomerular alterations using hematoxylin-eosin, trichrome, periodic acid–Schiff, and silver stains, with a minimum sample size of 10 glomeruli. Class I requires measurement of glomerular basement membranes (GBMs) by electron microscopy, however. Interstitial and vascular lesions are scored semiquantitatively, and the presence of coexistent nondiabetic renal disease is also noted.

This classification showed good reproducibility (intraclass correlation coefficient of 0.84) in an initial test cohort of 25 cases examined by 5 renal pathologists.[6] There are several areas of concern, however. Although the diagnosis of class IV (>50% global glomerulosclerosis) is straightforward, the definition of the other classes is more problematic. Specifically, class I requires direct measurement of GBM thickness by electron microscopy, which is not available in all centers. GBM thickening (defined as greater than the upper limit of normal plus 2 standard deviations) is dependent on patient age and must be individualized for each laboratory, not based on the values from a single laboratory that were used in the original article (see **Table 4**). GBM thickening may also be seen in nondiabetic patients, such as those with hypertension. For class II disease, mesangial expansion is defined as "an increase in extracellular material in the mesangium such that the width of the interspace exceeds 2 mesangial cell nuclei in at least 2 glomerular lobules." Class IIa requires mild mesangial expansion involving more than 25% of the total mesangium, whereas class IIb is defined

as severe mesangial expansion (defined as larger than the mean area of a capillary lumen) involving more than 25% of the total mesangium. This distinction appears arbitrary, complicated, and vague, and no instructions are provided for calculating the mean capillary lumen area. For class III, the definition of Kimmelsteil-Wilson lesion—"focal, lobular, round to oval mesangial lesions with an acellular, hyaline/matrix core, rounded peripherally by sparse, crescent-shaped mesangial nuclei" is based on a previous report[92] and could encompass a broad spectrum of changes, from a single small nodule to multiple large nodules. Finally, the assumption that these classes are progressive (ie, that diffuse mesangial disease progresses to sclerosing disease via nodular disease) remains unproved. There is some evidence that diffuse and nodular mesangial sclerosis may arise via distinct pathogenetic mechanisms.[93]

An independent validation study in 50 Korean patients with type 2 diabetes mellitus, all of whom had at least 1 g/d proteinuria, showed significantly different estimated 5-year survival rates among the classes by log rank analysis (100% class I and IIa, 75% class IIb, 66.7% class III, and 38.1% class IV).[94] Pathologic class correlated with estimated GFR (eGFR) and proteinuria at biopsy. On the other hand, a Japanese study of 69 patients with type 2 diabetes and diabetic glomerulosclerosis (class IIa, n = 11; class IIb, n = 15; class III, n = 36; and class IV, n = 7) found that severity of interstitial inflammation and tubulointerstitial scarring, but not glomerular class, predicted renal survival.[95] The investigators speculated that the lack of predictive value of glomerular class might reflect the small number of class IV cases and the high overall prevalence

Table 4
Renal Pathology Society classification of diabetic nephropathy

Class	Inclusion Criteria	Description
I	Biopsy does not meet criteria for class II, III, or IV. GBM >395 nm in female and >430 nm in male subject 9 y of age and older.	Mild or nonspecific light microsopic changes and GBM thickening by electron microscopy
IIa	Biopsy does not meet criteria for class III or IV. Mild mesangial expansion in >25% of the observed mesangium.	Mild mesangial expansion
IIb	Biopsy does not meet criteria for class III or IV. Severe mesangial expansion in >25% of the observed mesangium.	Severe mesangial expansion
III	Biopsy does not meet criteria for class IV. At least 1 convincing Kimmelstiel–Wilson lesion.	Nodular sclerosis (Kimmelstiel–Wilson lesion)
IV	Global glomerular sclerosis in >50% of glomeruli. Lesions from classes I through III.	Advanced diabetic glomerulosclerosis

of renal insufficiency (65% of patients), suggesting advanced nephropathy at time of biopsy. Based on an unpublished survey of RPS members, areas that need to be addressed in this classification include the definition of class I, the distinction of class IIa and IIb, and the proper scoring of tubulointerstitial lesions (eg, whether scoring of interstitial inflammation should be limited to areas with tubular atrophy and interstitial fibrosis).

A major concern with this classification is its relevance to clinical practice. As a general rule, patients with diabetes mellitus only undergo a renal biopsy when a diagnosis other than diabetic glomerulosclerosis is suspected (eg, those who have a rapidly progressive course, sudden onset of severe proteinuria, and/or serologic abnormalities). This reflects the fact that albuminuria and diabetic retinopathy are generally reliable clinical surrogates of diabetic glomerulosclerosis, at least in cases of type 2 diabetes mellitus.[96] In the study of Oh and colleagues,[94] nondiabetic kidney disease was identified in 60.9% of patients with type 2 diabetes undergoing renal biopsy. Similarly, at Columbia University Medical Center, New York, a retrospective study of 620 consecutive patients with diabetes who underwent renal biopsy in 2011 found that more than 60% had nondiabetic kidney disease.[97] Only 37% had findings of diabetic glomerulosclerosis alone, 36% had diabetic glomerulosclerosis plus nondiabetic disease, and 27% had nondiabetic disease alone.[97] The most common nondiabetic diseases (eg, acute tubular necrosis, hypertensive nephrosclerosis, and secondary FSGS), may have significant impact on management and clinical course in patients. The presence of coexistent conditions should be considered in future validation studies of the pathologic classification of diabetic glomerulosclerosis.

In summary, the classification of diabetic glomerulosclerosis requires further refinement of the criteria for distinguishing class IIa (mild) versus IIb (severe) mesangial disease, and reconsideration of the clinical utility of making a diagnosis of class I diabetic glomeruloscleorsis.

ANCA-ASSOCIATED GLOMERULONEPHRITIS

This classification was proposed by an international working group composed of renal pathologists using clinical data from the European Vasculitis Study Group, with the express purpose of providing prognostic information in cases of ANCA-associated glomerulonephritis.[7] Inclusion criteria include the presence of at least 1 glomerulus with necrotizing or crescentic features on light microscopy (with at least 10 glomeruli for adequacy) and pauci-immune staining on

> ### Key Features
> ### BERDEN CLASSIFICATION OF ANCA GLOMERULONEPHRITIS
>
> - Pathologic criteria are based on expert opinion, not empiric evidence.
> - Reproducibility has not been tested independently.
> - Validation studies show mixed outcomes for the mixed class.
> - Tubulointerstitial injury is not scored.
> - Clinical relevance is unclear.

immunofluorescence microscopy. The frequencies of proteinase 3 (PR3) and myeloperoxidase (MPO) ANCA were 46% and 48%, respectively; ANCA were negative in 2 patients and unavailable in the other 3; patients with Churg-Strauss syndrome were excluded.

Cases are divided into 4 categories based on the percentage of glomeruli showing either cellular crescents or global sclerosis by light microscopy: focal (≥50% of glomeruli are normal), crescentic (≥50% of glomeruli have cellular crescents), sclerotic (≥50% of glomeruli are globally sclerotic), or mixed (all other cases) (**Table 5**). In the initial cohort of 100 cases, these categories showed significant differences in renal survival at 1 year and 5 years (focal > crescentic > mixed > sclerotic).[7] Baseline eGFR and pathologic class were both independent predictors of outcome at 1 and 5 years in multivariate analyses, and patients with crescentic glomerulonephritis had significantly lower risk of developing ESRD compared with those with sclerotic disease. The addition of tubulointerstitial injury scores did not improve predictive value compared with glomerular classification alone.

Table 5
Classification schema for ANCA-associated glomerulonephritis

Light Microscopy Findings	Class
≥50% Normal glomeruli	Focal
≥50% Glomeruli with cellular crescents	Crescentic
<50% Normal, <50% crescentic, <50% globally sclerotic glomeruli	Mixed
≥50% Globally sclerotic glomeruli	Sclerotic

This classification has the merit of simplicity. Reproducibility was not tested in the original study set, but a prior study by the same investigators using these criteria did show good reproducibility.[11] Possible limitations include that the initial study population consisted of European patients who were enrolled in 1 of 2 therapeutic trials; whether these findings are generalizable to patients receiving other treatments outside of a study setting is unclear. The pathologic categories are empiric and their prognostic significance independent of clinical variables was not tested. Other criticisms include that the recognition of cellular crescents is somewhat subjective and tubulointerstitial lesions were not included. T-cell tubulitis and tubular atrophy have both been shown to significantly impact response to treatment in cases of ANCA-related glomerulonephritis.[98]

Seven retrospective validation studies have been performed, comprising Chinese,[99] Japanese,[100–102] Dutch,[103] Turkish,[104] and United States[105] populations. In a cohort of 54 Japanese patients, 100% of whom had MPO ANCA, Togashi and colleagues[101] found similar outcomes to the study of Berden and colleagues.[7] In a different study of 122 Japanese patients (84% MPO ANCA, 5% PR3 ANCA, and 11% ANCA negative), Iwakiri and colleagues[100] found that crescentic and mixed classes were indistinguishable and histologic class did not predict ESRD. Similarly, in a study of 87 Japanese patients (100% MPO ANCA), Muso and colleagues[102] found that ESRD was more common in the sclerotic group but was not significantly different in the other 3 groups. The investigators of the latter 2 studies speculated that this might reflect the higher frequency of MPO ANCA and less aggressive immunosuppressive therapy in the Japanese population. In a Chinese cohort of 121 cases, 89% of whom had MPO ANCA, crescentic class had worse outcomes than mixed class, perhaps reflecting less chronic lesions in the mixed group, less frequent plasmapheresis, and higher frequency of MPO ANCA.[99] In a study of 164 Dutch patients, 51% of whom had PR3 ANCA, there were significant overall differences in 5-year survival rates (91% for focal, 69% for mixed, and 64% for crescentic) but mixed and crescentic groups were indistinguishable and the sclerotic group was rare (only 1 subject).[103] The investigators noted that including the percentage of normal glomeruli led to improved predictive value. In the Turkish study of 141 patients (P ANCA 43.2%; C ANCA 42.6%; atypical ANCA 3.6%; and negative ANCA 17.7%), pathologic class correlated with need for dialysis but the presence of circumferential (full moon) crescents was the most significant pathologic predictor.[104] In a single-center

United States study of 76 cases (82% white; 30 cANCA+, 32 pANCA+, and 14 ANCA negative), age and baseline eGFR were predictive of eGFR at 1 year. Patients with crescentic, mixed, and sclerotic categories had worse eGFR at 1 year post-biopsy compared with those with focal disease.

In conclusion, validation studies of the Berden classification of ANCA vasculitis have consistently shown best outcomes for the focal class and generally worst outcomes for the sclerosing class, with variable findings for the mixed and crescentic classes. The use of 50% as the cutoff for defining sclerosing, crescentic, and focal classes ensures that the mixed class includes heterogeneous entities (eg, mainly but not predominantly crescentic or sclerosing disease), and this may explain some of the variability observed in outcomes for the mixed category. The prognostic impact of this classification in other ethnic groups (eg, African Americans) and the role of tubulointerstitial injury remain to be determined.

SUMMARY

Pathologic classifications provide a logical framework for standardizing renal pathologic diagnoses, allowing better communication among pathologists and with clinicians and facilitating collaborative studies between multiple centers. These classifications help identify distinct clinical-pathologic subgroups with different outcomes, but their role in guiding the management of individual patients is less certain. For example, current guidelines for the management of LN do not distinguish between class III and IV, or IV-S versus IV-G.[23,24] Similarly, the treatment of primary FSGS, IgA nephropathy, ANCA glomerulonephritis, and diabetic glomerulosclerosis is not predicated on pathologic subtypes, but nonspecific pathologic findings of advanced scarring (glomerulosclerosis and tubulointerstitial scarring) may influence the decision to withhold aggressive treatment. The prognostic significance of many pathologic classifications is inconsistent, reflecting problems related to sampling error and reproducibility, the interrelatedness of pathologic and clinical variables, difficulties inherent in retrospective validation studies, and the unknown causes and multifactorial pathogenesis of most kidney diseases. Despite these limitations, renal pathologic classifications are now well established and should be included in all future clinical trials, to better elucidate the relationship of pathologic variants and disease course. These classifications must be continually re-evaluated and updated, to incorporate new information emerging from clinical and experimental studies.

REFERENCES

1. McCluskey R. Lupus nephritis. East Norwalk (CT): Appleton-Century-Crofts; 1975.

2. Solez K, Axelsen RA, Benediktsson H, et al. International standardization of criteria for the histologic diagnosis of renal allograft rejection: the Banff working classification of kidney transplant pathology. Kidney Int 1993;44(2):411–22.

3. Cattran DC, Coppo R, Cook HT, et al. The Oxford classification of IgA nephropathy: rationale, clinico-pathological correlations, and classification. Kidney Int 2009;76(5):534–45.

4. Roberts IS, Cook HT, Troyanov S, et al. The Oxford classification of IgA nephropathy: pathology definitions, correlations, and reproducibility. Kidney Int 2009;76(5):546–56.

5. D'Agati VD, Fogo AB, Bruijn JA, et al. Pathologic classification of focal segmental glomerulosclerosis: a working proposal. Am J Kidney Dis 2004; 43(2):368–82.

6. Tervaert TW, Mooyaart AL, Amann K, et al. Pathologic classification of diabetic nephropathy. J Am Soc Nephrol 2010;21(4):556–63.

7. Berden AE, Ferrario F, Hagen EC, et al. Histopathologic classification of ANCA-associated glomerulonephritis. J Am Soc Nephrol 2010;21(10):1628–36.

8. Meehan SM, Chang A, Gibson IW, et al. A study of interobserver reproducibility of morphologic lesions of focal segmental glomerulosclerosis. Virchows Arch 2013;462(2):229–37.

9. Furness PN, Taub N. International variation in the interpretation of renal transplant biopsies: report of the CERTPAP Project. Kidney Int 2001;60(5): 1998–2012.

10. Furness PN, Taub N. Interobserver reproducibility and application of the ISN/RPS classification of lupus nephritis-a UK-wide study. Am J Surg Pathol 2006;30(8):1030–5.

11. Bajema IM, Hagen EC, Hansen BE, et al. The renal histopathology in systemic vasculitis: an international survey study of inter- and intra-observer agreement. Nephrol Dial Transplant 1996;11(10):1989–95.

12. Yu F, Wu LH, Tan Y, et al. Tubulointerstitial lesions of patients with lupus nephritis classified by the 2003 International Society of Nephrology and Renal Pathology Society system. Kidney Int 2010;77(9): 820–9.

13. Barber C, Herzenberg A, Aghdassi E, et al. Evaluation of clinical outcomes and renal vascular pathology among patients with lupus. Clin J Am Soc Nephrol 2012;7(5):757–64.

14. Wu LH, Yu F, Tan Y, et al. Inclusion of renal vascular lesions in the 2003 ISN/RPS system for classifying lupus nephritis improves renal outcome predictions. Kidney Int 2013;83(4):715–23.

15. D'Agati VD, Mengel M. The rise of renal pathology in nephrology: structure illuminates function. Am J Kidney Dis 2013;61(6):1016–25.

16. Weening JJ, D'Agati VD, Schwartz MM, et al. The classification of glomerulonephritis in systemic lupus erythematosus revisited. Kidney Int 2004; 65(2):521–30.

17. Churg J, Sobin L. Renal disease: classification and atlas of glomerular diseases. Tokyo: Igaku-Shoin; 1982.

18. Churg J, Bernstein J, Glassock R. Renal disease: classification and atlas of glomerular diseases. New York: Igaku-Shoin; 1995.

19. Yokoyama H, Wada T, Hara A, et al. The outcome and a new ISN/RPS 2003 classification of lupus nephritis in Japanese. Kidney Int 2004;66(6):2382–8.

20. Grootscholten C, Bajema IM, Florquin S, et al. Interobserver agreement of scoring of histopathological characteristics and classification of lupus nephritis. Nephrol Dial Transplant 2008;23(1):223–30.

21. Hiramatsu N, Kuroiwa T, Ikeuchi H, et al. Revised classification of lupus nephritis is valuable in predicting renal outcome with an indication of the proportion of glomeruli affected by chronic lesions. Rheumatology (Oxford) 2008;47(5):702–7.

22. Hill GS, Delahousse M, Nochy D, et al. Class IV-S versus class IV-G lupus nephritis: clinical and morphologic differences suggesting different pathogenesis. Kidney Int 2005;68(5):2288–97.

23. Hahn BH, McMahon MA, Wilkinson A, et al. American College of Rheumatology guidelines for screening, treatment, and management of lupus nephritis. Arthritis Care Res (Hoboken) 2012;64(6):797–808.

24. Bertsias G, Ioannidis JP, Boletis J, et al. EULAR recommendations for the management of systemic lupus erythematosus. Report of a Task Force of the EULAR Standing Committee for International Clinical Studies Including Therapeutics. Ann Rheum Dis 2008;67(2):195–205.

25. Bertsias GK, Tektonidou M, Amoura Z, et al. Joint European League Against Rheumatism and European Renal Association-European Dialysis and Transplant Association (EULAR/ERA-EDTA) recommendations for the management of adult and paediatric lupus nephritis. Ann Rheum Dis 2012; 71(11):1771–82.

26. Najafi CC, Korbet SM, Lewis EJ, et al. Significance of histologic patterns of glomerular injury upon long-term prognosis in severe lupus glomerulonephritis. Kidney Int 2001;59(6):2156–63.

27. Mittal B, Hurwitz S, Rennke H, et al. New subcategories of class IV lupus nephritis: are there clinical, histologic, and outcome differences? Am J Kidney Dis 2004;44(6):1050–9.

28. Haring CM, Rietveld A, van den Brand JA, et al. Segmental and global subclasses of class IV lupus

nephritis have similar renal outcomes. J Am Soc Nephrol 2012;23(1):149–54.

29. Kojo S, Sada KE, Kobayashi M, et al. Clinical usefulness of a prognostic score in histological analysis of renal biopsy in patients with lupus nephritis. J Rheumatol 2009;36(10):2218–23.

30. Yu F, Tan Y, Wu LH, et al. Class IV-G and IV-S lupus nephritis in Chinese patients: a large cohort study from a single center. Lupus 2009;18(12):1073–81.

31. Kim YG, Kim HW, Cho YM, et al. The difference between lupus nephritis class IV-G and IV-S in Koreans: focus on the response to cyclophosphamide induction treatment. Rheumatology (Oxford) 2008;47(3):311–4.

32. Schwartz MM, Korbet SM, Lewis EJ. The prognosis and pathogenesis of severe lupus glomerulonephritis. Nephrol Dial Transplant 2008;23(4):1298–306.

33. Song D, Wu LH, Wang FM, et al. The spectrum of renal thrombotic microangiopathy in lupus nephritis. Arthritis Res Ther 2013;15(1):R12.

34. Hertig A, Droz D, Lesavre P, et al. SLE and idiopathic nephrotic syndrome: coincidence or not? Am J Kidney Dis 2002;40(6):1179–84.

35. Kraft SW, Schwartz MM, Korbet SM, et al. Glomerular podocytopathy in patients with systemic lupus erythematosus. J Am Soc Nephrol 2005;16(1):175–9.

36. Nasr SH, D'Agati VD, Park HR, et al. Necrotizing and crescentic lupus nephritis with antineutrophil cytoplasmic antibody seropositivity. Clin J Am Soc Nephrol 2008;3(3):682–90.

37. Salvatore SP, Barisoni LM, Herzenberg AM, et al. Collapsing glomerulopathy in 19 patients with systemic lupus erythematosus or lupus-like disease. Clin J Am Soc Nephrol 2012;7(6):914–25.

38. Larsen CP, Beggs ML, Saeed M, et al. Apolipoprotein l1 risk variants associate with systemic lupus erythematosus-associated collapsing glomerulopathy. J Am Soc Nephrol 2013;24(5):722–5.

39. Howie AJ, Turhan N, Adu D. Powerful morphometric indicator of prognosis in lupus nephritis. QJM 2003;96(6):411–20.

40. Colvin RB, Cohen AH, Saiontz C, et al. Evaluation of pathologic criteria for acute renal allograft rejection: reproducibility, sensitivity, and clinical correlation. J Am Soc Nephrol 1997;8(12):1930–41.

41. Mueller A, Schnuelle P, Waldherr R, et al. Impact of the Banff '97 classification for histological diagnosis of rejection on clinical outcome and renal function parameters after kidney transplantation. Transplantation 2000;69(6):1123–7.

42. Tanaka T, Kyo M, Kokado Y, et al. Correlation between the Banff 97 classification of renal allograft biopsies and clinical outcome. Transpl Int 2004;17(2):59–64.

43. Cornell LD, Smith RN, Colvin RB. Kidney transplantation: mechanisms of rejection and acceptance. Annu Rev Pathol 2008;3:189–220.

44. Lefaucheur C, Loupy A, Vernerey D, et al. Antibody-mediated vascular rejection of kidney allografts: a population-based study. Lancet 2013;381(9863):313–9.

45. Haas M, Sis B, Racusen LC, et al. Banff 2013 meeting report: inclusion of c4d-negative antibody-mediated rejection and antibody-associated arterial lesions. Am J Transplant 2014;14(2):272–83.

46. Halloran PF, Reeve JP, Pereira AB, et al. Antibody-mediated rejection, T cell-mediated rejection, and the injury-repair response: new insights from the Genome Canada studies of kidney transplant biopsies. Kidney Int 2013;85:258–64.

47. Everly MJ, Rebellato LM, Haisch CE, et al. Incidence and impact of de novo donor-specific alloantibody in primary renal allografts. Transplantation 2013;95(3):410–7.

48. Vlad G, Ho EK, Vasilescu ER, et al. Relevance of different antibody detection methods for the prediction of antibody-mediated rejection and deceased-donor kidney allograft survival. Hum Immunol 2009;70(8):589–94.

49. Hill GS, Nochy D, Bruneval P, et al. Donor-specific antibodies accelerate arteriosclerosis after kidney transplantation. J Am Soc Nephrol 2011;22(5):975–83.

50. Mengel M, Sis B, Halloran PF. SWOT analysis of Banff: strengths, weaknesses, opportunities and threats of the international Banff consensus process and classification system for renal allograft pathology. Am J Transplant 2007;7(10):2221–6.

51. Suthanthiran M, Schwartz JE, Ding R, et al. Urinary-cell mRNA profile and acute cellular rejection in kidney allografts. N Engl J Med 2013;369(1):20–31.

52. Stokes MB, Valeri AM, Markowitz GS, et al. Cellular focal segmental glomerulosclerosis: Clinical and pathologic features. Kidney Int 2006;70(10):1783–92.

53. Thomas DB, Franceschini N, Hogan SL, et al. Clinical and pathologic characteristics of focal segmental glomerulosclerosis pathologic variants. Kidney Int 2006;69(5):920–6.

54. D'Agati VD, Alster JM, Jennette JC, et al. Association of histologic variants in FSGS clinical trial with presenting features and outcomes. Clin J Am Soc Nephrol 2013;8(3):399–406.

55. Sanna-Cherchi S, Burgess KE, Nees SN, et al. Exome sequencing identified MYO1E and NEIL1 as candidate genes for human autosomal recessive steroid-resistant nephrotic syndrome. Kidney Int 2011;80(4):389–96.

56. Huang J, Liu G, Zhang YM, et al. Plasma soluble urokinase receptor levels are increased but do

not distinguish primary from secondary focal segmental glomerulosclerosis. Kidney Int 2013; 84(2):366–72.

57. D'Agati V, Suh JI, Carbone L, et al. Pathology of HIV-associated nephropathy: a detailed morphologic and comparative study. Kidney Int 1989; 35(6):1358–70.

58. Moudgil A, Nast CC, Bagga A, et al. Association of parvovirus B19 infection with idiopathic collapsing glomerulopathy. Kidney Int 2001;59(6): 2126–33.

59. Thaunat O, Delahousse M, Fakhouri F, et al. Nephrotic syndrome associated with hemophagocytic syndrome. Kidney Int 2006;69(10):1892–8.

60. Markowitz GS, Appel GB, Fine PL, et al. Collapsing focal segmental glomerulosclerosis following treatment with high-dose pamidronate. J Am Soc Nephrol 2001;12(6):1164–72.

61. Markowitz GS, Nasr SH, Stokes MB, et al. Treatment with IFN-{alpha}, -{beta}, or -{gamma} is associated with collapsing focal segmental glomerulosclerosis. Clin J Am Soc Nephrol 2010;5(4):607–15.

62. Stokes MB, Davis CL, Alpers CE. Collapsing glomerulopathy in renal allografts: a morphological pattern with diverse clinicopathologic associations. Am J Kidney Dis 1999;33(4):658–66.

63. Kopp JB, Nelson GW, Sampath K, et al. APOL1 genetic variants in focal segmental glomerulosclerosis and HIV-associated nephropathy. J Am Soc Nephrol 2011;22(11):2129–37.

64. Najafian B, Kim Y, Crosson JT, et al. Atubular glomeruli and glomerulotubular junction abnormalities in diabetic nephropathy. J Am Soc Nephrol 2003;14(4): 908–17.

65. Howie AJ. Changes at the glomerular tip: a feature of membranous nephropathy and other disorders associated with proteinuria. J Pathol 1986;150(1): 13–20.

66. Kambham N, Markowitz GS, Valeri AM, et al. Obesity-related glomerulopathy: an emerging epidemic. Kidney Int 2001;59(4):1498–509.

67. Herlitz LC, Markowitz GS, Farris AB, et al. Development of focal segmental glomerulosclerosis after anabolic steroid abuse. J Am Soc Nephrol 2010; 21(1):163–72.

68. McGraw M, Poucell S, Sweet J, et al. The significance of focal segmental glomerulosclerosis in oligomeganephronia. Int J Pediatr Nephrol 1984;5(2): 67–72.

69. Bhathena DB, Julian BA, McMorrow RG, et al. Focal sclerosis of hypertrophied glomeruli in solitary functioning kidneys of humans. Am J Kidney Dis 1985;5(5):226–32.

70. Hodgin JB, Rasoulpour M, Markowitz GS, et al. Very low birth weight is a risk factor for secondary focal segmental glomerulosclerosis. Clin J Am Soc Nephrol 2009;4(1):71–6.

71. Harvey JM, Howie AJ, Lee SJ, et al. Renal biopsy findings in hypertensive patients with proteinuria. Lancet 1992;340(8833):1435–6.

72. Falk RJ, Jennette JC. Sickle cell nephropathy. Adv Nephrol Necker Hosp 1994;23:133–47.

73. Nagata M, Kriz W. Glomerular damage after uninephrectomy in young rats. II. Mechanical stress on podocytes as a pathway to sclerosis. Kidney Int 1992;42(1):148–60.

74. Howie AJ. Problems with 'focal segmental glomerulosclerosis'. Pediatr Nephrol 2011;26(8):1197–205.

75. Howie AJ, Brewer DB. The glomerular tip lesion: a previously undescribed type of segmental glomerular abnormality. J Pathol 1984;142(3):205–20.

76. Barisoni L, Schnaper HW, Kopp JB. A proposed taxonomy for the podocytopathies: a reassessment of the primary nephrotic diseases. Clin J Am Soc Nephrol 2007;2(3):529–42.

77. Haas M, Yousefzadeh N. Glomerular tip lesion in minimal change nephropathy: a study of autopsies before 1950. Am J Kidney Dis 2002;39(6):1168–75.

78. Stokes MB, Markowitz GS, Lin J, et al. Glomerular tip lesion: a distinct entity within the minimal change disease/focal segmental glomerulosclerosis spectrum. Kidney Int 2004;65(5):1690–702.

79. Gipson DS, Trachtman H, Kaskel FJ, et al. Clinical trial of focal segmental glomerulosclerosis in children and young adults. Kidney Int 2011;80(8): 868–78.

80. Chun MJ, Korbet SM, Schwartz MM, et al. Focal segmental glomerulosclerosis in nephrotic adults: presentation, prognosis, and response to therapy of the histologic variants. J Am Soc Nephrol 2004; 15(8):2169–77.

81. Roberts IS. Oxford classification of immunoglobulin A nephropathy: an update. Curr Opin Nephrol Hypertens 2013;22:281–6.

82. Haas M, Rastaldi MP, Fervenza FC. Histologic classification of glomerular diseases: clinicopathologic correlations, limitations exposed by validation studies, and suggestions for modification. Kidney Int 2013;85:779–93.

83. Coppo R, Troyanov S, Camilla R, et al. The Oxford IgA nephropathy clinicopathological classification is valid for children as well as adults. Kidney Int 2010;77(10):921–7.

84. Le W, Zeng CH, Liu Z, et al. Validation of the Oxford classification of IgA nephropathy for pediatric patients from China. BMC Nephrol 2012;13:158.

85. Katafuchi R, Ninomiya T, Nagata M, et al. Validation study of oxford classification of IgA nephropathy: the significance of extracapillary proliferation. Clin J Am Soc Nephrol 2011;6(12):2806–13.

86. Gutierrez E, Zamora I, Ballarin JA, et al. Long-term outcomes of IgA nephropathy presenting with minimal or no proteinuria. J Am Soc Nephrol 2012; 23(10):1753–60.

87. Alamartine E, Sauron C, Laurent B, et al. The use of the Oxford classification of IgA nephropathy to predict renal survival. Clin J Am Soc Nephrol 2011; 6(10):2384–8.

88. Herzenberg AM, Fogo AB, Reich HN, et al. Validation of the Oxford classification of IgA nephropathy. Kidney Int 2011;80(3):310–7.

89. Coppo R, Troyanov S, Bellur S, et al. Validation of the Oxford classification of IgA nephropathy in cohorts with different present ations and treatments. Kidney Int Apr 2, 2014. [Epub ahead of print].

90. El Karoui K, Hill GS, Karras A, et al. Focal segmental glomerulosclerosis plays a major role in the progression of IgA nephropathy. II. Light microscopic and clinical studies. Kidney Int 2011; 79(6):643–54.

91. Kiryluk K, Li Y, Sanna-Cherchi S, et al. Geographic differences in genetic susceptibility to IgA nephropathy: GWAS replication study and geospatial risk analysis. PLoS Genet 2012;8(6):e1002765.

92. Stout LC, Kumar S, Whorton EB. Focal mesangiolysis and the pathogenesis of the Kimmelstiel-Wilson nodule. Hum Pathol 1993;24(1):77–89.

93. Schwartz MM, Lewis EJ, Leonard-Martin T, et al. Renal pathology patterns in type II diabetes mellitus: relationship with retinopathy. The Collaborative Study Group. Nephrol Dial Transplant 1998;13(10): 2547–52.

94. Oh SW, Kim S, Na KY, et al. Clinical implications of pathologic diagnosis and classification for diabetic nephropathy. Diabetes Res Clin Pract 2012;97(3): 418–24.

95. Okada T, Nagao T, Matsumoto H, et al. Histological predictors for renal prognosis in diabetic nephropathy in diabetes mellitus type 2 patients with overt proteinuria. Nephrology (Carlton) 2012;17(1):68–75.

96. KDOQI clinical practice guidelines and clinical practice recommendations for diabetes and chronic kidney disease. Am J Kidney Dis 2007; 10(2 Suppl 2):S12–154.

97. Sharma SG, Bomback AS, Radhakrishnan J, et al. The modern spectrum of renal biopsy findings in patients with diabetes. Clin J Am Soc Nephrol 2013;8:1718–24.

98. Berden AE, Jones RB, Erasmus DD, et al. Tubular lesions predict renal outcome in antineutrophil cytoplasmic antibody-associated glomerulonephritis after rituximab therapy. J Am Soc Nephrol 2012;23(2):313–21.

99. Chang DY, Wu LH, Liu G, et al. Re-evaluation of the histopathologic classification of ANCA-associated glomerulonephritis: a study of 121 patients in a single center. Nephrol Dial Transplant 2012;27(6):2343–9.

100. Iwakiri T, Fujimoto S, Kitagawa K, et al. Validation of a newly proposed histopathological classification in Japanese patients with anti-neutrophil cytoplasmic antibody-associated glomerulonephritis. BMC Nephrol 2013;14(1):125.

101. Togashi M, Komatsuda A, Nara M, et al. Validation of the 2010 histopathological classification of ANCA-associated glomerulonephritis in a Japanese single-center cohort. Mod Rheumatol 2014; 24:300–3.

102. Muso E, Endo T, Itabashi M, et al. Evaluation of the newly proposed simplified histological classification in Japanese cohorts of myeloperoxidase-anti-neutrophil cytoplasmic antibody-associated glomerulonephritis in comparison with other Asian and European cohorts. Clin Exp Nephrol 2012;17: 659–62.

103. Hilhorst M, Wilde B, van Breda Vriesman P, et al. Estimating renal survival using the ANCA-Associated GN classification. J Am Soc Nephrol 2013;24(9):1371–5.

104. Unlu M, Kiremitci S, Ensari A, et al. Pauci-immune necrotizing crescentic glomerulonephritis with crescentic and full moon extracapillary proliferation: clinico-pathologic correlation and follow-up study. Pathol Res Pract 2013;209(2):75–82.

105. Ellis CL, Manno RL, Havill JP, et al. Validation of the new classification of pauci-immune glomerulonephritis in a United States cohort and its correlation with renal outcome. BMC Nephrol 2013; 14(1):210.

Renalomics
Molecular Pathology in Kidney Biopsies

Michael Mengel, MD

KEYWORDS

• Renal pathology • Kidney biopsies • Molecular diagnostics • Molecular pathology

ABSTRACT

In this article, various omics technologies and their applications in renal pathology (native and transplant biopsies) are reviewed and discussed. Despite significant progress and novel insights derived from these applications, extensive adoption of molecular diagnostics in renal pathology has not been accomplished. Further validation of specific applications leading to increased diagnostic precision in a clinically relevant way is ongoing.

OVERVIEW: MOLECULAR PATHOLOGY IN KIDNEY BIOPSIES

Empirically derived, descriptive consensus classifications for renal diseases are mostly based on morphology, immunopathology, and clinical correlates, but frequently without an etiologic basis. This approach is becoming increasingly insufficient in the era of personalized medicine, in which precise, mechanism-based diagnoses are the prerequisite for targeted treatment in the individual patient.[1] Thus, biology-based refinement of the taxonomy of diseases is necessary. With completion of the human genome project and rapid methodological advances in molecular biology, we expanded the scale from studying single genes, transcripts, proteins, or metabolites to studying all molecules simultaneously by using omics technologies.[2] The expectation is that such omics approaches will provide insights into disease mechanisms and through this identify diagnostic, prognostic, and theranostic

(ie, predicting response to treatment) biomarkers, not only for renal pathology.

In this article, various omics technologies and their applications in renal pathology (native and transplant biopsies) are reviewed and discussed. Despite significant progress and novel insights derived from these applications, extensive adoption of molecular diagnostics in renal pathology has not been accomplished. Further validation of specific applications leading to increased diagnostic precision in a clinically relevant way is ongoing.

TECHNIQUES, PLATFORMS, ANALYTICAL METHODS, AND PITFALLS

To date, most comprehensive data sets, including clinic-pathological correlations, are available for quantitative transcriptomics analysis from renal transplant biopsies and less extensively from urine or blood.[3–9] Fewer studies are available describing proteomic and metabolomics testing in renal patients, most likely because of methodological challenges and because these technologies are less suitable to be applied to tissue biopsies. Some promising results have been derived from urine specimens. Urine provides a potentially unique, noninvasive window on the kidney, especially for those molecules "leaking" into the urine in association with tubular injury.[10–12]

After initial euphoria,[13] genome-wide association studies for single nucleotide polymorphisms (SNPs) have been heavily criticized more recently,[14] mostly because of their inherent imbalance between huge number of detected polymorphisms and limited sample size and thus

Department of Laboratory Medicine and Pathology, University of Alberta Hospital, 4B1.18 Walter Mackenzie Center, 8440–112 Street, Edmonton T6G2S2, Canada
E-mail address: mmengel@ualberta.ca

Surgical Pathology 7 (2014) 443–455
http://dx.doi.org/10.1016/j.path.2014.04.005
1875-9181/14/$ – see front matter © 2014 Elsevier Inc. All rights reserved.

Diagnostic phenotypes and molecular correlates in kidney biopsies

Biopsy Type/ Clinical Phenotype	Morphologic Diagnostic Phenotype/Clinical Phenotype	Molecular Pathology	References
Native kidney biopsy			39
	FSGS	Point mutations in podocyte genes	34,35
	Advanced chronic kidney disease	Increased expression of injury-repair transcripts and embryonic genes (Wnt and Notch pathways). Decreased expression of solute carriers.	30,33,45
Renal transplant			9,23,104
	CMR per 2013 Banff consensus criteria, ie, interstitial infiltrate and tubulitis	Increased expression of transcripts expressed by cytotoxic T cells and macrophages. Transcripts induced by IFNγ.	8,28,67,105
	ABMR per 2013 Banff consensus criteria, ie, presence of DSA and microcirculation inflammation	Increased expression of transcripts expressed by endothelial cells and NK cells. Transcripts induced by IFNγ.	24,98,100,101
	Acute tubular injury	Increased (injury-repair molecules) and decreased (solute carriers) expression of transcripts expressed by tubular epithelial cells.	30,48,106
	Chronic allograft changes, ie, IFTA	Increased expression of transcripts expressed by B cells, plasma cells, and mast cells.	71
Clinical phenotype			
	Nephrotic syndrome	Point mutations in genes coding for glomerular basement membrane proteins	33,39
	Acute kidney failure	Increased expression of injury-repair transcripts.	30,92
	Renal transplant failure	Increased expression of injury-repair transcripts.	26

predisposition for accidentally finding statistically significant associations that are frequently biologically irrelevant.[15] New high-throughput technologies are emerging for the assessment of regulatory microRNA (miRNA), as well as sequencing technologies for DNA and RNA.[16,17]

For essentially all omics platforms, the biopsy material needs to be adequately stabilized for RNA extraction (ie, a separate specimen needs to be procured in RNALater or similar solutions).[18,19] But high-throughput gene expression platforms using formalin-fixed, paraffin-embedded (FFPE) samples have recently become available. For example, the NanoString nCounter Analysis System (Seattle, WA) is a molecular "barcode" probe-based technology that enables direct,

digital quantification of nucleic acids without amplification using low amounts of short fragments of total RNA, miRNA, or DNA. The nCounter Analysis System is a highly multiplexed platform to quantify up to 800 targets simultaneously.[20] Comparison of the NanoString nCounter gene expression system with microarrays and polymerase chain reaction (PCR) demonstrated that the nCounter system is more sensitive than microarrays and similar in sensitivity to real-time PCR.[20] Therefore, platforms like the NanoString system have the potential to enable the translation of multiparametric molecular signatures from omics discovery studies into clinical FFPE diagnostics using the same sample as reviewed under the microscope.

All omics approaches require sophisticated biostatistics as part of their application. The challenge lies in the fact that the number of omics results per specimen (tens of thousands) far exceeds the sample size in all to-date published studies. Thus, any statistical analysis is very susceptible to accidentally finding "significant" associations to clinic-pathological variables while not reflecting true biologic disease mechanisms. For example, the following are some of the common mistakes related to microarray data analysis[21]: (1) Insufficient exploratory data analysis, for example, to calculate correlations between high numbers of variables (eg, microarray results with pathologic lesions) that are not linearly related. Standard correlations like Spearman applied to thousands of variables will always find significant correlations even if no true biologic relationship exists. For instance, principal component analysis is superior for revealing the internal structure of the data. Principal component analysis can supply the user with a lower-dimensional picture of a complex data set. (2) Improper use and interpretation of the large variety of clustering algorithms. Clustering samples based on the genes differentially expressed between phenotypes is not supportive evidence for the clinical significance of the genes. Clustering generates treelike relationships within the data even when none truly exist. (3) Improper validation of results. No information derived from a test set (eg, differentially expressed genes from a class comparison, eg, rejection vs no-rejection) should leak into the validation procedure. (4) Weak experimental design (eg, limited challenge bias), meaning evaluating a diagnostic test using nonchallenging samples (eg, totally normal vs severely rejecting). By leaving out clinically relevant but diagnostically "difficult" samples (eg, borderline cases), reported accuracies, sensitivities, and so forth are inflated.[22]

Furthermore, high-dimensional data outputs from omics platforms are not feasible to be integrated into patient care and require postanalytical refinement to become clinically useful. To this end, several groups developed an approach through generating pathogenesis-related gene sets for an easy and rapid interpretation of complex cDNA microarray results.[23] Such gene sets provide annotation groups of related transcripts (sometimes several hundred) representing discrete biologic events relevant to specific biologic processes like various subtypes of inflammation (infiltration by T cells, B cells, or macrophages) and the injury-repair response in parenchyma, stroma, or microcirculation (endothelial cells). By the gene set approach, large-scale and cumbersome microarray gene expression results are collapsed into a small number of scores representing molecular measurements of the respective biologic processes.[24–26] A different approach toward high-dimensional omics data is to use sophisticated biostatistical tools and algorithms for a user-friendly refinement. For class prediction (eg, predicting the diagnosis of a new sample solely from the molecular assessment), frequently classifiers are used. Classifiers are mathematical algorithms/functions that assign probabilities to a new sample based on various input data (eg, the result of a microarray experiment) regarding its likelihood for belonging to a specific class/diagnosis. Classifiers are usually built using machine learning algorithms and supervised learning (ie, after training on a set of known classes/correctly diagnosed cases). Building a classifier represents a challenge if no true diagnostic gold standard is available for training, which is frequently the case and represents a significant obstacle for validating new "omics" diagnostics in clinical practice.[27] For example, any single classifier's predictions depend critically on the class labels it is given (ie, which pathologist assigns the "gold standard" for training the classifier). In addition, the variability resulting from applying different analytical methods/equations on the same high-dimensional data set can be similar to 2 pathologists reviewing the same histologic slide.[28]

MOLECULAR PATHOLOGY AND GENETIC ALTERATIONS OF NATIVE KIDNEY DISEASES

Although acute kidney injury (AKI) is a relevant problem in native kidneys, biopsies are rarely obtained, most likely because of the limited ability of histology to assess specific cause, extent, and recoverability of AKI. However, kidney transplantation offers in this regard a unique opportunity to study the molecular response of the tissue to acute injury because all transplants experience AKI to some extent (brain death, donation, reperfusion) and biopsies are obtained in great frequency.[29]

By comparing microarray mRNA expression profiles from renal allograft biopsies with histologic features of AKI and no rejection to time-matched pristine protocol biopsies, a molecular profile of AKI was identified in renal transplants.[30] This approach allowed subtraction of the ubiquitous injury changes every transplant is experiencing from clinically relevant AKI. Kidneys with AKI showed increased expression of 394 transcripts. This included among the top 30 transcripts many previously identified as AKI biomarkers in urine, blood, or kidney tissue[31]: epithelium-expressed injury molecules (FOS, EGR1, integrins β6 and β3), tissue-remodeling molecules (AKAP12, versican, ADAMTS1, ADAM9), and inflammation-associated transcripts (SERPINA3, lipocalin 2, FCGR3A).[30,32] Many other genes also correlated with the molecular phenotype, including the acute injury biomarkers HAVCR1 (KIM-1) and IL-18, but showed quantitatively less-extensive changes in expression. A molecular AKI score (= the geometric mean of all related transcripts) correlated with reduced graft function, future functional recovery, brain death, and need for dialysis. In contrast, histologic features of AKI did not correlate with function or with the molecular changes, indicating that a molecular AKI signature offers more precise assessment and quantification of tissue injury and its potential for recovery.

Similar observations were made in active and progressive diseases operating in native kidneys. Microarray analysis from biopsies of patients with chronic renal diseases revealed that different renal diseases share relatively large numbers of genes with a uniform concordance in the regulation of all genes in a network.[33] Glomeruli-specific (ie, after laser microdissection) genome-wide expression analysis in cases with primary and collapsing focal-segmental glomerulosclerosis (FSGS) compared with minimal change disease revealed in addition to dysregulated slit diaphragm and podocyte transcripts also differences in the biologic process of development, differentiation, cell motility, and signal transduction (ie, very similar to those involved in the injury response observed in renal allografts).[34,35]

A compelling illustration of how molecular insights can lead to more precise diagnoses in the area of nephropathology is the recently revised classification of membranoproliferative glomerulonephritis (MPGN). Since the 1970s, MPGN had been divided into types I, II, and III based on the location and ultrastructural appearance of deposits, rather than their immune composition and underlying disease mechanisms. It is now understood that the subset of type I and type III that contain C3 only, without immunoglobulin, are mediated by frequently genetically induced dysregulation of the alternative complement pathway. Accordingly, this subset of types I and III are now called C3 glomerulonephritis, and together with type II (dense deposit disease) comprise the umbrella of C3 glomerulopathies.[36,37]

Using mass spectrometry, renal amyloid can now be subtyped into immunoglobulin light and heavy chains, secondary reactive serum amyloid A protein, leukocyte cell-derived chemotaxin-2, fibrinogen-α chain, transthyretin, apolipoprotein A-I and A-IV, gelsolin, and β-2 microglobulin,[38] providing a diagnostic granularity that could not be accomplished by histochemical or immunohistochemical staining approaches. More precise typing of renal amyloidosis will guide genetic counseling and treatment in patients with amyloidosis, which is frequently first diagnosed in renal biopsies.

Fundamentally different molecular approaches apply to understanding the genetics underlying hereditary kidney diseases. Since the discovery of nephrin in 1998, major progress has been made in understanding FSGS as a major cause of nephrotic syndrome showing a common morphologic pattern, but actually representing a heterogeneous group of podocytopathies.[39] Numerous podocyte mutations are now described in familial and sporadic secondary FSGS and 20% to 35% of FSGS cases have some form of underlying mutations.[40] In up to 30% to 40% of FSGS cases, more uncommon, complex mutations are identified besides the classical high-penetration mutations in podocyte-specific genes like podocin, WT1, or nephrin. These classical gene mutations were identified by positional cloning and consecutive validation in mouse models (ie, through very labor intense and costly procedures). Now available high-throughput testing, like Next Generation Sequencing, allows identification of a significantly larger number of complex mutations underlying FSGS. It is likely that a cumulative burden of podocyte injury will lead to nonhereditary DNA damage causing FSGS and nephritic syndrome as the consequence of a multigene pathogenesis. Understanding the molecular pathology in these "acquired genetic" FSGS cases can provide targets for therapeutic intervention.

Similar novel insights thorough Next Generation Sequencing can be expected in complex genetic diseases sharing a common, nonspecific histologic phenotype, like cystic renal diseases and Alport syndrome. Complex mutations in the large COL4A3-5 genes can be very efficiently deciphered by using novel sequencing technologies and thus will provide better clinical stratification of patients with this heterogeneous and wide spectrum of Alport syndrome than morphology.[41,42]

MOLECULAR PATHOLOGY OF RENAL ALLOGRAFT BIOPSIES

MOLECULAR PATHOLOGY OF THE DONOR BIOPSY

Organ donation induces a significant molecular response in the donor tissue.[43,44] Assessing the quality of a donor organ and predicting its performance in the recipient represents a significant clinical need. Despite several histologic, clinical, and combined scoring systems for donor organs, a significant proportion of harvested donor kidneys is still discarded. At the transcriptional level, the response to tissue injuries presents as a decreased expression of functional genes (eg, solute carrier transcripts), and upregulation of cell cycle, repair, and tissue remodeling transcripts, and embryonic transcripts like *wnt* and *notch* pathways.[30,45] Donor kidneys from recipients with excellent transplant function at 1 year posttransplantation exhibited a distinctly different gene expression profile than matched subjects with impaired function: genes mainly belonging to the functional classes of immunity, signal transduction, and oxidative stress response were increased in donor biopsies from recipients with impaired function.[46] The mRNA expression of AKI biomarkers (LCN2 and HAVCR1/KIM-1) was significantly increased in recipients developing delayed graft function (DGF).[47] In a microarray study, 87 consecutive time-zero biopsies taken postreperfusion in 42 deceased and 45 living donor kidneys were compared with clinical and histopathology-based injury scores. Unsupervised analysis separated the kidneys into 3 groups: living donors, low-risk deceased donors, and high-risk deceased donors who showed the highest incidence of DGF. Clinical and histopathological risk scores did not discriminate high from low-risk deceased donors. A total of 1051 transcripts were differentially expressed between the 2 deceased donor risk groups.[43] In a subsequent study, the same group analyzed deceased donors only. The strongest correlate with early dysfunction in this high-risk subset was the mean expression of a set of 30 injury transcripts. Eleven transcripts of the 30 injury transcripts best predicted DGF and included well-known biomarkers of AKI, primarily expressed by tubular epithelial cells, like Osteopontin M receptor, Integrinβ6, LCN2 (lipocalin 2), versican, cathepsin S, and cadhorin 6.[48]

MOLECULAR PATHOLOGY OF CELL-MEDIATED REJECTION

The molecular phenotype found in renal allograft biopsies correlating with the characteristic histologic features of cell-mediated rejection (CMR) (ie, interstitial infiltration and tubulitis) primarily comprises transcripts expressed by subsets of T lymphocytes (cytotoxic T lymphocytes [CTLs], effector memory T cells, T-helper cells, regulatory T cells[49–52]), macrophages,[53,54] and transcripts regulated by interferon-gamma (IFNγ).[55,56] Earlier PCR studies already identified in biopsies with CMR prototypical cytotoxic T lymphocyte (CTL)

transcripts: granzyme B, perforin, and Fas ligand.[8,19,57–62]

IFNγ mRNA has been described as being detectable in fine-needle aspirate samples taken 1 week before the clinical onset of rejection, consistent with the view that IFNγ is synthesized early in rejection and that IFNγ mRNA is upregulated very rapidly on T-cell receptor engagement[63–65] and therefore in many studies distinguishes acute rejection from controls.[5,8,57,63,66,67] Among the numerous IFNγ-regulated cytokines and chemokines associated with acute rejection were transforming growth factor beta (TGFβ), tumor necrosis factor alpha (TNFα), RANTES, MIP-1α, HLA class I and II molecules, CXCL9, CXCL10, and CXCL11.[8,67,68]

To date, comprehensive microarray studies confirmed earlier PCR-based results on a genome-wide level, but also revealed that in addition to the hypothesis-derived PCR targets (eg, single T-cell–associated transcripts), numerous other transcripts show similar expression patterns under the same condition.[3,23,67,69] First, Sarwal and colleagues[7] at Stanford provided a systematic screening of genes expressed in rejecting grafts. In addition to confirming the expression of T-cell transcripts in rejecting allografts, they also found a signature associated with subsequent graft failure. Interestingly, this turned out to be B-cell transcripts. In another microarray study, B-cell–associated transcripts were increased in late allograft biopsies and associated with the extent of interstitial fibrosis and tubular atrophy (IFTA). Late allograft biopsies per se are associated with a higher risk for failure due to advanced disease stages.[70,71] Different results have been reported in small microarray series, probably related to the problem of the very small ratio of samples to parameters,[4] highlighting the still existing need for considerable collaborative effort to define robust transcription patterns from the myriad of idiosyncratic results, influenced by timing, patient population, control groups, and therapy.

Recently the Edmonton group used their comprehensive collection of human renal allograft biopsies mRNA microarray data to build a predictive CMR-classifier.[28,68] The CMR classifier assigns to each individual biopsy a probability score in percent indicating its likelihood of having CMR according to its molecular phenotype. Interestingly, the transcripts the CMR classifier used most often to render a molecular diagnosis of rejection, were IFNγ inducible or cytotoxic T-cell associated, for example, CXCL9, CXCL11, GBP1, and INDO.[68]

Several groups accessed publically available microarray data sets and did meta-analysis or applied existing gene sets and classifiers to new biopsy series from other centers. In one study, a comparative analysis was performed across 4 different microarray datasets of heterogeneous sample collections. A common transcriptional profile of 70 genes was identified, comprising transcripts related to antigen presentation (eg, MHC, CD163), T-cell activation (eg, CD8, granzyme A), and IFNγ-regulated transcripts (eg, GBP1, CXCL9). The expression of the 70 gene set is significantly upregulated in all rejection samples as compared with stable allografts or healthy kidneys, and strongly correlates with the severity of Banff rejection classes.[72]

Interestingly, the individual members in the described gene sets change their expression in a coordinated, highly correlated, stereotyped fashion and thus move in large groups reflecting the major biologic processes operating in renal allografts.[9,23,67] This observation was recently expanded in a comprehensive meta-analysis of human gene expression studies in allograft rejection across all organ types.[73] The investigators postulate the "Immunologic Constant of Rejection" hypothesis based on the observation that different immune-mediated processes (ie, allograft

rejection, autoimmunity, infection, cancer, graft-versus-host disease, acute cardiovascular events, chronic-obstructive pulmonary diseases, placental villitis) share common convergent final molecular mechanisms. Molecular features consistently described through all these different immune-mediated tissue destruction processes include the activation of interferon-γ–regulated genes, the recruitment of cytotoxic cell through massive production of respective chemokine ligands (primarily through CXCR3/CCR5 ligand pathways), and the activation of immune effector function genes (ie, genes expressed by CD8 cells and natural killer [NK] cells on activation). **Fig. 1** shows the networks of related molecules involved in these central pathways jointly representing the "Immunologic Constant of Rejection."[73] Because these biologic pathways operate diffusely in the tissue, respective changes in the transcriptome can be detected by assessing few representative "top" transcripts in tissue specimens that are otherwise inadequate for histology.

Only a few studies are published describing the expression of regulatory miRNA in a small series of human biopsies with rejection. Preliminary data suggest that miRNA expression patterns tightly

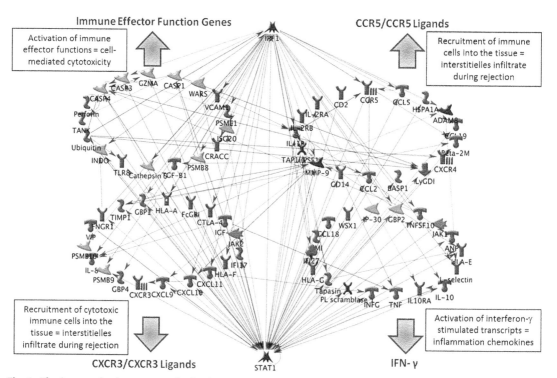

Fig. 1. The immunologic constant of rejection: common molecular phenotype between autoimmunity, pathogen infection, cancer immunity, and allograft rejection. (*Adapted from* Spivey TL, Uccellini L, Ascierto ML, et al. Gene expression profiling in acute allograft rejection: challenging the immunologic constant of rejection hypothesis. J Transl Med 2011;9:174.)

correlate with mRNA expression patterns but may serve as better biomarkers of the human renal allograft status due to their greater stability, especially in body fluids and after formalin fixation and paraffin embedding of tissue biopsies.[74,75]

MOLECULAR PATHOLOGY OF ALLOGRAFT URINE

It is obvious to expect that significant components of the molecular phenotype in the allograft tissue are transferred to the nephrons and are thus excreted with the urine. Among the mRNA species first described in the urine and correlated with acute rejection are the inhibitor of granzyme B,[76] serine protease inhibitor-9 (PI-9),[77] IP-10 and CXCR3,[78] CD103,[79] and granulysin.[80] These were described to have good sensitivity and to rise before clinical evidence of rejection and thus have potential as screening tests. Using enzyme-linked immunosorbent assay testing increased amounts of IFNγ-inducible chemokines CXCL9/10/11 were detected in urine of patients with clinical and subclinical CMR, similar to mRNA findings in the biopsy.[81] In a consecutive validation study, CXCL10 turned out to be the most robust urine protein marker for noninvasive rejection screening, including for subclinical rejection (ie, without detectable rise in creatinine).[82]

Several studies applied high-throughput proteomics to urine specimens with the aim of discovering new noninvasive biomarkers of allograft rejection. Using biostatistics, most of these studies (reviewed in Refs.[83–85]) revealed long lists of proteins discriminating between stable and dysfunctional/rejecting allografts. Most frequently, the proteins identified by mass spectrometry were not sequenced and thus not functionally annotated. Among those proteins frequently identified were β2 microglobulin, TNFα, various integrins, collagens, uromodulin, matrix metalloproteinases, and CD44.[85–87] Small-scale urine metabolomics is performed since the first days of transplantation by measuring creatinine and glucose in urine. Only a few groups applied high-throughput metabolomics platforms to human urine specimens.[88] Often metabolomics and proteomics studies do not identify specific compounds per se. The notion is that specific patterns of unknown or unidentified metabolites or peptides, rather than specific compounds, can be used to diagnose rejection from urine.[89] However, the limited metabolomics and proteomic data still await further validation in humans, which is hampered by the fact that the necessary equipment is not standard in diagnostic laboratories, and is very large, complex, and expensive. Furthermore, because large parts of the urine metabolome correlate with clinically well-established, cheap-to-measure metabolites like creatinine and β2 microglobulin require that for new omics-based markers and patterns an added value still needs to be demonstrated.

MOLECULAR PATHOLOGY OF CHRONIC ALLOGRAFT DAMAGE

Early application of targeted PCR mRNA expression analysis to late allograft biopsies showed that increased TGFβ, but not IL-2, IFNγ, IL-4, IL-10, or granzyme B or perforin, correlates with concurrent fibrosis.[61,90] Using microarrays for assessing late biopsies, the strongest molecular correlate of the extent of interstitial fibrosis and tubular atrophy were mast cell and B-cell–associated transcripts.[71] In addition, the expression of plasma cell associate transcripts (ie, immunoglobulin heavy chain transcripts) and also Foxp3 showed a significant positive correlation with time posttransplantation.[70,71,91]

A molecular classifier for the prediction of allograft failure in clinically indicated biopsies taken more than 1 year posttransplantation was superior to all known clinical (creatinine, proteinuria, glomerular filtration rate) and morphologic (Banff lesion scores) risk factors for allograft failure. Interestingly, the classifier includes genes part of the molecular injury response as the main source for prediction, suggesting that an ongoing, active molecular injury response of the tissue due to progressive diseases like rejection or glomerular diseases is the main correlate for functional deterioration in late allograft biopsies.[26] Increased expression of a gene set reflecting the acute injury response in the kidney parenchyma correlated with poor function and with inflammation in areas of fibrosis, but not with fibrosis without inflammation.[92] Many individual transcripts expressed in late biopsies were shared between the injury gene set[30,92] and the molecular risk score; for example, integrin β6 (ITGB6), versican (VCAN), nicotinamide N-methyltransferase (NNMT).

Using miRNA sequencing in 8 human kidney allograft biopsies (4 IFTA and 4 normal) guided selection of miRNAs accompanying IFTA, which were quantified in 18 biopsies using real-time quantitative PCR. Total miRNA content was 50% lower in IFTA compared with normal biopsies. Several miRNAs, including miR-21, 142-3p, and 5p and the cluster comprising miR-506 on chromosome X, had twofold to sevenfold higher expression in IFTA compared with normal biopsies, whereas miRNA miR-30b and 30c were lower in IFTA biopsies. However, no specific diagnoses were assigned to the IFTA cases, allowing further understanding of potential specific disease mechanisms.[93]

Suthanthiran and colleagues[94] describe a noninvasive diagnostic test for fibrosis based on mRNA measurements in urine by RT-PCR. The following urine mRNAs were significantly associated with IFTA: vimentin, hepatocyte growth factor, α-smooth muscle actin, fibronectin 1, perforin, plasminogen activator inhibitor 1, TGFβ1, TIMP1, granzyme B, fibroblast-specific protein 1, CD103, and collagen 1A1. A 4-gene model composed of the levels of mRNA for vimentin, NKCC2, and E-cadherin and of 18S ribosomal RNA provided the most accurate diagnostic model of IFTA.[94]

Thus, a stereotyped acute molecular injury signal, comprising numerous individual transcripts identical to those observed during acute kidney injury, is present in late biopsies with many different diseases as a reflection of parenchymal stress. On a molecular level, progression to failure is primarily a function of ongoing parenchymal injury caused by various specific diseases, and not nonspecific fibrogenesis.

MOLECULAR PATHOLOGY OF ANTIBODY-MEDIATED REJECTION

Recent findings suggest that increased diagnostic specificity in renal allografts can be accomplished for antibody-mediated tissue injury through gene expression studies. Accordingly, the 2013 revised international Banff classification for allograft rejection now includes molecular assessment of antibody-mediated injury as a potential diagnostic criterion for antibody-mediated rejection (ABMR), independent of C4d staining.[95] Over the past couple of years, considerable evidence emerged that previous Banff criteria for ABMR, due to its dependence on C4d, missed a significant proportion of ABMR cases. In parallel, underlying mechanisms of antibody-mediated tissue injury are now better understood.[96] In the vast majority of ABMRs, anti-HLA antibodies find their target in the microcirculation of the allograft. This interaction between antibodies and the endothelial cell causes stress to the microcirculation, either mediated through complement activation, or direct interaction of the antibody with the endothelium, or through cell-dependent cytotoxicity mediated through Fc receptors on neutrophils, NK cells, or macrophages.[97] Such interactions between antibody and antigen lead to significant molecular changes in the endothelium of the microcirculation (ie, peritubular capillaries and glomeruli). Sis and colleagues[98] were the first to develop a literature-based set of transcripts with primary expression in endothelial cells. The investigators found a significant upregulation of endothelium-specific molecules, such as factor VIII (VWF), melanoma cell adhesion molecule (CD146/MCAM), Cadherin 5 (CDH5), selectin E (SELE/CD62e), platelet/endothelial cell adhesion molecule 1 (PECAM1/CD31), CD34 molecule, and caveolin 1 (CAV1) in human renal allograft biopsies with histologic features of antibody-mediated tissue injury and simultaneous presence of donor-specific antibodies (DSAs). Furthermore, as the correlate of antibody binding to the endothelium facilitating cell-dependent cytotoxicity with adhesion of inflammatory cells and interaction with Fc receptors of NK cells, molecules specific for NK infiltration have been demonstrated to be associated with respective pathology of the microcirculation (capillaritis and glomerulitis) and the presence of DSAs.[99,100] By comparing the intragraft gene expression from patients with DSAs to those without DSAs, the following NK-cell–specific transcripts were identified: fractalkine receptor (CX3CR1), myeloblastosis viral oncogene homolog (MYBL1), fibroblast growth factor binding protein 2 (FGFBP2, also known as KSP37), killer cell lectinlike receptor F1 (KLRF1, also known as NKp80) and SH2 domain containing 1B (SH2D1B, also known as EAT2). Both increased expression of endothelial and NK cell transcripts in the presence of DSAs and ABMR pathology, and were independent of C4d staining results. Thus, adding quantitative molecular assessments to cases with DSAs has the potential to increase diagnostic precision for C4d-negative antibody-mediated rejection. The Mayo group studied intragraft gene expression profiles of positive crossmatch (+XM) kidney transplant recipients who develop transplant glomerulopathy (TG) and those who did not. Comparing protocol renal allograft biopsies +XM/TG+ and control groups, significantly altered expression was seen for up to 3200 genes. Pathway analyses revealed inflammatory genes, NK cell transcripts and numerous endothelial cell transcripts.[24]

Using microarray data, a classifier was developed that assigned diagnostic ABMR probability scores to each biopsy. Again the transcripts distinguishing ABMR from other diagnoses were mostly expressed in endothelial cells or NK cells, or were IFNγ inducible. The classifier scores correlated with the presence of microcirculation injury according to Banff lesion scores and DSA levels.[101] The fact that the classifier independently uses endothelial and NK cell-associated transcript for diagnosing ABMR corroborates the previous, hypothesis-driven observations by others, that such transcripts are specifically increased in renal allografts with ABMR.

MOLECULAR PATHOLOGY OF POLYOMAVIRUS NEPHROPATHY (PVN)

Only a few studies have examined intragraft gene expression profiles in polyomavirus nephropathy (PVN). Similar to histopathology in which lesions significantly overlap between CMR and PVN, one study also demonstrated similar gene expression profiles in PVN and CMR. Expression of transcripts described in CMR, including CD8, IFNγ, CXCR3, and perforin, were higher in PVN than CMR. In addition, transcription of molecules associated with extracellular matrix turnover, including collagens, TGFβ, and matrix metalloproteinases, were significantly higher in PVN than CMR.[102] Still, identification of specific antiviral responses of the renal tubular epithelium has not been accomplished, neither on the morphologic nor on the molecular level.

SUMMARY

The results obtained from genome-wide expression studies in kidney biopsies suggest that the vast majority of differentially expressed molecules represent a stereotyped response of the tissue to disease of any kind. But underneath this non-specific injury and inflammation response, to which extent corresponds to disease activity and prognosis, disease-specific information can be discovered. Finding diagnostic specificity in large-scale molecular changes is obviously as challenging as with nonspecific morphologic features.

Deriving a diagnostic molecular signature from large-scale, high-dimensional omics data represents a challenge if no true diagnostic gold standard is available for training and validation of the new molecular diagnostic. This is frequently the case in pathology, as numerous diagnostic classification systems are empirically derived and consensus-based but not necessarily the pathogenetic and biologic correct disease mechanisms.[103] This represents a significant obstacle for implementing new "omics" diagnostics into clinical practice.

Thus, with the exception of diseases with a strong genotype-phenotype association (ie, hereditary diseases) it is unlikely that even comprehensive molecular assessments will provide absolute diagnostic precision. Although in some areas, the molecules are superior, for example, the assessment of tissue injury, which is essentially invisible to morphology, histopathology will always carry greater specificity and sensitivity in other areas (eg, focal glomerular diseases). More likely is that an integrated diagnostic system comprising molecular, morphologic, serologic, and clinical variables will provide the greatest diagnostic precision. The adoption of such refined, integrated diagnostic systems into clinical practice will require ongoing interdisciplinary and iterative efforts and well-designed prospective validation studies.

The primary aim for such studies has to be an increased diagnostic precision in the biopsy before new noninvasive diagnostic markers (eg, urine proteomics and metabolomics) can be validated against the biopsy as a *true* gold standard.

REFERENCES

1. Mirnezami R, Nicholson J, Darzi A. Preparing for precision medicine. N Engl J Med 2012;366(6): 489–91.
2. Ewis AA, Zhelev Z, Bakalova R, et al. A history of microarrays in biomedicine. Expert Rev Mol Diagn 2005;5(3):315–28.
3. Halloran PF, Einecke G. Microarrays and transcriptome analysis in renal transplantation. Nat Clin Pract Nephrol 2006;2(1):2–3.
4. Akalin E, Hendrix RC, Polavarapu RG, et al. Gene expression analysis in human renal allograft biopsy samples using high-density oligoarray technology. Transplantation 2001;72(5):948–53.
5. Stegall M, Park W, Kim D, et al. Gene expression during acute allograft rejection: novel statistical analysis of microarray data. Am J Transplant 2002;2(10):913–25.
6. Scherer A, Krause A, Walker JR, et al. Early prognosis of the development of renal chronic allograft rejection by gene expression profiling of human protocol biopsies. Transplantation 2003;75(8):1323–30.
7. Sarwal M, Chua MS, Kambham N, et al. Molecular heterogeneity in acute renal allograft rejection identified by DNA microarray profiling. N Engl J Med 2003;349(2):125–38.
8. Hoffmann SC, Hale DA, Kleiner DE, et al. Functionally significant renal allograft rejection is defined by transcriptional criteria. Am J Transplant 2005;5(3): 573–81.
9. Halloran PF, de Freitas DG, Einecke G, et al. An integrated view of molecular changes, histopathology and outcomes in kidney transplants. Am J Transplant 2010;10(10):2223–30.
10. Muthukumar T, Dadhania D, Ding R, et al. Messenger RNA for FOXP3 in the urine of renal-allograft recipients. N Engl J Med 2005;353(22): 2342–51.
11. Suthanthiran M, Schwartz JE, Ding R, et al. Urinary-cell mRNA profile and acute cellular rejection in kidney allografts. N Engl J Med 2013;369(1):20–31.
12. Keslar KS, Lin M, Zmijewska AA, et al. Multicenter evaluation of a standardized protocol for

noninvasive gene expression profiling. Am J Transplant 2013;13(7):1891–7.

13. Hoffmann S, Park J, Jacobson LM, et al. Donor genomics influence graft events: the effect of donor polymorphisms on acute rejection and chronic allograft nephropathy. Kidney Int 2004;66(4):1686–93.

14. Manolio TA. Genomewide association studies and assessment of the risk of disease. N Engl J Med 2010;363(2):166–76.

15. Salomon DR. Challenges to doing genetic association studies in transplantation. Am J Transplant 2012;12(12):3173–5.

16. Wang Z, Gerstein M, Snyder M. RNA-Seq: a revolutionary tool for transcriptomics. Nat Rev Genet 2009;10(1):57–63.

17. Marguerat S, Wilhelm BT, Bahler J. Next-generation sequencing: applications beyond genomes. Biochem Soc Trans 2008;36(Pt 5):1091–6.

18. Mengel M, Bock O, Priess M, et al. Expression of pro- and antifibrotic genes in protocol biopsies from renal allografts with interstitial fibrosis and tubular atrophy. Clin Nephrol 2008;69(6):408–16.

19. Allanach K, Mengel M, Einecke G, et al. Comparing microarray versus RT-PCR assessment of renal allograft biopsies: similar performance despite different dynamic ranges. Am J Transplant 2008;8(5):1006–15.

20. Geiss GK, Bumgarner RE, Birditt B, et al. Direct multiplexed measurement of gene expression with color-coded probe pairs. Nat Biotechnol 2008;26(3):317–25.

21. Allison DB, Cui X, Page GP, et al. Microarray data analysis: from disarray to consolidation and consensus. Nat Rev Genet 2006;7(1):55–65.

22. Mengel M, Campbell P, Gebel H, et al. Precision diagnostics in transplantation: from bench to bedside. Am J Transplant 2013;13(3):562–8.

23. Halloran PF, de Freitas DG, Einecke G, et al. The molecular phenotype of kidney transplants. Am J Transplant 2010;10(10):2215–22.

24. Dean PG, Park WD, Cornell LD, et al. Intragraft gene expression in positive crossmatch kidney allografts: ongoing inflammation mediates chronic antibody-mediated injury. Am J Transplant 2012;12(6):1551–63.

25. Hayde N, Bao Y, Pullman J, et al. The clinical and molecular significance of C4d staining patterns in renal allografts. Transplantation 2013;95(4):580–8.

26. Einecke G, Reeve J, Sis B, et al. A molecular classifier for predicting future graft loss in late kidney transplant biopsies. J Clin Invest 2010;120(6):1862–72.

27. Waikar SS, Betensky RA, Emerson SC, et al. Imperfect gold standards for kidney injury biomarker evaluation. J Am Soc Nephrol 2012;23(1):13–21.

28. Reeve J, Sellares J, Mengel M, et al. Molecular diagnosis of T cell-mediated rejection in human kidney transplant biopsies. Am J Transplant 2013;13(3):645–55.

29. Mengel M, Chang J, Kayser D, et al. The molecular phenotype of 6-week protocol biopsies from human renal allografts: reflections of prior injury but not future course. Am J Transplant 2011;11(4):708–18.

30. Famulski KS, de Freitas DG, Kreepala C, et al. Molecular phenotypes of acute kidney injury in kidney transplants. J Am Soc Nephrol 2012;23(5):948–58.

31. Vaidya VS, Ozer JS, Dieterle F, et al. Kidney injury molecule-1 outperforms traditional biomarkers of kidney injury in preclinical biomarker qualification studies. Nat Biotechnol 2010;28(5):478–85.

32. Einecke G, Kayser D, Vanslambrouck JM, et al. Loss of solute carriers in T cell-mediated rejection in mouse and human kidneys: an active epithelial injury-repair response. Am J Transplant 2010;10(10):2241–51.

33. Bhavnani SK, Eichinger F, Martini S, et al. Network analysis of genes regulated in renal diseases: implications for a molecular-based classification. BMC Bioinformatics 2009;10(Suppl 9):S3.

34. Skoberne A, Konieczny A, Schiffer M. Glomerular epithelial cells in the urine: what has to be done to make them worthwhile? Am J Physiol Renal Physiol 2009;296(2):F230–41.

35. Hodgin JB, Borczuk AC, Nasr SH, et al. A molecular profile of focal segmental glomerulosclerosis from formalin-fixed, paraffin-embedded tissue. Am J Pathol 2010;177(4):1674–86.

36. Sethi S, Fervenza FC. Membranoproliferative glomerulonephritis—a new look at an old entity. N Engl J Med 2012;366(12):1119–31.

37. Pickering MC, D'Agati VD, Nester CM, et al. C3 glomerulopathy: consensus report. Kidney Int 2013;84(6):1079–89.

38. Sethi S, Vrana JA, Theis JD, et al. Laser microdissection and mass spectrometry-based proteomics aids the diagnosis and typing of renal amyloidosis. Kidney Int 2012;82(2):226–34.

39. Hildebrandt F. Genetic kidney diseases. Lancet 2010;375(9722):1287–95.

40. Santin S, Bullich G, Tazon-Vega B, et al. Clinical utility of genetic testing in children and adults with steroid-resistant nephrotic syndrome. Clin J Am Soc Nephrol 2011;6(5):1139–48.

41. Liapis H, Jain S. The interface of genetics with pathology in Alport nephritis. J Am Soc Nephrol 2013;24(12):1925–7.

42. Storey H, Savige J, Sivakumar V, et al. COL4A3/COL4A4 mutations and features in individuals with autosomal recessive Alport syndrome. J Am Soc Nephrol 2013;24(12):1945–54.

43. Mueller TF, Reeve J, Jhangri GS, et al. The transcriptome of the implant biopsy identifies donor kidneys at increased risk of delayed graft function. Am J Transplant 2008;8(1):78–85.

44. Hauser P, Schwarz C, Mitterbauer C, et al. Genome-wide gene-expression patterns of donor

kidney biopsies distinguish primary allograft function. Lab Invest 2004;84(3):353–61.

45. Einecke G, Broderick G, Sis B, et al. Early loss of renal transcripts in kidney allografts: relationship to the development of histologic lesions and alloimmune effector mechanisms. Am J Transplant 2007; 7(5):1121–30.

46. Kainz A, Perco P, Mayer B, et al. Gene-expression profiles and age of donor kidney biopsies obtained before transplantation distinguish medium term graft function. Transplantation 2007; 83(8):1048–54.

47. Korbely R, Wilflingseder J, Perco P, et al. Molecular biomarker candidates of acute kidney injury in zero-hour renal transplant needle biopsies. Transpl Int 2011;24(2):143–9.

48. Kreepala C, Famulski KS, Chang J, et al. Comparing molecular assessment of implantation biopsies with histologic and demographic risk assessment. Am J Transplant 2013;13(2):415–26.

49. Einecke G, Melk A, Ramassar V, et al. Expression of CTL associated transcripts precedes the development of tubulitis in T-cell mediated kidney graft rejection. Am J Transplant 2005;5(8):1827–36.

50. Famulski KS, Einecke G, Reeve J, et al. Changes in the transcriptome in allograft rejection: IFN-gamma-induced transcripts in mouse kidney allografts. Am J Transplant 2006;6(6):1342–54.

51. Hidalgo LG, Einecke G, Allanach K, et al. The transcriptome of human cytotoxic T cells: similarities and disparities among allostimulated CD4(+) CTL, CD8(+) CTL and NK cells. Am J Transplant 2008;8(3):627–36.

52. Hidalgo LG, Einecke G, Allanach K, et al. The transcriptome of human cytotoxic T cells: measuring the burden of CTL-associated transcripts in human kidney transplants. Am J Transplant 2008;8(3): 637–46.

53. Famulski KS, Einecke G, Sis B, et al. Defining the canonical form of T-cell-mediated rejection in human kidney transplants. Am J Transplant 2010; 10(4):810–20.

54. Famulski KS, Kayser D, Einecke G, et al. Alternative macrophage activation-associated transcripts in T-cell-mediated rejection of mouse kidney allografts. Am J Transplant 2010;10(3):490–7.

55. Famulski K, Einecke G, Halloran PF. IFN-g inducible transcripts are increased in T cell mediated rejection (TCMR), but some are also increased in tissue injury. Am J Transplant 2005;5(s11): 448–9.

56. Famulski KS, Einecke G, Reeve J, et al. Changes in the transcriptome in allograft rejection: IFN-gamma-induced transcripts in mouse kidney allografts. Am J Transplant 2006;6(6):1342–54.

57. Strehlau J, Pavlakis M, Lipman M, et al. Quantitative detection of immune activation transcripts as

a diagnostic tool in kidney transplantation. Proc Natl Acad Sci U S A 1997;94:695–700.

58. Sharma VK, Bologa RM, Li B, et al. Molecular executors of cell death—differential intrarenal expression of Fas ligand, Fas, granzyme B, and perforin during acute and/or chronic rejection of human renal allografts. Transplantation 1996;62(12):1860–6.

59. Lipman ML, Stevens AC, Strom TB. Heightened intragraft CTL gene expression in acutely rejecting renal allografts. J Immunol 1994;152(10):5120–7.

60. Strehlau J, Pavlakis M, Lipman M, et al. The intragraft gene activation of markers reflecting T-cell-activation and -cytotoxicity analyzed by quantitative RT-PCR in renal transplantation. Clin Nephrol 1996;46(1):30–3.

61. Suthanthiran M. Molecular analyses of human renal allografts: differential intragraft gene expression during rejection. Kidney Int Suppl 1997;58:S15–21.

62. Desvaux D, Schwarzinger M, Pastural M, et al. Molecular diagnosis of renal-allograft rejection: correlation with histopathologic evaluation and antirejection-therapy resistance. Transplantation 2004;78(5):647–53.

63. Nast CC, Zuo XJ, Prehn J, et al. Gamma-interferon gene expression in human renal allograft fine-needle aspirates. Transplantation 1994;57(4): 498–502.

64. Halloran PF, Miller LW, Urmson J, et al. IFN-gamma alters the pathology of graft rejection: protection from early necrosis. J Immunol 2001;166(12): 7072–81.

65. Hidalgo LG, Halloran PF. Role of IFN-gamma in allograft rejection. Crit Rev Immunol 2002;22(4): 317–49.

66. Kirk AD, Bollinger RR, Finn OJ. Rapid, comprehensive analysis of human cytokine mRNA and its application to the study of acute renal allograft rejection. Hum Immunol 1995;43(2): 113–28.

67. Mueller TF, Einecke G, Reeve J, et al. Microarray analysis of rejection in human kidney transplants using pathogenesis-based transcript sets. Am J Transplant 2007;7(12):2712–22.

68. Reeve J, Einecke G, Mengel M, et al. Diagnosing rejection in renal transplants: a comparison of molecular- and histopathology-based approaches. Am J Transplant 2009;9(8):1802–10.

69. Flechner SM, Kurian SM, Head SR, et al. Kidney transplant rejection and tissue injury by gene profiling of biopsies and peripheral blood lymphocytes. Am J Transplant 2004;4(9):1475–89.

70. Einecke G, Reeve J, Mengel M, et al. Expression of B cell and immunoglobulin transcripts is a feature of inflammation in late allografts. Am J Transplant 2008;8:1434–43.

71. Mengel M, Reeve J, Bunnag S, et al. Molecular correlates of scarring in kidney transplants: the

emergence of mast cell transcripts. Am J Transplant 2009;9(1):169–78.

72. Saint-Mezard P, Berthier CC, Zhang H, et al. Analysis of independent microarray datasets of renal biopsies identifies a robust transcript signature of acute allograft rejection. Transpl Int 2009;22(3): 293–302.

73. Spivey TL, Uccellini L, Ascierto ML, et al. Gene expression profiling in acute allograft rejection: challenging the immunologic constant of rejection hypothesis. J Transl Med 2011;9:174.

74. Anglicheau D, Sharma VK, Ding R, et al. MicroRNA expression profiles predictive of human renal allograft status. Proc Natl Acad Sci U S A 2009; 106(13):5330–5.

75. Mas VR, Dumur CI, Scian MJ, et al. MicroRNAs as biomarkers in solid organ transplantation. Am J Transplant 2013;13(1):11–9.

76. Dadhania D, Muthukumar T, Ding R, et al. Molecular signatures of urinary cells distinguish acute rejection of renal allografts from urinary tract infection. Transplantation 2003;75(10):1752–4.

77. Muthukumar T, Ding R, Dadhania D, et al. Serine proteinase inhibitor-9, an endogenous blocker of granzyme B/perforin lytic pathway, is hyperexpressed during acute rejection of renal allografts. Transplantation 2003;75(9):1565–70.

78. Tatapudi RR, Muthukumar T, Dadhania D, et al. Noninvasive detection of renal allograft inflammation by measurements of mRNA for IP-10 and CXCR3 in urine. Kidney Int 2004;65(6):2390–7.

79. Ding R, Li B, Muthukumar T, et al. CD103 mRNA levels in urinary cells predict acute rejection of renal allografts. Transplantation 2003;75(8): 1307–12.

80. Kotsch K, Mashreghi MF, Bold G, et al. Enhanced granulysin mRNA expression in urinary sediment in early and delayed acute renal allograft rejection. Transplantation 2004;77(12):1866–75.

81. Schaub S, Nickerson P, Rush D, et al. Urinary CXCL9 and CXCL10 levels correlate with the extent of subclinical tubulitis. Am J Transplant 2009;9(6): 1347–53.

82. Ho J, Rush DN, Karpinski M, et al. Validation of urinary CXCL10 as a marker of borderline, subclinical, and clinical tubulitis. Transplantation 2011;92(8): 878–82.

83. Schaub S, Wilkins JA, Nickerson P. Proteomics and renal transplantation: searching for novel biomarkers and therapeutic targets. Contrib Nephrol 2008;160:65–75.

84. Schaub S, Wilkins JA, Rush D, et al. Developing a tool for noninvasive monitoring of renal allografts. Expert Rev Proteomics 2006;3(5):497–509.

85. Bohra R, Klepacki J, Klawitter J, et al. Proteomics and metabolomics in renal transplantation—quo vadis? Transpl Int 2013;26(3):225–41.

86. Schaub S, Wilkins JA, Antonovici M, et al. Proteomic-based identification of cleaved urinary beta2-microglobulin as a potential marker for acute tubular injury in renal allografts. Am J Transplant 2005;5(4 Pt 1):729–38.

87. Metzger J, Chatzikyrkou C, Broecker V, et al. Diagnosis of subclinical and clinical acute T-cell-mediated rejection in renal transplant patients by urinary proteome analysis. Proteomics Clin Appl 2011;5(5–6):322–33.

88. Wishart DS. Metabolomics: the principles and potential applications to transplantation. Am J Transplant 2005;5(12):2814–20.

89. Lindon JC, Holmes E, Bollard ME, et al. Metabonomics technologies and their applications in physiological monitoring, drug safety assessment and disease diagnosis. Biomarkers 2004;9(1):1–31.

90. Sharma VK, Bologa RM, Xu GP, et al. Intragraft TGF-beta 1 mRNA: a correlate of interstitial fibrosis and chronic allograft nephropathy. Kidney Int 1996; 49(5):1297–303.

91. Bunnag S, Allanach K, Jhangri GS, et al. FOXP3 expression in human kidney transplant biopsies is associated with rejection and time post transplant but not with favorable outcomes. Am J Transplant 2008;8(7):1423–33.

92. Famulski KS, Reeve J, de Freitas DG, et al. Kidney transplants with progressing chronic diseases express high levels of acute kidney injury transcripts. Am J Transplant 2013;13(3):634–44.

93. Ben-Dov IZ, Muthukumar T, Morozov P, et al. MicroRNA sequence profiles of human kidney allografts with or without tubulointerstitial fibrosis. Transplantation 2012;94(11):1086–94.

94. Anglicheau D, Muthukumar T, Hummel A, et al. Discovery and validation of a molecular signature for the noninvasive diagnosis of human renal allograft fibrosis. Transplantation 2012;93(11):1136–46.

95. Haas M, Sis B, Racusen LC, et al. Banff 2013 meeting report: inclusion of c4d-negative antibody-mediated rejection and antibody-associated arterial lesions. Am J Transplant 2014;14(2):272–83.

96. Colvin RB. Antibody mediated rejection: diagnosis and pathogenesis. J Am Soc Nephrol 2007;18(4): 1046–56.

97. Akiyoshi T, Hirohashi T, Alessandrini A, et al. Role of complement and NK cells in antibody mediated rejection. Hum Immunol 2012;73:1226–32.

98. Sis B, Jhangri GS, Bunnag S, et al. Endothelial gene expression in kidney transplants with alloantibody indicates antibody-mediated damage despite lack of C4d staining. Am J Transplant 2009;9(10):2312–23.

99. Hidalgo LG, Sellares J, Sis B, et al. Interpreting NK cell transcripts versus T cell transcripts in renal transplant biopsies. Am J Transplant 2012;12(5): 1180–91.

100. Hidalgo LG, Sis B, Sellares J, et al. NK cell transcripts and NK cells in kidney biopsies from patients with donor-specific antibodies: evidence for NK cell involvement in antibody-mediated rejection. Am J Transplant 2010;10(8):1812–22.

101. Sellares J, Reeve J, Loupy A, et al. Molecular diagnosis of antibody-mediated rejection in human kidney transplants. Am J Transplant 2013; 13:971–83.

102. Mannon RB, Hoffmann SC, Kampen RL, et al. Molecular evaluation of BK polyomavirus nephropathy. Am J Transplant 2005;5(12):2883–93.

103. Mengel M, Sis B, Halloran PF. SWOT analysis of Banff: strengths, weaknesses, opportunities and threats of the international Banff consensus process and classification system for renal allograft pathology. Am J Transplant 2007;7(10):2221–6.

104. Hsu YH, Sis B. Molecular transplantation pathology: the interface between molecules and histopathology. Curr Opin Organ Transplant 2013;18(3): 354–62.

105. Mengel M, Reeve J, Bunnag S, et al. Scoring total inflammation is superior to the current Banff inflammation score in predicting outcome and the degree of molecular disturbance in renal allografts. Am J Transplant 2009;9(8):1859–67.

106. Bunnag S, Einecke G, Reeve J, et al. Molecular correlates of renal function in kidney transplant biopsies. J Am Soc Nephrol 2009;20(5): 1149–60.

Emerging Concepts and Controversies in Renal Pathology

C4d-Negative and Arterial Lesions as Manifestations of Antibody-Mediated Transplant Rejection

Mark Haas, MD, PhD

KEYWORDS

- Renal transplant • Transplant rejection • Antibody-mediated rejection • Transplant glomerulopathy
- Transplant glomerulitis • Transplant arteriopathy • Intimal arteritis • Complement C4d

ABSTRACT

The consensus classification of antibody-mediated rejection (AMR) of renal allografts developed at the Sixth Banff Conference on Allograft Pathology, in 2001, identified three findings necessary for the diagnosis of active AMR: histologic evidence, antibodies against the graft, and capillary C4d deposition. Morphologic and molecular studies have noted evidence of microvascular injury, which, in the presence of donor-specific antibodies (DSAs) but the absence of C4d deposition, is associated with development of transplant glomerulopathy and graft loss. Recent studies suggest that intimal arteritis may in some cases be a manifestation of DSA-induced graft injury. These newly recognized lesions of AMR have now been incorporated into a revised Banff diagnostic schema.

INTRODUCTION

During the past 2 decades there has developed an increasing awareness of antibody-mediated rejection (AMR) as an important cause of both short- and long-term injury to renal allografts.[1–3] Part of the difficulty in recognizing the importance of AMR was related to the lack of specific morphologic findings that could be used to identify changes of AMR on allograft biopsies. Acute rejection in the presence of donor-specific anti-HLA antibodies (DSAs) shows histologic changes very different from those of acute T cell–mediated rejection (CMR), characterized by microvascular injury and inflammation, including margination of neutrophils and mononuclear leukocytes (later documented as monocytes/macrophages[4]) in peritubular and glomerular capillaries, thrombotic microangiopathy (TMA), and, in severe cases, fibrinoid necrosis of arterioles and small arteries.[5] Antibody usually cannot be detected in the microvasculature by immunofluorescence microscopy, however.[5] Furthermore, these morphologic changes are not specific for AMR and can be seen with other causes of endothelial injury, including acute calcineurin inhibitor nephrotoxicity and recurrent TMA.[6–9]

The use of staining for C4d by immunofluorescence or immunohistochemistry (IHC) has been an important development in allowing pathologists to more accurately diagnose acute AMR in allograft biopsies and in recognizing the contribution of humoral immunity to lesions of chronic renal allograft rejection.[10–18] Although C4d, formed on cleavage of complement factor C4, a component of the classical complement pathway, is itself biologically inactive, it binds covalently at the site of C4 cleavage, rendering it a long-lived marker for

Department of Pathology and Laboratory Medicine, Cedars-Sinai Medical Center, 8700 Beverly Boulevard, Los Angeles, CA 90048, USA
E-mail address: mark.haas@cshs.org

Surgical Pathology 7 (2014) 457–467
http://dx.doi.org/10.1016/j.path.2014.04.003
1875-9181/14/$ – see front matter © 2014 Elsevier Inc. All rights reserved.

surgpath.theclinics.com

humoral immunity.[19] At the Sixth Banff Conference on Allograft Pathology, in 2001,[20] consensus diagnostic criteria for acute AMR in renal allografts were adopted that require immunopathologic evidence in the form of C4d deposition in peritubular capillaries (ptc) as well as morphologic evidence (microvascular lesions as discussed previously) and the presence of DSAs.

During the past several years, however, limitations of these diagnostic criteria have been recognized. It is now well documented that DSAs may cause graft injury in the absence of C4d deposition. Furthermore, there is now evidence that intimal, non-necrotizing arteritis, previously thought to represent acute CMR, may in the presence of DSAs be (at least in part) humorally mediated. This review focuses on evidence supporting these paradigm shifts within the morphologic spectrum of AMR and reviews new consensus diagnostic criteria for AMR developed at the 12th Banff Conference on Allograft Pathology in 2013.[21]

C4D-NEGATIVE ANTIBODY-MEDIATED REJECTION

Sis and coworkers[22] used gene expression microarrays done on tissue from 173 indication renal allograft biopsies (performed for acute or persistent graft dysfunction or for proteinuria) to examine expression of a set of known endothelial-associated transcripts (ENDATs). They found that the combination of DSAs and high ENDAT expression (but not DSAs alone) was associated with a significantly increased rate of graft loss, even in the absence of C4d, although diffuse ptc C4d staining further increased the rate of graft loss.[22] They found that overexpression of 12 individual ENDATs was correlated with an increased risk of graft loss; the gene with the highest associated risk was that for von Willebrand factor.[22] A second key study supporting the existence of C4d-negative AMR and its association with development of graft scarring came from Loupy and colleagues.[23] These investigators examined clinical and pathologic findings at 1 year posttransplantation in 45 recipients of deceased donor renal allografts with known DSAs, based on findings observed on protocol biopsies done 3 months posttransplantation. Based on these 3-month biopsies, the patients of Loupy and colleagues[23] fell into 3 groups: those with no evidence of AMR, those with subclinical AMR characterized by both ptc C4d staining and histologic features of AMR (glomerulitis, peritubular capillaritis, or both), and those with histologic features of AMR

but no ptc C4d staining. At 1 year posttransplantation, patients whose 3-month biopsy had no evidence of AMR had good graft function and interstitial fibrosis/tubular atrophy (IF/TA) in only one-third of cases. These 1-year biopsies also showed no evidence of transplant glomerulopathy (TG), a lesion that is most often a manifestation of chronic AMR. TG is characterized histologically by duplication of glomerular basement membranes (GBMs), best demonstrated on sections stained with periodic acid–Schiff (PAS) or Jones methenamine silver stains to highlight GBMs. Patients whose 3-month biopsy showed subclinical AMR had reduced graft function, IF/TA in all cases, and TG in approximately half. Patients whose 3-month biopsy showed glomerulitis and/or peritubular capillaritis but no C4d had a mean creatinine clearance and frequencies of IF/TA and TG intermediate between the no AMR and C4d-positive subclinical AMR cohorts.[23] These findings are highly consistent with those of Sis and colleagues,[22] supporting the existence of a C4d-negative form of antibody-mediated graft injury that is less severe than C4d-positive AMR but is nonetheless associated with the development of chronic changes within the graft, including TG. **Fig. 1** illustrates the key microvascular lesions of AMR: glomerulitis, peritubular capillaritis, and TG.

Although TG is most often a manifestation of chronic AMR, approximately 25% of cases of TG occur in DSA-negative patients and are likely due to other causes (see Key Points).[24–27] Diagnosis of TG is important because this lesion is associated with poor graft outcome,[28] regardless of cause, although lesions associated with hepatitis C (rather than those associated with DSAs) were found to have the fastest rate of progression to graft loss.[26] In diagnosing TG, however, it is important to differentiate this from other lesions that also show GBM duplication, notably membranoproliferative glomerulitis (MPGN) type I and forms of C3 glomerulopathy (C3G), including dense deposit disease (formerly termed MPGN type II), both of which frequently recur in renal allografts.[29] MPGN type I is often associated with hepatitis C[30]; in addition to GBM double contours, the glomeruli appear hypercellular and hyperlobular due to mesangial cell proliferation and matrix expansion as well as endocapillary hypercellularity that is in part due to mononuclear leukocytes within the glomerular tuft. Although MPGN type I is easily distinguished from TG without glomerulitis by light microscopy due to a lack of glomerular hypercellularity in the latter, the distinction by light microscopy alone can be more difficult when TG is accompanied by moderate or severe glomerulitis.[31] MPGN type I, however, shows immune

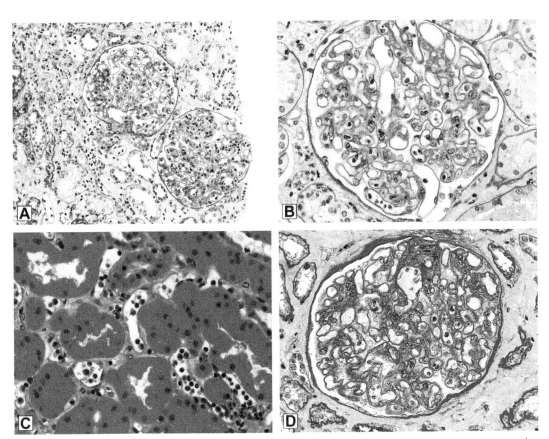

Fig. 1. Histopathologic lesions of AMR. (*A*) Glomerulitis and peritubular capillaritis. There are many mononuclear leukocytes as well as a small number of neutrophils in glomerular capillaries and ptc, with endothelial swelling and partial occlusion of some glomerular capillary lumens (PAS, original magnification ×200). (*B*) Glomerulitis. Marginated mononuclear leukocytes are present in multiple glomerular capillaries, in some associated with endothelial cell swelling and partial or nearly complete occlusion of the capillary lumen (PAS ×400). (*C*) Peritubular capillaritis. The ptc of the renal cortex (note that most tubules present are proximal tubules) contain prominent numbers of leukocytes, many of which have the typical appearance of monocytes (hematoxylin-eosin stain ×400). (*D*) TG. Several GBM double contours are evident on the PAS stain, notably at the lower portion of the glomerulus. Segmental glomerulitis is also present, consistent with chronic, active AMR in this patient who had circulating DSAs (see **Box 2**) (PAS ×400).

complex deposits (most often containing IgG and C3, sometimes with IgM and C1q) by immunofluorescence and electron microscopy (EM), and using these modalities it is readily distinguished from TG, which lacks such deposits. C3G is not associated with hepatitis C but results from abnormal activation of the alternative pathway of complement, due to mutations in complement regulatory proteins, including factor H and factor H–related proteins, autoantibodies against factor H, and/or C3 nephritic factor, an IgG autoantibody that binds to and prevents the inactivation of C3 convertase, resulting in the persistent cleavage of C3.[32–34] The histology of C3G is variable; GBM double contours may be present and in some cases glomerular

hypercellularity may be mild, resembling that in **Fig. 1**D. Glomeruli in C3G, however, show strong C3 staining by immunofluorescence (with the intensity of C3 staining exceeding that of any immunoglobulin by at least 2+ on a 0–3+ scale[35]) and deposits (although not true immune complexes per se) by EM that may include highly electron-dense, elongated intramembranous deposits (typical of dense deposit disease), less electron-dense subendothelial or intramembranous/transmembranous deposits, and even subepithelial hump-like deposits resembling those of acute postinfectious glomerulonephritis (see Pickering and colleagues[34] for a description of morphologic findings in C3G).

Key Points
MAJOR CAUSES OF TRANSPLANT GLOMERULOPATHY

- Chronic (or chronic, active) AMR
  - Accounts for approximately 75% of cases of TG[24]
  - In chronic, active AMR, there is frequently concurrent glomerulitis (see **Fig. 1D**).
- Chronic or persistent TMA
  - May be recurrent (eg, recurrent hemolytic-uremic syndrome) or de novo (eg, due to calcineurin inhibitor nephrotoxicity)
- Changes related to hepatitis C virus infection
  - May be related to TMA associated with anticardiolipin antibodies[25]
  - Associated with worse prognosis for graft survival than TG secondary to AMR or TMA in hepatitis C–negative patients[26]
  - Must be distinguished from MPGN type I, which may also be related to hepatitis C. In MPGN type I, the glomeruli show immune complex deposits by immunofluorescence and EM, although this is not the case with TG, even when glomerulitis is also present.
- Changes related to T-cell activation
  - A recent study showed that in cases of TG without C4d deposition or DSAs, there was increased expression of cytotoxic T cell–associated transcripts.[27]

Although TG, as evident by light microscopy on PAS and silver-stained sections, is rarely observed during the first 6 months posttransplantation,[36] Wavamunno and colleagues[37] showed that morphologic changes associated with the subsequent development of overt TG may be seen during the first 1 to 3 months posttransplantation by EM. These ultrastructural changes include swelling and vacuolization of glomerular endothelial cells, subendothelial electron-lucent widening (or widening of the lamina rara interna), and early duplication/multilayering of GBMs (**Fig. 2**). Recently, it was shown that one or more of these ultrastructural findings are seen in most biopsies with microvascular injury in DSA-positive patients during the first 3 months posttransplantation, whether or not C4d is present.[38]

ROLE OF ANTIBODY IN ARTERIAL LESIONS

Certain arterial lesions in renal allografts are well accepted as having a pathogenesis that often involves humoral immunity. As discussed previously, transmural necrosis in one or more arteries is included among those lesions satisfying the histologic component for diagnosis of acute AMR in the Banff classification.[20] Some recent studies provide evidence, however, for expanding the range of arterial lesions associated with antibody-mediated graft injury.

Intimal arteritis is currently classified as a lesion of CMR and defines type 2 acute rejection according to the Banff classification of CMR.[39] There is emerging evidence, however, that intimal arteritis may in some cases be, at least in part, humorally mediated. In some cases, such as that shown in **Fig. 3**, lesions of intimal arteritis contain a predominance of CD68-positive macrophages, which are also highly prominent in glomerulitis and peritubular capillaritis,[4,40] as opposed to CD3-positive T lymphocytes that typically predominate in the tubulointerstitial lesions of acute CMR.[41–43] Most recently, Lafaucheur and colleagues[44] reported on 64 cases of intimal arteritis in DSA-positive patients. They found that compared with cases of AMR without intimal arteritis, those with intimal arteritis had a 3-fold higher rate of graft loss. Although a majority of cases of intimal arteritis with DSAs also showed interstitial inflammation and tubulitis, indicating a combined lesion of AMR and CMR, it was also noteworthy that intimal arteritis with DSAs was associated with a significantly (and approximately 6-fold) higher rate of graft loss than intimal arteritis without DSAs, the latter representing pure CMR.[44] These findings suggest an association of lesions of intimal arteritis with AMR when DSAs are present and may account

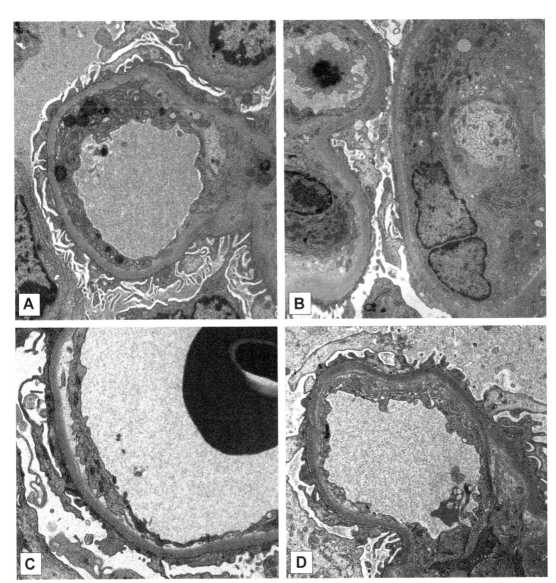

Fig. 2. Early ultrastructural lesions of glomerular capillaries in patients with acute/active AMR. (*A*) Glomerular endothelial swelling and vacuolization in a biopsy showing C4d-positive AMR, done on posttransplantation day (PTD) 9. Uranyl acetate and lead citrate stain (original magnification ×7200). (*B*) Severe glomerular endothelial swelling and segmental subendothelial electron-lucent widening in a biopsy showing C4d-negative AMR, PTD 29 (uranyl acetate and lead citrate ×7200). (*C*) Subendothelial electron-lucent widening in a biopsy showing C4d-positive AMR, PTD 10 (uanyl acetate and lead citrate ×10,000). (*D*) Subendothelial electron-lucent widening and early GBM duplication in a biopsy showing C4d-negative AMR, PTD 52 (uranyl acetate and lead citrate ×7500).

in part for the frequent lack of a complete response of lesions reported as Banff type 2 acute CMR to therapy directed at T cells.[45,46]

The data of Lefaucheur and colleagues[44] argue that testing for DSAs is indicated in renal allograft recipients with a biopsy showing intimal arteritis, even if C4d staining is negative. Likewise, treatment in these cases should include measures to

remove DSAs if the latter are present, because persistence of DSAs, microvascular inflammation, and intimal arteritis is associated with poor graft outcomes in patients with AMR.[47] Still, although these findings suggest that the presence of intimal arteritis may identify a more severe form of AMR than those cases without intimal arteritis, the evidence directly linking intimal arteritis to humoral

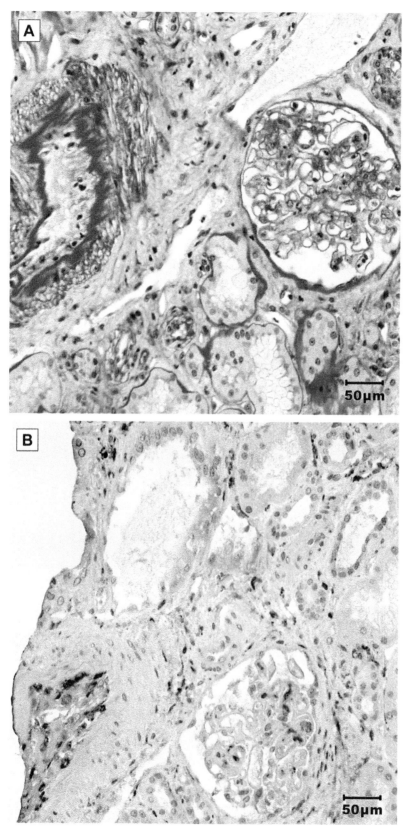

Fig. 3. Macrophages in a case of acute rejection with intimal arteritis, microvascular inflammation, and DSAs. The biopsy was performed 2 months posttransplantation for an acute rise in serum creatinine level. The PAS stain (*A*) shows glomerulitis and an artery with intimal arteritis. There is only very mild interstitital inflammation and minimal tubulitis. An IHC stain for CD68 (*B*) shows many CD68-positive macrophages within glomerular capillaries and ptc as well as within the lesion of intimal arteritis (lower left of the photomicrograph). Only small numbers of CD3-positive T cells were seen in the artery with intimal arteritis (not shown). Immunofluorescence staining of tissue from this biopsy for C4d was negative, although the patient had anti-HLA class II DSAs at the time of biopsy. (Original magnification of both photomicrographs ×200; bar = 50 μm.)

immunity is indirect and still preliminary. Of the 64 DSA-positive cases studied by Lefaucheur and colleagues,[44] only 8 showed intimal arteritis as an isolated finding, in the absence of glomerulitis and/or peritubular capillaritis, and isolated intimal arteritis may also be an infrequent manifestation of acute CMR.[21] Also, as discussed previously, 72% and 63% of these 64 cases had interstitial inflammation and tubulitis, respectively, consistent with earlier findings of a strong association between glomerulitis and intimal arteritis[48] and suggesting the presence of CMR as well as AMR. Finally, the link between predominance of CD68-positive cells in lesions of intimal arteritis and AMR is hypothetical, and one study found no difference in clinical outcomes in patients having biopsies with intimal arteritis with a predominance of CD68-positive cells compared with intimal arteritis with primarily CD3-positive T cells.[49] Thus, it is important that additional studies be undertaken to determine if lesions of intimal arteritis containing mainly CD68-positive cells (see **Fig. 3**) are significantly associated with the presence of DSAs and other histologic lesions of active AMR and if these lesions respond to treatment of AMR, particularly in those cases where initial treatment with agents used for the treatment of acute CMR fail to produce a return of graft function to baseline level.

The association of arterial lesions with humoral immunity also seems to extend to intimal fibrosis. Lesions of arterial intimal fibrosis with multiple intimal leukocytes (sometimes termed transplant arteriopathy), such as that shown in **Fig. 4**, have been shown to be associated with DSAs and C4d.[17,18] Furthermore, in a study of protocol biopsies done at 3 and 12 months posttransplantation, Hill and colleagues[50] found that in renal transplant recipients with DSAs, but not those without, the mean Banff intimal fibrosis (cv) score increased significantly from month 3 to month 12. At later times, the mean cv score continued to increase at a faster rate in DSA-positive patients. By contrast, hypertension was not significantly associated with the increase in cv score. Although intimal fibrosis in a majority of DSA-positive patients did show a hypercellular zone close to the endothelium that was not observed (or was much less pronounced) in those arteries from DSA-negative patients with intimal fibrosis, there were DSA-positive patients with a prior history of acute AMR whose biopsies showed bland intimal fibrosis, indistinguishable from banal arteriosclerosis.[50] It is possible that those lesions of bland intimal fibrosis in DSA-positive patients represent a late, quiescent stage of the more cellular lesions, because biopsies from DSA-positive patients showing bland arterial intimal fibrosis showed no

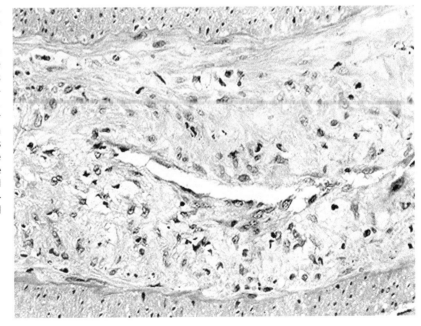

Fig. 4. Transplant arteriopathy. This arcuate artery shows marked intimal thickening and narrowing of the lumen. There are leukocytes as well as activated-appearing fibroblasts within the intima, especially portions closer to the lumen, although there are no leukocytes directly beneath the endothelium to indicate acute rejection (intimal arteritis) (hematoxylineosin stain, original magnification ×200).

glomerulitis or peritubular capillaritis to suggest an active component of AMR.[50]

REVISED (2013) BANFF CRITERIA FOR ANTIBODY-MEDIATED REJECTION

A consensus reached during and after the most recent Banff Conference, held in August 2013, has resulted in modification of the Banff criteria for diagnosis of both acute/active (**Box 1**) and chronic, active AMR (**Box 2**) in renal allografts.[21] These revised criteria include C4d-negative lesions. Lesions of intimal arteritis are also included, although, as discussed previously, intimal arteritis as the sole histologic manifestation of AMR is uncommon and the current evidence directly linking intimal arteritis to humoral immunity is indirect and somewhat preliminary. Still, Banff criteria are (and have always been) a working classification open to future revision if warranted by new data. Revised portions of the classification are indicated in boldface type in **Boxes 1** and **2**. Biopsies showing AMR should be designated as C4d positive or without evident C4d deposition (see **Boxes 1** and **2**) and, in the absence of C4d, more stringent evidence of current or recent antibody interaction with the vascular endothelium must be present; this helps avoid overdiagnosis of AMR. Such evidence may be morphologic, in the form of at least moderate microvascular inflammation, or molecular, provided the latter is based on a thoroughly validated test. The latter was mainly included to allow the classification to adapt to emerging data, because at present the only validated molecular marker of antibody-mediated endothelial injury is ENDAT expression,[22] and even this has been validated only at a single center.

Box 1

Revised (Banff 2013) classification of acute/active antibody-mediated rejection in renal allografts (all 3 features must be present for diagnosis[a,b])

- Histologic evidence of acute tissue injury, including one or more of the following:
  - Microvascular inflammation (g score >0[c] and/or ptc score >0)
  - Intimal or transmural arteritis (v score >0)[d]
  - Acute TMA, in the absence of any other cause
  - Acute tubular injury, in the absence of any other apparent cause
- **Evidence of current/recent antibody interaction with vascular endothelium, including at least one of the following:**
  - **Linear C4d staining in ptc (involving at least 10% of ptc by immunofluorescence on frozen sections or any ptc by IHC on paraffin sections)**
  - **At least moderate microvascular inflammation (sum of g and ptc scores ≥2)[e]**
  - **Increased expression of gene transcripts in the biopsy tissue indicative of endothelial injury, if thoroughly validated[f]**
- Serologic evidence of DSAs (HLA or other antigens)

[a] For all AMR diagnoses, it should be specified in the report whether the lesion is C4d positive (involving ≥10% of ptc by immunofluorescence on frozen sections or any ptc by IHC on paraffin sections) or without evident C4d deposition (<10% of ptc by immunofluorescence on frozen sections; completely negative by IHC on paraffin sections).

[b] These lesions may be clinically acute, smoldering, or subclinical. Biopsies showing 2 of the 3 features, except those with DSAs and C4d without histologic abnormalities potentially related to AMR or CMR (the latter seen mainly in ABO-incompatible renal allografts) may be designated as "suspicious" for acute/active AMR.

[c] Recurrent/de novo glomerulonephritis should be excluded.

[d] These arterial lesions may be indicative of AMR, CMR, or mixed AMR/CMR. Arterial lesions are only scored in arteries having a continuous media with 2 or more smooth muscle layers.

[e] In the presence of acute CMR, borderline infiltrates, or evidence of infection, ptc score ≥2 alone is not sufficient to define moderate microvascular inflammation, and glomerulitis must be present (g score ≥1).

[f] At present, the only validated molecular marker meeting this criterion is ENDAT expression,[22] and this has only been validated in a single center (University of Alberta). The use of ENDAT expression at other centers or other test(s) of gene expression within the biopsy as evidence of AMR must first undergo independent validation as was done for ENDAT expression by Sis and colleagues.[22]

Box 2
Revised (Banff 2013) classification of chronic, active antibody-mediated rejection in renal allografts (all 3 features must be present for diagnosis[a,b])

- Morphologic evidence of chronic tissue injury, including one or more of the following:
  - TG (cg score >0)[c], if no evidence of chronic TMA
  - Severe peritubular capillary basement membrane multilayering (requires EM)[d]
  - Arterial intimal fibrosis of new onset, excluding other causes[e]
- **Evidence of current/recent antibody interaction with vascular endothelium, including at least one of the following:**
  - **Linear C4d staining in ptc (involving at least 10% of ptc by immunofluorescence on frozen sections, or any ptc by IHC on paraffin sections)**
  - **At least moderate microvascular inflammation (sum of g and ptc scores ≥2)[f]**
  - **Increased expression of gene transcripts in the biopsy tissue indicative of endothelial injury, if thoroughly validated[g]**
- Serologic evidence of DSAs (HLA or other antigens)

[a] For all AMR diagnoses, it should be specified in the report whether the lesion is C4d positive (involving ≥10% of ptc by immunofluorescence on frozen sections or any ptc by IHC on paraffin sections) or without evident C4d deposition (<10% of ptc by immunofluorescence on frozen sections; completely negative by IHC on paraffin sections).
[b] Lesions of chronic, active AMR can range from primarily active lesions with early TG evident only by EM to those with advanced TG and other chronic changes in addition to active microvascular inflammation. In the absence of evidence of current/recent antibody interaction with the endothelium, the term, *active*, should be omitted; in such cases, DSAs may be present at the time of biopsy or at any previous time posttransplantation.
[c] Includes GBM duplication by EM only or GBM double contours by light microscopy.
[d] ≥7 Layers in 1 cortical peritubular capillary and ≥5 in 2 additional capillaries, avoiding portions cut tangentially.[51]
[e] Although leukocytes within the fibrotic intima favor chronic rejection, these are seen with chronic CMR as well as chronic AMR and are, therefore, helpful only if there is no history of CMR. An elastic stain may be helpful as absence of elastic lamellae is more typical of chronic rejection and multiple elastic lamellae are most typical of arteriosclerosis, although these findings are not definitive.
[f] In the presence of acute CMR, borderline infiltrates, or evidence of infection, ptc score ≥2 alone is not sufficient to define moderate microvascular inflammation, and glomerulitis must be present (g score ≥1).
[g] At present, the only validated molecular marker meeting this criterion is ENDAT expression,[22] and this has only been validated in a single center (University of Alberta). The use of ENDAT expression at other centers or other test(s) of gene expression within the biopsy as evidence of AMR must first undergo independent validation as was done for ENDAT expression by Sis and colleagues.[22]

ACKNOWLEDGMENTS

The author has no commercial or other relationships that have influenced, could be perceived as having influenced, or give the appearance of potentially influencing any of the material presented in this article. I thank Bill Pollard for assistance in preparation of figures.

REFERENCES

1. Terasaki PI, Cai J. Human leukocyte antigen antibodies and chronic rejection: from association to causation. Transplantation 2008;86:377–83.

2. Colvin RB. Antibody-mediated renal allograft rejection: diagnosis and pathogenesis. J Am Soc Nephrol 2007;18:1046–56.

3. Sis B, Mengel M, Haas M, et al. Banff '09 meeting report: antibody mediated graft deterioration and implementation of Banff working groups. Am J Transplant 2010;10:464–71.

4. Magil AB, Tinckam K. Monocytes and peritubular capillary C4d deposition in acute renal allograft rejection. Kidney Int 2003;63:1888–93.

5. Trpkov K, Campbell P, Pazderka F, et al. Pathologic features of acute renal allograft rejection associated with donor-specific antibody: analysis using the Banff grading schema. Transplantation 1996; 61:1586–92.

6. Noris M, Remuzzi G. Thrombotic microangiopathy after kidney transplantation. Am J Transplant 2010;10:1517–23.

7. Randhawa PS, Shapiro R, Jordan ML, et al. The histopathological changes associated with allograft rejection and drug toxicity in renal transplant

recipients maintained on FK506. Am J Surg Pathol 1993;17:60–8.

8. Trimarchi HM, Truong LD, Brennan S, et al. FK506-associated thrombotic microangiopathy. Transplantation 1999;67:539–44.

9. Meehan SM, Baliga R, Poduval R, et al. Platelet CD61 expression in vascular calcineurin inhibitor toxicity of renal allografts. Hum Pathol 2008;39:550–6.

10. Feucht HE, Felber E, Gokel MJ, et al. Vascular deposition of complement-split products in kidney allografts with cell-mediated rejection. Clin Exp Immunol 1991;86:464–70.

11. Collins AB, Schneeberger EE, Pascual MA, et al. Complement activation in acute humoral renal allograft rejection: diagnostic significance of C4d deposits in peritubular capillaries. J Am Soc Nephrol 1999;10:2208–14.

12. Regele H, Exner M, Watschinger B, et al. Endothelial C4d deposition is associated with inferior kidney allograft outcome independently of cellular rejection. Nephrol Dial Transplant 2001;16:2058–66.

13. Mauiyyedi S, Crespo M, Collins AB, et al. Acute humoral rejection in kidney transplantation: II. Morphology, immunopathology, and pathologic classification. J Am Soc Nephrol 2002;13:779–87.

14. Bohmig GA, Exner M, Habicht A, et al. Capillary C4d deposition in kidney allografts: a specific marker of alloantibody-dependent graft injury. J Am Soc Nephrol 2002;13:1091–9.

15. Herzenberg AM, Gill JS, Djurdjev O, et al. C4d deposition in acute rejection: an independent long-term prognostic factor. J Am Soc Nephrol 2002;13:234–41.

16. Nickeleit V, Zeiler M, Gudat F, et al. Detection of the complement degradation product C4d in renal allografts: diagnostic and therapeutic implications. J Am Soc Nephrol 2002;13:242–51.

17. Mauiyyedi S, Pelle PD, Saidman S, et al. Chronic humoral rejection: identification of antibody-mediated chronic allograft rejection by C4d deposits in peritubular capillaries. J Am Soc Nephrol 2001;12:574–82.

18. Regele H, Bohmig GA, Habicht A, et al. Capillary deposition of complement split product C4d in renal allografts is associated with basement membrane injury in peritubular and glomerular capillaries: a contribution of humoral immunity to chronic allograft rejection. J Am Soc Nephrol 2002;13:2371–80.

19. Zwirner J, Felber E, Herzog V, et al. Classical pathway of complement activation in normal and diseased human glomeruli. Kidney Int 1989;36:1069–77.

20. Racusen LC, Colvin RB, Solez K, et al. Antibody-mediated rejection criteria – an addition to the Banff '97 classification of renal allograft rejection. Am J Transplant 2003;3:708–14.

21. Haas M, Sis B, Racusen LC, et al. Banff 2013 meeting report: inclusion of C4d-negative antibody-mediated rejection and antibody-associated arterial lesions. Am J Transplant 2014;14:272–83.

22. Sis B, Jhangrl GS, Bunnag S, et al. Endothelial gene expression in kidney transplants with alloantibody indicates antibody-mediated damage despite lack of C4d staining. Am J Transplant 2009;9:2312–23.

23. Loupy A, Suberbielle-Boissel C, Hill GS, et al. Outcome of subclinical antibody-mediated rejection in kidney transplant recipients with preformed donor-specific antibodies. Am J Transplant 2009;9:2561–70.

24. Sis B, Campbell PM, Mueller T, et al. Transplant glomerulopathy, late antibody-mediated rejection and the ABCD tetrad in kidney allogtaft biopsies for cause. Am J Transplant 2007;7:1743–52.

25. Baid S, Pascual M, Williams WW Jr, et al. Renal thrombotic microangiopathy associated with anti-cardiolipin antibodies in hepatitis C-positive renal allograft recipients. J Am Soc Nephrol 1999;10:146–53.

26. Baid-Agrawal S, Farris AB III, Pascual M, et al. Overlapping pathways to transplant glomerulopathy: chronic humoral rejection, hepatitis C infection, and thrombotic microangiopathy. Kidney Int 2011;80:879–85.

27. Hayde N, Bao Y, Pullman J, et al. The clinical and genomic significance of donor-specific antibody-positive/C4d-negative and donor-specific antibody-negative/C4d-negative transplant glomerulopathy. Clin J Am Soc Nephrol 2013;8:2141–8.

28. Cosio FG, Gloor JM, Sethi S, et al. Transplant glomerulopathy. Am J Transplant 2008;8:492–6.

29. Choy BY, Chan TM, Lai KN. Recurrent glomerulonephritis after kidney transplantation. Am J Transplant 2006;6:2535–42.

30. Johnson RJ, Gretch DR, Yamabe H, et al. Membranoproliferative glomerulonephritis associated with hepatitis C virus infection. N Engl J Med 1993;328:465–70.

31. Haas M. Transplant glomerulopathy: it's not always about chronic rejection. Kidney Int 2011;80:801–3.

32. Servais A, Noel LH, Roumenina LT, et al. Acquired and genetic complement abnormalities play a critical role in dense deposit disease and other C3 glomerulopathies. Kidney Int 2012;82:454–64.

33. Sethi S, Fervenza FC, Zhang Y, et al. C3 glomerulonephritis: clinicopathologic findings, complement abnormalities, glomerular proteomic profile, treatment, and follow-up. Kidney Int 2012;82:465–73.

34. Pickering MC, D'Agati VD, Nester CM, et al. C3 glomerulopathy: consensus report. Kidney Int 2013;84:1079–89.

35. Hou J, Markowitz GS, Bomback AS, et al. Toward a working definition of C3 glomerulopathy by immunofluorescence. Kidney Int 2014;85:450–6.

36. Gloor JM, Sethi S, Stegall MD, et al. Transplant glomerulopathy: subclinical incidence and association with alloantibody. Am J Transplant 2007;7: 2124–32.

37. Wavamunno MD, O'Connell PJ, Vitalone M, et al. Transplant glomerulopathy: ultrastructural abnormalities occur early in longitudinal analysis of protocol biopsies. Am J Transplant 2007;7:1–12.

38. Haas M, Mirocha J. Early ultrastructural changes in renal allografts: correlation with antibody-mediated rejection and transplant glomerulopathy. Am J Transplant 2011;11:2123–31.

39. Racusen LC, Solez K, Colvin RB, et al. The Banff 97 working classification of renal allograft pathology. Kidney Int 1999;55:713–23.

40. Hidalgo LG, Sis B, Sellares J, et al. NK cell transcripts and NK cells in kidney biopsies from patients with donor-specific antibodies: evidence for NK cell involvement in antibody-mediated rejection. Am J Transplant 2010;10:1812–22.

41. Hancock WW, Thomson NM, Atkins RC. Composition of interstitial cellular infiltrate identified by monoclonal antibodies in renal biopsies of rejecting human allografts. Transplanation 1983;35:458–63.

42. Kolbeck PC, Tatum AH, Sanfilippo F. Relationships among the histologic pattern, intensity, and phenotypes of T cells infiltrating renal allografts. Transplantation 1984;38:709–13.

43. Einecke G, Melk A, Ramassar V, et al. Expression of CTL associated transcripts precedes the development of tubulitis in T cell mediated kidney graft rejection. Am J Transplant 2005;5:1827–36.

44. Lefaucheur C, Loupy A, Vernerey D, et al. Antibody-mediated vascular rejection of kidney allografts: a population-based study. Lancet 2013;381:313–9.

45. Minervini MI, Torbenson M, Scantlebury V, et al. Acute renal allograft rejection with severe tubulitis (Banff 1997 grade IB). Am J Surg Pathol 2000;24: 553–8.

46. Haas M, Kraus ES, Samaniego-Picota M, et al. Acute renal allograft rejection with intimal arteritis: histologic predictors of response to therapy and graft survival. Kidney Int 2002;61:1516–26.

47. Lefaucheur C, Nochy D, Hill GS, et al. Determinants of poor graft outcome in patients with antibody-mediated acute rejection. Am J Transplant 2007; 7:832–41.

48. Messias NC, Eustace JA, Zachary AA, et al. Cohort study of the prognostic significance of acute transplant glomerulitis in acutely rejecting renal allografts. Transplantation 2001;72:655–60.

49. Kozakowski N, Bohmig GA, Exner M, et al. Monocytes/macrophages in kidney allograft intimal arteritis: no association with markers of humoral rejection or with inferior outcome. Nephrol Dial Transplant 2009;24:1979–86.

50. Hill GS, Nochy D, Bruneval P, et al. Donor-specific antibodies accelerate arteriosclerosis after kidney transplantation. J Am Soc Nephrol 2011;22: 975–83.

51. Liapis G, Singh HK, Derebail VK, et al. Diagnostic significance of peritubular capillary basement membrane multilaminations in kidney allografts. Old concepts revisited. Transplantation 2012;94:620–9.

Index

Moving?

Make sure your subscription moves with you!

To notify us of your new address, find your **Clinics Account Number** (located on your mailing label above your name), and contact customer service at:

Email: journalscustomerservice-usa@elsevier.com

800-654-2452 (subscribers in the U.S. & Canada)
314-447-8871 (subscribers outside of the U.S. & Canada)

Fax number: 314-447-8029

Elsevier Health Sciences Division
Subscription Customer Service
3251 Riverport Lane
Maryland Heights, MO 63043

*To ensure uninterrupted delivery of your subscription, please notify us at least 4 weeks in advance of move.